Third Edition

Conceptual Models For Nursing Practice

Third Edition

Conceptual Models For Nursing Practice

Joan P. Riehl-Sisca

APPLETON & LANGE
Norwalk, Connecticut/San Mateo, California

0-8385-1210-0

Prentice-Hall International (UK) Limited, *London*
Prentice-Hall of Australia Pty. Limited, *Sydney*
Prentice-Hall Canada, Inc., *Toronto*
Prentice-Hall Hispanoamericana, S.A., *Mexico*
Prentice-Hall of India Private Limited, *New Delhi*
Prentice-Hall of Japan, Inc., *Tokyo*
Simon & Schuster Asia Pte. Ltd., *Singapore*
Editora Prentice-Hall do Brasil Ltda., *Rio de Janeiro*
Prentice-Hall, *Englewood Cliffs, New Jersey*

Library of Congress Cataloging-in-Publication Data

Conceptual models for nursing practice.

  Includes bibliographies and index.
  1. Nursing—Philosophy. I. Riehl-Sisca, Joan.
[DNLM: 1. Models, Theoretical. 2. Nursing. WY 100 C744]
RT84.5.C663 1988   610.73'01   88-24222
ISBN 0-8385-1210-0

Production Editor: Mary Beth Miller
Designer: Lynn M. Luchetti
Cover Designer: Michael J. Kelly

PRINTED IN THE UNITED STATES OF AMERICA

To My Family

Experience without theory is blind
but theory without experience is mere intellectual play

Kant

Reviewers

Olga Andruskiw, R.N., Ed.D., FAAN
Formerly Chairperson
Department of Nursing
Russell Sage College
Troy, New York

Juanita Fleming, R.N., Ph.D., FAAN
Professor of Nursing
Associate Vice Chancellor of Academic Affairs
College of Nursing
University of Kentucky
Lexington, Kentucky

Margaret Hardy, R.N., Ph.D.
Professor
College of Nursing
The University of Rhode Island
Kingston, Rhode Island

Betty Neuman, R.N., Ph.D.
Consultant/Counselor
Beverly, Ohio

Lorraine Walker, R.N., Ed.D., FAAN
Professor
Center for Health Care Research and Evaluation
School of Nursing
The University of Texas at Austin
Austin, Texas

Contents

PART III: DEVELOPMENTAL MODELS FOR NURSING PRACTICE / 179

PART IV: INTERACTION MODELS FOR NURSING PRACTICE / 323

Contributors

Peter Aggleton, M.A., M.Ed., Ph.D., A.B.P.S.S.
Senior Lecturer in Education
Bristol Polytechnic
Bristol, England

Heather A. Andrews, Ph.D., R.N.
Sherwood Park, Alberta, Canada

Utharas Arumugam, Dip.N., R.M.N.
School of Nursing
North Manchester General Hospital
Crumpsall, Manchester, England

Elizabeth Ann Manhart Barrett, Ph.D., R.N.
Associate Professor of Nursing
Hunter-Bellevue School of Nursing
Hunter College of the City of New York

Susan Burd, B.S.N., R.N.
Westmoreland Hospital
Greensburg, Pennsylvania
M.S.N. student, Indiana University of Pennsylvania
Indiana, Pennsylvania

Vicki Campbell, M.S.N., R.N.
Nursing Department
University of Minnesota Hospital and Clinics
Minneapolis, Minnesota

Karen Cerilli, B.S.N., R.N.
Educator
Jeannette District Memorial Hospital
Jeannette, Pennsylvania
M.S.N. student, Indiana University of Pennsylvania
Indiana, Pennsylvania

Helen Chalmers, S.R.N., Dip.N., R.N.T., B.A.
Senior Nurse Tutor
Bath District Health Authority
Bath, England

Marilyn K. Chrisman, M.N., R.N.
Respiratory Clinical Nurse Specialist in private practice
and consultant in respiratory care
Visalia, California

Gloria M. Clayton, Ed.D., R.N.
Associate Professor and Associate Dean
School of Nursing
Medical College of Georgia
Augusta, Georgia

Ivory Coleman, M.S.N., R.N.
Department of Nursing
Community College of Philadelphia
Philadelphia, Pennsylvania

M. Jean Daubenmire, R.N., M.S.
The Ohio State University
College of Nursing
Columbus, Ohio

Patricia B. DiNardo, B.S.N., R.N.
M.S.N. Student
Indiana University of Pennsylvania
Indiana, Pennsylvania

John English, R.N., M.H.Sc.
Department of Nursing and Health Studies
Brandon University
Brandon, Manitoba, Canada

Rebecca Lynn Feathers, M.S.N., R.N.
Professor
School of Nursing
Mercy Hospital
Pittsburgh, Pennsylvania

Helen M. Ference, Ph.D., R.N.
Nursing Consultation and Research
Pebble Beach, California

Rose Marie Foster, M.S.N., R.N.
Administrative Department Head
Family Medical Center
Conamough Valley Memorial Hospital
Johnstown, Pennsylvania

Elizabeth Geden, Ph.D., R.N.
University of Missouri-Columbia
School of Nursing
Columbia, Missouri

Janet L. Glass, M.S.N., R.N.
Western Pennsylvania Hospital School of Nursing
Pittsburgh, Pennsylvania

Ella B. Gross, M.S.N., R.N.
School of Nursing
Neumann College
Aston, Pennsylvania

Marguerite Hessian, R.N., M.Ed.
Assistant Professor and Chairperson
Department of Nursing
The College of St. Catherine
St. Paul, Minnesota

Margaret C. Jopp, Ed.D., R.N.
Assistant Professor
University of Delaware
Newark, Delaware

Kathryn Buchanan Keller, R.N., M.S.N., C.C.R.N.
Critical Care Educator
Mercy Hospital
Miami, Florida

Imogene M. King, Ed.D., R.N.
College of Nursing
University of South Florida Medical Center
Tampa, Florida

Donna G. Knauth, M.S., R.N.
Perinatal Clinical Nurse Specialist and Clinical Coordinator in Maternity
Riverview Medical Center
Red Bank, New Jersey

Myra Estrin Levine, R.N., M.S.N., FAAN
Emeritus Professor of Nursing and Adjunct Professor of
Humanistic Studies
College of Nursing
University of Illinois at Chicago
Chicago, Illinois

Margaret Louis, Ph.D., R.N.
Associate Professor
School of Nursing
University of Nevada
Las Vegas, Nevada

Lois W. Lowry, D.N.Sc., R.N.
Professor and Director of Nursing
Cecil Community College
North East, Maryland

Andrea Mengel, Ph.D., R.N.
Department of Nursing
Community College of Philadelphia
Philadelphia, Pennsylvania

Marilee Woehning Miller, R.N.C., Ph.D.
Professor and Chairperson
Department of Nursing
Gustavus Adolphus College
St. Peter, Minnesota

Dorothy Evanson Mrkonich, R.N., Ph.D.
Professor and Chairperson
Department of Nursing
St. Olaf College
Northfield, Minnesota

Eileen Nahigian, M.S.N., R.N.
Inservice Education Department
Childrens Hospital of Buffalo
Buffalo, New York

M. Janice Nelson, Ed.D., R.N.
Dean, College of Nursing
Health Science Center
State University of New York
Syracuse, New York

Betty Neuman, Ph.D., R.N.
Author, Lecturer, and Consultant
Beverly, Ohio

Rosemarie Rizzo Parse, Ph.D., R.N.
Discovery International, Inc.
Pittsburgh, Pennsylvania

Cynthia Deibert Pioli, M.S.N., R.N.
School of Nursing
Conamough Valley Memorial Hospital
Johnstown, Pennsylvania

Louise Pugliese, M.S.N., R.N.
School of Nursing
St. Francis Medical Center
Pittsburgh, Pennsylvania

Joan Riehl-Sisca, Ph.D., R.N.
Coordinator, Graduate Nursing Program
Indiana University of Pennsylvania
Indiana, Pennsylvania

Martha E. Rogers, Sc.D., R.N., FAAN
New York University
Division of Nursing
School of Education, Health, Nursing, and Arts Professions
New York, New York

Sister Callista Roy, Ph.D., R.N.
Boston College
Boston, Massachusetts

Lynn G. Ryan, B.S.N., R.N.
M.S.N. Student
University of Pittsburgh
Pittsburgh, Pennsylvania

Janet Kwarta Sandor, M.S.N., R.N.
School of Nursing
Conamough Valley Memorial Hospital
Johnstown, Pennsylvania

Susan Sherman, M.A., R.N.
Director, Nursing Program
Community College of Philadelphia
Philadelphia, Pennsylvania

Mary Jane Smith, Ph.D., R.N.
Professor of Nursing
West Virginia University
Morgantown, West Virginia

Jeanne Steele, Ph.D., R.N.
Department of Nursing
Indiana University of Pennsylvania
Indiana, Pennsylvania

Linda R. Stumpf, R.N., M.S.N.
Case Manager
Forbes Health System
Monroeville, Pennsylvania

Joyce Waterman Taylor, M.S.N., C.S., R.N., FAAN
Clinical Nurse Specialist, Neuroscience
Kaiser Permanente
Fontana, California

Jean Watson, Ph.D., R.N., FAAN
Dean and Professor of Nursing
Associate Director of Nursing Service
University of Colorado Health Sciences Center
Denver, Colorado

Doris J. Wiegand, R.N., M.S.C.
School of Nursing
Conamough Valley Memorial Hospital
Johnstown, Pennsylvania

Preface

In this text nursing models are classified into three groups: systems, developmental, and interaction models. Although these designations were determined for the first edition, printed in 1974, they still hold today. Contributing authors of models were asked to classify their frameworks according to one of these three categories. Some did so, some did not respond to the request, and some were uncertain about which group would be most appropriate. This is understandable, because as models are developed they may assume a somewhat different perspective, although the primary principles remain unchanged. When an author of a model indicated her preference, her model was placed in the requested group. The other determinations were made by this author. The decision was based on the model's philosophy, its primary focus, or its nursing domain.

The scenario for this text is that in each unit the original model is presented by its author first. The model presentation is followed by a critique utilizing Stevens' evaluation criteria.* The subsequent chapters are reports of the use of the model in various situations or research done employing the model as a theoretical base. Research on each model was included whenever such information was located. This was considered important because along with critiques, research on nursing models should be available to verify their validity and reliability.

As with the first two editions, this book is intended to be used by students, nurse educators, and administrators who are interested in learning more about nursing theory and its implementation. The research done to date is included to serve as guidelines and encouragement to those pursuing this line of endeavor. Nurses new to research sometimes have difficulty conceptualizing the relationship between a theoretical framework and a problem area they wish to study. Because the purpose of research is to contribute to a body of knowledge, it is essential that new nurse researchers learn this process. It remains for nurse educators, administrators, and books of this nature to show the way.

It has been my good fortune to know many of the nursing theorists who are

---

*Stevens, B. J. (1984). *Nursing theory: Analysis, application, evaluation* (2nd ed.). Boston: Little, Brown.

writing today and others who are contributing to the promotion of nursing science. Although the list is too numerous to mention, I am also indebted to the many peers and former students who have graciously given their time and thoughtful consideration that is evident in the papers included in this text. Their ideas are their own. Only editorial guidance was provided to ensure some continuity in the overall format of the book. Thanks is also given to the publishing staff for their patience while this manuscript was being completed.

Joan P. Riehl-Sisca
October, 1988

Prologue: An Historical Perspective

Because epistemology and praxis in nursing are the general concerns in this text, it seemed advisable to examine these relationships from a broad perspective. In establishing a body of nursing knowledge, we might ask what other disciplines and history have to offer. Prior to the 1920s, epistemology tended to be accepted without question. However, after that time at least three changes occurred that had an impact. One change was that knowledge was not as certain as thought previously. A second change was that academicians became more and more isolated and had few new insights to offer. Finally, it was thought that one could study knowledge and yet ignore the natural sciences.[1]

In considering the historical development of knowledge, traditional relationships between the rationality and progressiveness concepts of science were accepted for a long time. Recently, these also have been questioned and alternatives have been offered. However, the newer options pose problems as well. One is the mistake of jumping to premature conclusions, which should also be a concern in nursing. There are numerous nursing models available today and some taxonomies for nursing diagnoses. An example of the latter is the North American Nursing Diagnosis Association (NANDA) Taxonomy I. Perhaps in our eagerness to establish our science of nursing knowledge, we too are jumping to premature closure. Laudan suggests that we start anew and ask elementary questions about science for a different perspective on knowledge. For example, science fundamentally aims at solving problems. Little has been done to explore this in detail. We can identify what types of problems need study and what makes some more important than others.

The traditional relationship between rationality (an atemporal concept) and progress (a temporal concept) is that the former is of primary importance. Laudan proposes that this assumption be inverted so that rationality, which is more obscure, be explained by progress, which is easily understood. He states that "rationality consists in making the most progressive theory choices, not that progress consists in accepting successively the most rational theories (p. 6)." He proposes that the best link between rationality and the progressiveness

---

[1]Laudan, L. (1977). *Progress and its problems: Toward a theory of scientific growth*. Berkeley, CA: University of California Press.

of a theory is its problem-solving effectiveness. Historically, most scientific philosophers have mistakenly focused on an individual theory rather than on research, which is what is needed. There is an echo of this in nursing. Fortunately, some heed the message, as evidenced by proliferating research conferences and publications. However, inroads are few in the match between research and our nursing models. More and more nurses are receiving their doctorates. Their dissertations are based on theoretical frameworks. As conceptual maps are developed in nursing, as in other fields, our science will be delineated. Progress is not just the accretion of knowledge. It needs to be selectively directed and yet be broad in scope. From this perspective, moral and cognitive, social, spiritual, and material progress are some of the concepts that could be pursued within a nursing framework. Most of these variables impinge on nursing and are addressed in some manner in many nursing models, which provides sufficient latitude for research.

An example of such a framework is the Riehl Interaction Model. It incorporates these variables in its structural and funtional concepts. To remain at the grass-roots level of scientific endeavor, problem solving was selected for its operational methodology in the nurse-other decision-making process. In this model, there is expansiveness and room for change as the underlying thread of dialecticism broadens. As this occurs, the emerging synthesis results in greater insights into knowledge. Problem-solving methodology is a natural initial fit for this model. It is based on symbolic interaction theory, in which inherent precepts are communication and dialogue. As difficult as it is to avoid emotive overtones that pervade interaction, effort must be made to direct energy into objectivity for progress to be accomplished in nursing theory and practice. A complete presentation of this model is provided later in this text. For an interesting and informative discussion on the perspective of some other models, the reader is referred to Meleis' book entitled *Theoretical Nursing: Development and Progress.*[2]

Several nursing leaders are surely among the good and great thinkers of our time and can hold a candle (no pun intended) to similar persons in other fields. They are well read and keep abreast of scientific developments and research in general. They guide us with their wisdom. It is to them and others pursuing the identification of the body of nursing knowledge that this commentary is directed. It is not meant to be a finished piece of work, for much has yet to be said in nursing theory, research, and practice. The chapters in this book are offered as a cooperative venture and a continuing dialogue with the community of interested others in nursing.

---

[2]Meleis, A. (1985). *Theoretical nursing: Development and progress.* Philadelphia: Lippincott.

Part I_____

Setting the Stage: Application of Theory in Education, Administration, and Research

Three topics have been selected for this first section representing three general positions in nursing: education, administration of nursing services, and research. The first chapter, written by Jeanne Steele, a nurse educator with vast experience, illustrates how general education and nursing theories are applied in curriculum development. This process is important to show how theory building occurs and is utilized. The total content is not learned in one course but is a part of the progression in a masters degree program. A beginning of the synthesis of knowledge is illustrated as well. Chapter 2 identifies and discusses models used by nurse administrators. When she wrote the chapter, M. Janice Nelson was a nurse administrator and had held the position for several years. This is obvious in the well-informed material presented and the authority with which she speaks. Chapter 3, a research report by Margaret Jopp, examines nursing conceptual themes related to the common terms addressed in all models. Perspectives from the three different types of nursing programs are analyzed.

Learning to Be an Educator in Today's World

Theory and Model Application

Jeanne Steele

> If one is to be an educator one must be a
> learner and if one is to educate in a
> democracy one must live by its principles.
> Education then is not just a job—it is a
> way of life.
>
> *J. Lanier and P. Cusik (1985, p. 711)*

Educating graduate nursing students to become teachers of nursing is addressed in this chapter. The heart of this process is curriculum development. The essentials needed to develop a curriculum include identification of the philosophy, concepts, models, and educational theories. Once these are accepted by all the faculty involved, implementation of the curriculum is facilitated.

PHILOSOPHY

Philosophy is commonly defined to mean the conceptions, beliefs, or assumptions one holds about life, human behavior, and education. More strictly defined, philosophy is a search for an understanding of human nature with its realities, meanings, values, and standards of behavior as they relate to the nature of society and education.

The areas of study encompassed by philosophy are epistemology, logic, ethics, aesthetics, and metaphysics, all of which center on the search for truth. Epistemology focuses on the origin, nature, methods, and limits of knowledge—that is, what humans know. Logic is concerned with the normative formal principles of reasoning in the argument, justification, and explanation of a theory. Ethics deals with the study of standards of human conduct and the underlying morals and values of a theory. Aesthetics concentrates on the study of art and beauty, its sources, forms, and effects. Metaphysics is the study seeking to explain the nature of being or reality, which is associated with epistemology, cosmology, ontology, and phenomenology. Ontology involves the study of the nature of being, reality, or ultimate substance; cosmology the origin and structure of the world; and phenomenology the description and classification of phenomena without attempt at metaphysical explanation (Ennis, 1969; Green, 1971).

The scholarly movements in philosophy have resulted in the formation of several systems of philosophical approach. Some of the traditional systems are pragmatism, existentialism, positivism, idealism, and realism. Pragmatism is a philosophical system associated with C.S. Pierce and William James that determines the meaning and truth of all concepts by testing their validity with the results obtained. Existentialism, stemming from the work of Kierkegaard (1941), Sartre (1966), and Heidegger (1972), is based on the doctrine that existence takes precedence over essence, holding the position that humans are totally free and responsible for their acts and that this responsibility is the source of an encompassing dread and anguish. Positivism, which emerged from the efforts of Auguste Comte, is a system of philosophy that bases knowledge solely on the data of sense experience and relies on scientific facts and their relationship to each other. Idealism is that system that views objects of perception as being actually ideas that the mind knows directly and not existing as objects in and of themselves. Realism is the doctrine that considers universal or abstract terms as objectively actual, so that material objects exist in and of themselves.

Whichever system of philosophy is employed, in general philosophy provides the knowledge about the nature of humanity and the universe and the tools for theory development or logical analysis of the principles underlying thought. Among those areas of philosophy that have been most heavily relied on in the development of knowledge for the professions are epistemology and logic.

Epistemology seeks to explain the basic premises about the nature of human beings, reality, and knowledge. During the explication process, concepts that are believed to be relevant to each discipline are identified. These concepts relate to the nature, reality, purpose, goals, focus, obligations, norms, and values of the discipline under study.

Logic is the area of philosophy providing the means of pursuing correct reasoning in the advancement of theoretical argument. The accepted forms of reasoning are deductive and inductive.

CONCEPTS

Theoretical knowledge begins with a concept, which may be defined in a variety of ways. For example, a concept may be defined as a label or a word symbol used to classify objects, events, or behavioral phenomena that share common characteristics. Norris (1982) defines a concept as an abstraction of concrete events representing ways of perceiving a phenomenon. As Norris points out, however, a single concept cannot stand alone because it is insufficient in and of itself to represent the totality of a phenomenon. Therefore, the full meaning of a concept is dependent upon its relationship to a key concept in a discipline. This key concept may have several subconcepts or minor concepts that are logically related to and are supportive of it. When this key concept is related to other major concepts that have been logically developed along with an operational definition reflecting their relationship, a basis for theory development results and emergence of a theory begins.

Concepts have the greatest utility if they meet two conditions. First, they need to be labeled with terms that have agreed-upon meanings or meanings that have common usage in definitions. Second, concepts should be measurable in concrete situations. Both conditions require continued efforts toward the achievement of precision in the evolution of concepts. Without these conditions being met it is doubtful that the concepts developed can be validated.

Brunner, Goodnow, and Austin (1976) studied the manner in which individuals form concepts and the reason for concept formation. Based on their assumption that people live in an extraordinarily diverse environment, they concluded that individuals use the process of categorization and concept formation to cope with the environment and manipulate the world about them. These theorists also identified three types of concepts: conjunctive, disjunctive, and relational. A conjunctive concept is defined by the simultaneous presence of several attributes or characteristics. An example is a "male nurse," a concept in which the attributes of *male* and *nurse* are joined. In the disjunctive category, members share the presence or absence of attributes. An example is a male nurse who is not registered. Lastly, the relational concept defines relations such as wife, husband, daughter, and son.

Thus, to conceptualize requires one to identify common characteristics or elements of objects, events, and behaviors that have been observed in numerous and separate circumstances. Once developed, the concepts can be used in statements to describe the actual world and human existence.

To teach students to form concepts and understand the nature of concepts is crucial to understanding the nature of knowledge, because concepts are the basis of personal and scientific knowledge (Hyman, 1968). To assist nurse educators in teaching concepts, King (1986) has provided a precise approach to the development of a concept. She delineates the following steps as components of this process:

1. A literature review of the previous work done on the concept in terms of investigations and theories using a general literature search.
2. A review of the nursing literature for studies related to the concept.
3. An analysis and identification of the nature or characteristics of the concept from the exploration of the literature.
4. Derivation of an operational definition for the concept.

Using this process, subconcepts related to the major concept are delineated and explained with their relationship to each other and the major concept. The result is fashioned into an operational definition to establish the meaning of the concept according to its intended usage (King, 1986, p. 4).

According to Ausubel, each academic discipline has a hierarchically organized set of concepts that provide a framework or structure that shapes the information-processing system of that discipline. The most inclusive concepts are viewed as holding the position at the top of the apex of a hierarchial structure, and increasingly differentiated, less inclusive concepts developed from factual data are found at the lower levels (Joyce & Weil, 1972).

Advantages of Concepts

Smith (1969) contends that one of the most essential areas of teaching is the teaching of concepts, which are the bricks and mortar of knowledge and a top priority in all subjects. We not only use them to interpret the world as we perceive it, but we also use them to build all theoretical knowledge, rules, and laws.

Most educators value analysis of concepts as a useful strategy for promoting critical thinking in the teaching process. In addition, the teacher finds concepts a systematic approach to organizing teaching content, facilitating the development of logical reasoning in students, and increasing the students' ability to see patterns of meaning in the subject matter they are learning. Finally, utilizing the strategy of students developing concepts fosters their creativity (Joyce & Weil, 1972).

Disadvantages of Concepts

As Griffiths (1959) observed, theories are not built for eternity but to help in the identification and clarification of current problems and those in the immediate future. This same observation applies to concepts which, like theories, suffer from obsolescence. An example of the continued use of an obsolescent concept central to nursing and the consequences of the decision made in the selection of the concept is described by Hall and Allan (1986). They analyzed and compared the effects on nursing when the concepts of disease and health were used in nursing education. Using the disease concept, which allies nursing with medical practice, the consequences were that the focus was on the dependent functions of nursing within the nurse-physician relationship, which aimed at producing a technocrat. These writers contended that focusing on the concept of disease could not be used to study people as an entity. They reasoned that disease could not be separated from the person or the person's environment. Further, they argued that health could not be separated from disease, the person, or the environment. By using the disease model, with its technological approach to nursing, the result was that nursing's focus was on technology as an end in itself rather than as providing a means to a better life (Hall & Allan,

1986). Both concepts (health and disease) cannot exist together in nursing for each gives different directions to theory development, research, and clinical practice. An attempt to use both concepts, either in the same class or in the same educational program as a primary focus, creates a dualism in nursing education that results in confusion, nonproductive conflict within the profession, and a reduction in the total health care that is provided.

MODELS

Models are developed using related concepts which have not yet progressed toward theory. In general, models may be defined as structural designs consisting of organized and related concepts. However, in the strictest sense models are defined as pictorial representations that show the simplified details of a concept or concepts considered relevant to measuring specific outcomes of a discipline.

Torres (1986) advances the notion that models are developed to give some meaning to the relationships between concepts, enabling the user to visualize diagramatically how one concept logically or causally influences and connects with another. She further categorizes models into four types according to their structure: (1) linear and directional models; (2) circular models; (3) core identification models; and (4) foundational models.

Joyce and Weil (1972) view models as varying in their amount of structure and level of complexity, ranging from low to high levels with each model having a different focus. They provide an in-depth discussion of models for teaching. Among these models are those based on information processing, development of creativity, behavioral modification, and human development.

The increase over the past two decades in the development and use of nursing models reflects a substantial change in the attitudes of professional nurses toward nursing practice and education. An example is the model for problem solving developed by Predham, Hansen, and Conrad for the purpose of encouraging critical thinking and inquiry and incorporated into the nursing process by Nehring, Durham, and Macek (1986).

Propositions Developed from Models

Statements expressing the relationship of concepts contained within models can be developed into propositions to be tested by research for truthfulness. These propositions are considered to be simple statements of the relationship. If research shows that the proposition is true, then theory development is ready to proceed.

Although some authorities equate propositions with assumptions, others define the terms differently. Thus, assumptions are defined according to conventional use as anything taken for granted that does not require validation. Assumptions so defined can be explicit and specified or implicit and unspecified.

In the more scholarly efforts of theory building from models and concepts, efforts have been directed toward the development of conditional propositions. Conditional propositions are those statements specifying that if a particular condition or situation exists and prevails, then a specified consequence will result. Conditional propositions take the form of "if x then y." Thus, a conditional proposition contains the element of an antecedent and a consequent. An example frequently experienced in teaching is that if the student is intrinsically motivated, then he or she will learn more rapidly. As can be seen in this example, two concepts that are related are motivation and learning. From this type of proposition a hypothesis can be generated to test and research. From concepts stated in conditional propositions and tested through the research process, theories can be developed that may result in the establishment of laws or facts.

Advantages of Models

The nursing models used in nursing education are those that provide the framework for the process and the content of nursing curricula. The educational models are used in the actual teaching or implementation of curricula.

Although all individuals throughout the life span engage in educational activity either through planned, sequential learning or through incidental learning of an experiential nature, the higher education setting fosters a prolonged period of intellectual and psychological development. Within this setting planned use of models empowers the teacher to assist students during the learning process to achieve problem-solving and critical thinking skills.

The primary advantage of teaching or learning models is that they provide a conceptual framework for the direction, analysis, and evaluation of the teaching and learning process. Concepts related to these models can be used to provide the teacher with several ways of thinking about how students learn. Integrating this knowledge into practice enables the teacher to more effectively clarify the content being taught.

Some models are more suitable than others for the selection and development of instructional materials. An example is the behavioral modification model, which is the most appropriate model for programmed instruction. Other models are more appropriate for fostering personal interaction, development of inquiry, or group investigation efforts (Joyce & Weil, 1972).

Disadvantages of Models

Disadvantages in the use of models primarily result from inappropriate decisions in the selection of models. It is important to have more than a superficial or tenuous grasp of the concepts contained within models. If the concepts and their attributes are not fully understood, the outcome of teaching and learning will be characterized by confusion and ineffectiveness. It is impossible to convey its meaning to the learner. Therefore, a systematic analysis of models is a prerequisite for their use. Also, in this way, the teacher avoids the trap of instant and premature adoption of one model to the exclusion of others while ignoring the focus, setting, logic, and completeness of the model adopted.

THEORY

Underlying all theoretical knowledge about teaching and learning are the assumptions or philosophy about human beings. Therefore, every theorist begins as a philosopher whose assumptions about the nature of humans and their relationship with the environment influence the approach taken in the development of theory. Because of the differing assumptions there has been and continues to be a wide variation in the theories which have been developed or are in the process of development. Bigge (1971) used three models to demonstrate opposing assumptions that influence the development of theoretical knowledge (Fig. 1-1). The models represented view people as mind or organism, organism, and person, in relation with the external environment. In the first model, humans are presented as passive. In the second model, people are active; and in the third, interactive.

The definition of theory often differs according to the focus of the theorists defining the term. In the past confusion has resulted in the definition of theory that is related to semantics. *Conceptual models, conceptual frameworks, theories,* and *paradigms* were and in some cases still are terms that are used interchangeably. An in-depth study of theory, however, clearly shows that theories are not conceptual frameworks, models, or paradigms. Theories consist of concepts organized in a systematic, logically connected manner to explain their relationship. Conceptual frameworks, models, and paradigms serve as a link in theory development by being prototypes of theory.

Exploration of the efforts to define theory has resulted in clarifying its nature and characteristics. The nature of a theory is that it either specifies or implies a set of operations; is cyclic; and is always in the process of development. It emanates from significant problems in practice and includes the work and

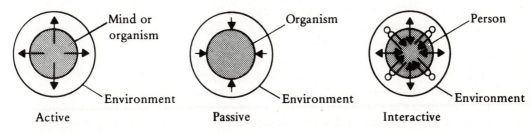

Active   Passive   Interactive

Figure 1-1. Models of theoretical knowledge development. (*Reproduced with permission from Bigge [1971], p. 16.*)

definitions of previous theorists, taking into account the themes and emergent issues resulting from their theory construction.

The characteristics of theories are that they differ in structure, practice goals, research, specific domain or multiple uses, and their tenativeness in status.

The definition of theory that appears to have the most utility for teaching and nursing is that developed by Chinn and Jacobs (1983): "a set of concepts, definitions, and propositions that projects a systematic view of phenomena by designating specific inter-relationships among concepts for the purpose of describing, explaining, predicting, and/or controlling phenomena (p. 70)." As Meleis (1985) points out in her discussion of theory, this definition leaves the decision for the uses of theory up to the consumer of theory.

Advantages of Theory

As the root of knowledge in all disciplines, theory is essential for a profession because it provides the focus on the profession's goals of practice. It establishes a definition of the boundaries of the profession and a description of the nature of the profession in relation to the people it serves. Perhaps one of the most significant contributions of theory to a practice profession is that it identifies appropriate behaviors for members of that profession.

With professional autonomy and accountability being a major concern of the professional organizations, nursing leaders in the profession take the position that both autonomy and accountability are heightened by the use of theory in practice. They view theory as providing the theory's user with control over the practice situation and promoting relationships among nurses involved in the component roles in nursing practice.

Disadvantages of Theory

If theory does not provide terms for effective communication to the practice discipline, it is rendered useless. Too often a theory is selected for use without taking this into account. This results in alienation of those people in practice from those educating students *for* practice.

More often the disadvantages in the use of theory are due to the competing theories in both nursing and education. These theories provide different answers to the questions raised in practice. Unfortunately, decisions made in the selection of a theory often rely on an authority who is a proponent or originator of a specific theory. Obviously, the prominence of the authority in and of itself does not guarantee reliability and validity in the use of the theory. Even top theorists disagree. Whether the consumer intends to use the theory for the curriculum process, clinical practice, research, or administrative purposes, a decision about the use of a specific theory necessitates comparative thinking in the selection process. Attention needs to be directed toward the theory to evaluate whether it is specific, general, or tentative in its development.

If no investment is made in this type of investigation, unreal expectations of the theory are likely to result, creating frustration on the part of the consumer.

Theories cannot be expected to be prescriptive because they generally address practice in its broadest sense. Many theories are linked to research for validation prior to being linked to practice. In the majority of instances, however, the research evidence to support theoretical efforts remains scant at best. Beyond this limitation, theories are occasionally biased in terms of the cultural practices and climates of the educational and health care settings. As a result, certain theories may not be congruent with societal views of health care and education.

Fads in the adoption of theories due to their popularity at certain phases in the development of a discipline often result in premature closure on the evaluation and applicability of the theory. As a consequence, the nature of the theory is overlooked, and rigid support of the theory with popular appeal may result in a disservice to the practice discipline.

DEVELOPMENT OF THE NURSE EDUCATOR

For the neophyte teacher to navigate the chasm between pupilhood and teacherhood and to develop a concept of teaching requires active involvement in the analysis of philosophies, concepts, models, theories, and research about teaching and learning. The primary focus of theory building has been on learning theory, instructional models, and research on teacher effectiveness. There is still a need for a theory that focuses on the process of change that occurs in the development of a teacher.

Fuller and Brown (1975) identified three stages of learning based on their research that focused on teacher concerns related to the task of teaching, the teacher, and students. These three stages of learning to teach with clusters of behaviors were identified as:

1. *The survival stage* in which the teacher has concerns about adequacy and survival in the role of teacher. Emphasis is on control of the class and being liked by pupils.
2. *The mastery stage* in which the teacher is trying to perform so that teaching behaviors are effective. Concerns are on the time pressures, lack of instructional support, materials, and having too many students.
3. *The pupil counts stage* in which the social and emotional needs of the student become the teacher's focus. In this stage the inappropriate nature of some curriculum materials becomes evident, and concerns shift to teaching or reaching the individual students (p. 37).

In the third stage teachers are described as either settling into stable routines and becoming resistant to change or becoming consequence oriented. In being consequence oriented teachers are concerned about their impact on pupils and are responsive, perhaps, to feedback from students about their teaching (Fuller & Brown, 1975).

These stages provide insight into the development of the teacher. Further, they are useful as means of describing the stage of development of the individual learning to teach.

OVERVIEW OF SELECTED LEARNING THEORIES FOR NURSING EDUCATION

Impetus was given to the development of learning theories during the twentieth century by the emergence of the disciplines of psychology and education, the movement toward the utilization of scientific thought rather than continued reliance on authority, and the change in the settings in which learning occurred. Theorists and researchers have centered their efforts on the exploration and clarification of what, how, and when learning becomes evident. The traditional learning theories resulting from these efforts are generally classified into two broad categories: (1) the stimulus-response conditioning theories, which are linked to the behaviorist school of thought; and (2) the cognitive-field theories linked to the Gestalt school of thought.

A brief review of selected learning theories reveals that each theory has contributed to the development of later theories and each theory rests upon an extensive body of knowledge and research. Therefore, an in-depth analysis is required to avoid the oversimplification and misuse of individual theories.

Stimulus-Response Theory

Edward L. Thorndike's theory of learning was a precursor of the stimulus-response (S-R) conditioning theories of the behaviorist school of thought. This theory was called the S-R bond theory, which was labeled connectionism. Thorndike's assumptions upon which his theory is based were strongly influenced by the new physiological psychology emerging at the time of his work. His major assumptions were:

1. The learner plays a passive role in learning.
2. Through conditioning, specific responses become linked with specific stimuli, and these links or bonds are products of a biological change.
3. There are both physical and mental events involved in learning. A mental unit or event is something sensed or perceived. A physical unit is a stimulus or response. The two units can be connected in various combinations.
4. Humans are neutral passive or reactive organisms capable of many S-R connections (Bigge, 1971, p. 53).

From his research with cats, Thorndike formulated the concept that the principle way S-R connections were formed was through random trial-and-error-learning. Continuing with a rather loose collection of rules and suggestions, Thorndike set down some "laws" of learning. His primary laws were identified as those related to readiness, exercise, and effect. The secondary laws were classified as laws related to multiple response, set or attitude, prepotency of elements, response by analogy, and associative shifting.

Thorndike's primary laws are those that have received the most attention from scholars interested in learning theory. The law of readiness related to the conduction unit or connection of the neurons and synapses involved in establishing a bond. The law stated that for a conduction unit to conduct was satisfying and failure to conduct was annoying. The law of exercise or repetition stated that the more times a stimulus-response pair was repeated the longer it would be retained—the bond was strengthened by exercise. The law of effect stated that if the S-R connection was followed by satisfaction, there was an increase in the strength of the S-R bond or connection. In the event that the S-R connection went with or followed an annoyance, the result was a decrease in the strength of the connection (Bigge, 1971). This law related to positive and negative reinforcement, concepts still used by many engaged in teaching.

For the most part these laws leave little room for insight into the thought processes and appear mechanical in nature. They also do not deal with the psychological concept of purposiveness.

Although behaviorists rejected some of Thorndike's ideas, the law of associative shifting became the keystone for the behaviorist movement toward theory development. This law stated that a response elicited from a learner was that which he or she was capable of and was associated with any situation to which the learner was sensitive.

Behaviorist Theory

Prominent among the S-R theorists who followed Thorndike was B.F. Skinner, who developed the theory of conditioning through reinforcement. His assumptions about humans were:

1. A human being is a neutral-passive organism.
2. Human behavior is lawful and subject to external variables outside the organism in its immediate environment or personal history.
3. Human behavior is an observable phenomenon (Joyce & Weil, 1972, pp. 269–270).

Skinner defined learning as a change in the probability of a response in most cases of operant conditioning. Reinforcement served as the basis for operant conditioning and response was the unit of behavior involved in this theoretical approach. A set of acts were identified as operants that were reinforced to increase the probability of their recurrence in the future. In addition to Skinner's primary concepts of reinforcement and operant conditioning, he established two types of operant reinforcements: stimulus discrimination and response differentiation.

Relating his theory to classroom practice, Skinner saw operant conditioning as an answer to some of the weaknesses in educational practices. He made several salient observations in supporting his view of these weaknesses. The most serious criticism he offered about classroom procedures was the infrequency of reinforcement during the learning process. He stated that although it was not possible for one teacher to provide an adequate number of reinforcement contingencies to a class of 30 or more students, this problem could be overcome by the use of programmed instruction. A second criticism was that student behaviors were frequently dominated by aversion stimulation. These aversion stimuli were a series of minor distasteful events such as teacher criticism or demonstrated displeasure and peer ridicule. According to Skinner, distasteful events could be avoided if teaching and learning were centered on operant conditioning. He explained that with the conditioning approach the teacher would utilize control and stimulus discrimination, which were fundamental to learning, rather than permit unplanned aversion stimulation. The third criticism noted by him was the excessive time lapse between a response and its reinforcement, which destroyed most of the effect of reinforcement on learning. An example given by Skinner related to material studied and tested at the beginning of the week not being graded until the end of the week; the consequence was that the learning experience was obstructed or diminished.

Cognitive-Field Theory

In an attempt to resolve the active-passive dilemma among learning theorists, Kurt Lewin and other cognitive-field theorists moved toward the development of an emergent synthesis for understanding learning. To them an emergent synthesis was achieved by the selection and modification of knowledge from incompatible positions, adding new thinking when necessary, and developing a new position more adequate than its precursors. Thus, it could not be equated with an eclectic compromise, in which aspects of opposing theories were selected and a position somewhere among them taken.

Contrary to S-R theories, cognitive-field psychology does not consider learning as an expression of inner urges or "unfoldment." Learning is defined as the development of insight into the nature of a person's world.

Among the key concepts in Lewin's cognitive-field theory were life space, foreign hull, goal, and cognitive structure. A person's life space did not refer to physical entities but represented his or her psychological world or contemporaneous situation. The foreign hull of life space was that part of one's physical and social environment that limited behavioral possibilities. Goal was defined as that region of life space toward or away from which the person was psychologically drawn. Cognitive structure represented insight or under-standing.

From these theoretical formulations life space was used as a model that en-abled one to consider the total life of a person. Interaction of the person within his or her life space was characterized according to the nature of the person's perception. Subsequently, it was the cognitive experiential processes by which a person psychologically and simultaneously reached out of his or her environ-ment, making something of it and seeing the consequences of action. Learning in accordance with this position was defined as a dynamic process through in-teractive experiences, insights, or cognitive structures of life spaces, wherein life spaces were changed to become more serviceable for future guidance (Bigge, 1971).

Information-Processing Theory

One of the most prominent among contemporary theorists is Robert Gagné whose theory emerged from efforts to overcome the limitations of traditional learning theories. Influenced by system, information, and cybernetic theory and basing his theoretical work only on manifest human behavior and per-formance, he identified eight types and phases of learning.

The underlying philosophy in this theory is that human beings are active agents who interact with their environment. A self-regulatory feedback system generates its own activities in order to detect and control specific stimulus characteristics of the environment.

Learning is viewed as an attempt to change the manifest behavior and performance of the learner. The learning process itself consists of sequen-tial achievement of learning tasks moving from the simple to the more complex.

The eight types of learning identified by Gagné were:

1. *Signal learning*, the simplest of learning tasks, in which the learner learns to make a diffuse, general response to a signal or stimulus.
2. *Stimulus-response learning*, in which the learner acquires a well-defined response to a specific stimulus or stimuli.
3. *Chaining*, in which the learner acquires a chain of two or more stim-ulus-response connections.
4. *Verbal association*, in which the learning is acquired in verbal chains for naming a thing or object.
5. *Discriminate learning*, by which the learner learns to make different re-sponses to different stimuli that may resemble each other in physical ap-pearance. Naming of objects is developed prior to discrimination. Through this learning concept development begins.
6. *Concept learning*, in which the learner acquires the ability to make a common response to a class of stimuli that differs widely from each other in appearance.

7. *Rule learning,* in which learning simple to complex rules, and being able to apply these rules, is accomplished.
8. *Problem solving,* in which learning to combine two or more previously learned rules produces a new capacity for resolving problems.

The learning process organized in Gagne's sequential stages provides a framework for the selection of teaching strategies at each level to facilitate progress of students toward the achievement of desired objectives.

Cognitive Moral Development Theory

Refining Piaget's developmental stages and researching cross-cultural values and structures of moral judgment, Lawrence Kohlberg (1977) developed a theory of moral development. In the developmental sense, this theory is a cognitive theory. Learning is viewed as the transformations that occur in a person's form or structure of thought as that person's moral autonomy and conception of justice increases.

Implicit assumptions underlie Kohlberg's theory. One assumption is that people are interactive with their social environment. The second is that people are the psychological product of educational systems that in the past have separated themselves from any responsibility for a moral education of students to avoid conflict with other social systems.

Kohlberg's (1977) stages of cognitive development, which he uses to formulate a structure of moral reasoning, are organized into six sequential stages, which are subsumed under three major levels of moral development. These levels, stages, and accompanying behaviors are as follows:

I. Preconventional level
 Stage 1. Punishment-orientation, with unquestioned deference to power and avoidance of punishment.
 Stage 2. Instrumental-relativist orientation, with satisfaction of one's own needs and occasionally the needs of others.
II. Conventional level
 Stage 3. "Good boy—nice girl" orientation, with conformity to stereotypical images for approval of behaviors.
 Stage 4. Law and order orientation, with respect for maintaining social order and doing one's duty. Adherence to personal expectations and social order. Support and justification for social order and identification with those groups that are similar in behavior.
III. Postconventional, autonomous, or principles level
 Stage 5. Social-contract, legalistic orientation, in which right actions tend to be viewed in terms of general individual rights and standards critically examined and agreed on by society. Clear awareness of relativism of personal values.
 Stage 6. Universal-ethical-principle orientation, in which right is defined by the decision of conscience, adhering to self-chosen ethical

principles related to universal principles of justice, reciprocity, and equality in human rights. Respect for the dignity of human beings as individual persons is demonstrated.

There are three primary characteristics of the stages described in Kohlberg's theory. These characteristics are as follows:

1. The stages are organized systems of thought wherein individuals are consistent in their level of moral judgment.
2. Under all but the most extreme conditions individuals move forward toward the next stage in the sequence of development, never skipping a stage.
3. The stages form a hierarchial integration in that thinking at a higher stage includes all that is comprehended at lower stages.

In addition to these characteristics, an individual's tendency is to function at the highest level achieved in his or her moral development.

Kohlberg's theory provides the means to focus on the holistic development of nursing students. With the dilemma faced by nurses, who have to function at both dependent and independent levels of practice in health care systems that emphasize obedience to authority, the need for nursing educators to attend to the moral development of students is evident. Assessing the moral development level of students and generating teaching strategies to assist them in their moral development are courses of action necessary to producing morally mature, committed, and self-directed professionals.

Implications of Kohlberg's theory of moral development for education are twofold. First, moral development needs to be diagnosed if learners are to move toward greater skills in analysis and increased independence in thinking and performing tasks. Second, the method of choice in teaching moral education is that of exposing learners to conflict situations and introducing them to new levels of reaction to these situations.

A THEORETICAL MODEL FOR TEACHING

The relationship between teaching and learning remains unsettled. We have yet to discover how and to what extent teaching causes learning. As previously discussed, Joyce and Weil (1972) have presented a number of models for teaching based on numerous theories of learning. Green (1971) however, developed his model for teaching from an analysis and an exploration of the concept of teaching and its related concepts.

In the development of his model, Green first organized the activities of teaching into the logical, strategic, and institutional acts. The logical acts primarily related to the elements of thinking and reasoning practiced in the conduct of teaching. The strategic activities related to the teacher's plan or strategy for teaching and included the ways in which materials were organized and how students were directed during the teaching process. The first two acts within Green's categories are as follows:

Logical Acts	*Strategic Acts*
1. Explaining	1. Motivating
2. Concluding	2. Counseling
3. Inferring	3. Evaluating
4. Giving reasons	4. Planning
5. Assessing evidence	5. Encouraging
6. Demonstrating	6. Disciplining
7. Defining	7. Questioning
8. Comparing	

The third category of teacher acts, which Green labels the institutional acts of teaching, are not discussed here because these acts were not found necessary in the strictest sense to the activity of teaching. They included such acts as making reports, keeping records, and taking attendance.

The categorization of teaching acts is useful for two reasons. First, it described what teachers do in the role of teaching. Second, it led to Green's analysis of the forms that teaching takes, resulting in the development of his model for teaching.

Beginning with an analysis of the concept of *teaching* and an exploration of related concepts, Green discovered considerable ambiguity existing in the meaning of the term. The terms he found related to teaching were *indoctrination, conditioning, training,* and *instructing* (Green, 1971), which to some degree appeared to overlap in meaning. However, in organizing these terms as subconcepts of teaching, he developed a model showing their relationship to teaching and correlated them with specific goals of teaching. Training and conditioning are shown in his model as the subconcepts of teaching used for shaping behavior. Instructing and indoctrinating were identified as the subconcepts of teaching which are used for shaping knowledge and belief. Each of these related subconcepts is placed on a continuum that extends in opposite directions from the center of the model. The progression from conditioning to indoctrinating represents increasing degrees of the manifestation of intelligence required from the student who is being taught. The model is shown in Figure 1-2.

Green explains all of the subconcepts as ways of teaching that depend on the circumstances facing the teacher. In conditioning, a student responds to external stimuli in a predictable manner. In training, people acquire knowledge and beliefs, and habits and behaviors are formed. Teaching is viewed as beginning at the point where students go beyond the fundamental skills they have learned. Teaching is primarily centered on the subconcept of instructing in which the goal is concerned with enlarging the manifestation of intelligence. And finally, indoctrinating relates to teaching someone that specific beliefs and knowledge are valued.

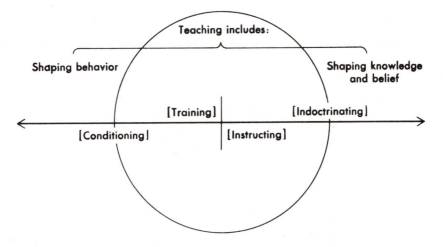

Figure 1-2. Green's model of teaching. (*Reproduced with permission from Green [1971], p. 33.*)

THE INFLUENCE OF THE TEACHER'S CONCEPTS OF EDUCATION, TEACHING, AND LEARNING

The teaching role primarily involves the functions of assisting students in learning subject matter and skills specific to nursing practice and facilitating interpersonal relationships aimed at self-awareness and working with others. The way in which the teacher conceptualizes education, teaching, and learning influences the selection of the theory or model used to guide the teacher in the performance of these functions.

The development of these concepts requires an analysis of the literature with an examination of the underlying assumptions or philosophy of education expressed by the theorist or writer who formulates the concept. Criteria for the selection of the concepts are that:

1. The philosophy or assumptions are consistent with the teacher's own philosophy.
2. A particular meaning in the form of a definition is provided, which indicates or includes a corresponding set of operations.

A teacher's concept of education is usually based on his or her identification of the purposes of education. According to educators at the national level, the purpose of education is to make learners more functionally competent and employable. To achieve this in an environment of technological change a major purpose of education is to instill in the learner the value of pursuing lifelong learning. This requires teachers to teach students to think analytically, examine information critically, challenge assumptions, and think creatively (Danner, 1986).

Definitions of learning that have been developed deal either with the scope of teaching or the relation of teaching to learning. A definition that is generally accepted by educators and encompasses both of these aspects has not yet emerged. Perhaps one of the most accepted definitions that relates to the scope of teaching is the one developed by Scheffler. He states that teaching may be characterized as an activity aimed at the achievement of learning and practiced in such a manner as to respect the student's intellectual integrity and capacity for independent judgment (Hyman, 1968).

There are many learning theorists who have developed theories that include definitions of learning. King (1986) is among the nursing theorists who have provided an example of clarity and comprehensiveness in the definition of learning. She defines learning as "a process of sensory perception, conceptualization, and critical thinking involving multiple experiences in which changes in concepts, skills, symbols, habits, and values can be evaluated in observable behaviors and inferred from behavioral manifestations (p. 24)." The assumptions about the learner that accompany this definition are well organized and generally accepted by educators in nursing and other disciplines.

SELECTION OF A THEORY OR MODEL FOR TEACHING

Although one may wish that teaching could be simplified by reliance on one comprehensive theory to guide the teaching process, such a theory does not yet exist. Differences in the developmental level, cognitive style, personality, and natural ability of teachers and students add to the complexity of teaching and learning. Due to this complexity, no one learning theory is adequate for consistent use and attention must be directed to the selection of appropriate theories and models for the tasks of teaching and learning.

The steps that are necessary in the selection of a theory or model are the following:

1. Exploration of a theory, its underlying philosophy, and major concepts.
2. Identification of the theory's significant features and the relationship of these features to the types of learning required to meet the goals of teaching.
3. Evaluation of the theory's relevance to the goals of the curriculum.

In the process of selection, three facts become evident. One is that each theory relates to and explains learning from a different vantage point. The second is that each theory explicitly or implicitly contains varying and specific sets of operations related to its use. The third is that teaching one theory is not sufficient to cover all situations or areas of practice.

The Eclectic Use of Theory

Throughout their teaching careers, many educators have become victims of fads in learning theory and the research supporting it. Thus, they have frequently adopted an array of theories that have conflicting features and cannot be blended for effective teaching. These theories differ not only in their philosophical underpinnings and the nature of their concepts but also in the set of teaching practices implied by each theory.

Since any learning theory is able to account only for certain aspects of the learning phenomenon and unable to account for other aspects, the eclectic approach to the use of theory is viewed as essential by many educators. This approach to teaching and learning is possible in many instances only through the resolution of philosophical differences between the theory and the teacher for whose use the theory was intended. This is not an easy task, for some of the philosophical positions about human beings are still subject to debate. This is not to say, however, that it is impossible to find philosophies of certain theories that are consistent with the teacher's own philosophy.

In the eclectic approach to teaching, the educator needs to keep in touch with the connections between theories in their continued development. Further, it is necessary to keep abreast of what is currently known about learning and to continue the integration of learning principles derived from this knowledge into practice.

IMPLEMENTATION OF THEORY INTO PRACTICE

In the implementation of theory into practice, several critical factors require consideration. These factors are the individual differences in learning, the variations in the cognitive styles of the learner, the developmental level of the learner, and his or her goals and motives.

An example of these considerations is given by Kohlberg, who cautions that teaching should be geared to the appropriate moral level of the learner. As he suggests, it would be inappropriate to provide a learner who is at Stage 1 with a Stage 5 task. He also issues an imperative for the successful use of his model: the teacher must be well grounded in the needs and developmental stages of the learners, irrespective of the diversity encountered in the group of learners.

In addition to the aforementioned considerations and imperative, it is important to remember that knowledge of teaching and learning theories are not all a teacher needs to know in the implementation of theory. An in-depth theoretical background and well-developed skills in communication, leadership, motivation, and change are also essential.

The teacher's search for the body of knowledge about and related to teaching and learning that enables him or her to select effective teaching strategies and instructional methods may be frustrating, and at times may require a considerable expenditure of time and effort. However, having once explored the theoretical knowledge that provides the foundation for teaching, the teacher discovers many routes are available for development of teaching strategies to approach the tasks of teaching and learning.

REFERENCES

Berlyn, D.E. (1966) *Problem solving, research, method, and theory.* New York: Wiley.

Bigge, M.L. (1971). *Learning theories for teaching* (2nd ed.). New York: Harper & Row.

Brunner, J., Goodnow, J., & Austin, G. (1976). *A study of thinking.* New York: Science Editions.

Chinn, P., & Jacobs, M. (1983). *Theory and nursing: A systematic approach.* St. Louis: Mosby.

Danner, M.D. (moderator). (1986, Feb. 19). National Commission on Excellence in Education. Forum: How not to fix the schools—A nation at risk. *Harper's, 272,* 39–51.

Ennis, R.H. (1969). *Logic in teaching.* Englewood Cliffs, NJ: Prentice-Hall.

Fuller, F., & Brown, O. (1975). Becoming a teacher. In K. Ryan (Ed.), *Teacher education.* Chicago: National Society for the Study of Education.

Green, T.F. (1971). *The activities of teaching.* New York: McGraw-Hill.

Griffiths, D.E. (1959). *Administrative theory.* New York: Appleton-Century-Crofts.

Hall, B., & Allan, J. (1986, June). Sharpening nursing's focus by focusing on health. *Nursing and Health Care, 7,* 315–320.

Heidegger, M. (1972). *On time and being.* New York: Harper & Row.

Hyman, R.T. (Ed.). (1968). *Teaching: Vantage points for study.* New York: Lippincott.

Joyce, B., & Weil, M. (1972). *Models of teaching.* Englewood Cliffs, NJ: Prentice-Hall.

Kierkegaard, S. (1941). *Sickness into death.* Translated by W. Laurie. Princeton: Princeton University Press. (Originally published in 1849.)

King, I.M. (1986). *Curriculum and instruction in nursing: Concepts and process.* Norwalk, CT: Appleton-Century-Crofts.

Kohlberg, L., & Hersh, R. (1977, April). Moral development: A review of the theory. In *Theory in practice, 16,* 53–59.

Lanier, J., & Cusik, P. (1985, June). An oath for professional educators. *Phi Delta Kappa, 66,* 711.

Meleis, A.I. (1985). *Theoretical nursing: Development and progress.* New York: Lippincott.

Nehring, W., Durham, J., & Macek, M. (1986, May/June). Effective teaching: A problem-solving paradigm. *Nursing Educator, 11,* 23–26.

Norris, C. (1982). *Concept clarification in nursing.* Rockville, MD: Aspen.

Sartre, J.-P. (1966). *Being and nothingness: A principles text of modern existentialism.* Translated by Hazel Barnes. Boulder, CO: University of Colorado Philosophical Library.

Smith, B.O. (1969). *Teachers for the real world.* Washington, DC: American Association of Colleges for Teacher Education.

Torres, G. (1986). *Theoretical foundations of nursing.* Norwalk, CT: Appleton-Century-Crofts.

Utilizing Conceptual Models in Nursing Service

M. Janice Nelson

> And thus, the new endowment would swell with those structural elements that form the institutional context for nursing practice and the driving forces to their attainment.
>
> *M.M. Styles (1982, p. 212)*

Conceptual models have been used in nursing service for nearly three decades. Although longevity is not at issue, it is important to note that *service* is the culminating arena where the nursing phenomenon occurs and where validation of theories takes place—hopefully through empirical research.

The development of theories and models has long been the domain of academicians and scholars. Indeed, it is that scholarly thrust that gives meaning and impetus to practice as well as to the profession as a whole.

CONCEPTUAL MODELS

In defining conceptual models, Fawcett (1984) tells us that models present diverse views of certain phenomena in the world, but represent only an approximation or simplification of those concepts considered relevant to understanding the phenomena.

Fawcett further elucidates that models must be "placed within a structural hierarchy of knowledge within a discipline (p. 5)." Clearly, since we all inhabit the world and the disciplines we define are of that same world, phenomena are shared and often overlap. Thus "each discipline singles out certain phenomena with which it will deal in a unique manner (p. 5)." These singled-out phenomena, taken in their entirety as they relate to a discipline form the "metaparadigm"—that which encapsulates these selected concepts from a global or broad vantage point and is perceived in some manner to be the focus of a particular discipline. Thus, nursing encompasses four central concepts that have been agreed on by the experts to constitute nursing's world, or its metaparadigm. These are the person, the environment, health, and nursing acts or interventions taken in themselves (Fawcett, 1984, pp. 5-6).

If one considers the multiple theories of nursing that currently exist, be they developmental, systems, or interactive, they do indeed encompass these four concepts in the practice arena. It is the purpose of this chapter to focus on a dimension that considers conceptual models from a functional and structural perspective dealing with the environment or milieu in which the phenomenon of nursing takes place.

Thus, it can be said that these functional or structural models deal more with *broad patterns* of relationships as opposed to the modular conceptualization of the *nature* of relationships between nurse and client, or attempting to describe how these relationships occur.

The conceptual models for clinical nursing practice presented in this text are sufficiently elaborated on and dealt with as a package. To select one of these as *the* model for nursing service would be a serious oversight—nor can a practice model be eclectically selected by the individual practitioner. Rather, selection of a particular model for a particular setting is entirely dependent upon the organizational "fit"—that is, it depends upon the congruence between organizational philosophy and goals and the practice model interface. In other words, in the interest of consistency and continuity, it is essential that the elements of the model are reflected in the philosophy and goals of the department, and that the structural environment is one that facilitates the process.

Conceptual models utilized in nursing service describe functional modalities or organizational structures that enhance the professional roles of nursing, taking into consideration those bona fide professional components of administration, education, research, and clinical practice.

The models are rooted in a collective, personal, and corporate philosophy that best expresses the aggregate belief in the individual, the family and society, the environment, health, nursing, and responsibilities of the profession in general. The philosophy sets the stage for the model to emerge, and the model in turn becomes the paradigm that sets the tone for the environment or setting in which the dynamics of nursing operate. For example, the primary nursing model, most recently of the care delivery systems in the acute care setting, clearly underscores and enhances professional autonomy, accountability, and clinical decision making within a professional organizational matrix while clearly lending itself to supporting broad criteria of a profession. This model is anchored in an organizational philosophy that speaks to beliefs about the professional role of the nurse, the nurse-patient relationship, consistency and continuity of care, patient education, and the structural milieu that facilitates the process.

The primary nursing model—although relatively new to the acute and perhaps long-term setting—is not new to nursing. Rather, it is an adaptation of the professional nursing model that has traditionally been the norm in public health nursing. The notion of districts and total patient care being planned, pro-vided, and evaluated by the registered professional nurse was introduced to the acute care setting by Hall and Alfano at Loeb Center for Nursing and Rehabili-tation in the Bronx (New York) during the late 1950s and early 1960s. Thanks to Hall (1963) and her professional practice vision, the primary nurse has become the role model for professional practice across a variety of health care settings, and very effectively serves as a connecting link between education and service at the staff nurse level—with the primary nurse serving as undergraduate stu-dent preceptor in the clinical practicum.

In contrast, the not yet extinct (although clearly obsolete) model of functional nursing within the hospital setting long served a purpose of ef-ficiency. Supporting the bureaucratic model and its divisions of labor, the functional method reflected a philosophy that had little to do with corporate beliefs about humanity, society, or professional nursing. The model promoted fragmentation, quantification, task orientation and identification, and cost-effectiveness with little or no attention paid to quality of patient care or pro-fessional growth and reward of the nurse. Designed in the Weberian tradition, it was a simple structure. In most instances it was (and continues to be) divorced from and devoid of creativity, critical thinking, or educational input. Alive and well today for all its tradition, the model asks for nothing and it gives nothing, merely lending itself to the maintenance of the status quo.

Contemporarily with Hall's "Center for Nursing" model at Loeb Center, "team nursing" also emerged in the 1950s. Although not identified as a model per se, the method of delivery of care developed, tested, and implemented by Lambertsen (1953) and her colleagues at Teachers College, Columbia Univer-sity in concert with the nursing administration of Frances Delafield Hospital in New York City, reflected a dramatic change in philosophy that was instrumen-tal in shifting the focus of hospital nursing away from fragmented hierarchy and "nursing the system" to a patient-centered approach. Lambertsen, and certainly Hall, as leaders in the field, might well be credited as having set the stage and provided the thrust for the emergence of better-defined and more sophisticated conceptual modes applied to nursing service as we know them today.

STRUCTURAL MODELS

In addition to the evolution of models that determine the mode of delivery of care, others have emerged that address parameters of structure—that is, they present a paradigm that speaks to the structural environment and patterns of relationships within which administration, education, research, and clinical practice function.

Although perhaps more architectural than scientific in some respects, these models clearly reflect a philosophy relevant to the interrelatedness of nursing education, nursing practice, administration, and research.

Although gradually on the increase, the fact that there continues to be relatively few nursing service models (in relation to the numbers of academic and service settings nationally) across a 25-year span tells us that the feat is easier said than done. Many nurse educators who have tried to formulate an organizational design can identify with Pannell (1982) when she so aptly states that "organizational designs that unite research, service, and education demand maturity and commitment from all participants and are not without attendant stresses and strains (p. 61)."

Many administrative and practice issues are difficult to reconcile, therefore increased role strain on many of the principles involved, and a decided amount of disparity rooted in the prevalent lack of agreement on standards of nursing education has an incredible impact on the multiple issues at hand. According to MacPhail (1972),

> nurse educators, in general, had not, and still have not, assumed responsibility for ensuring high standards of nursing in the health care agencies used as laboratories for students' learning opportunities . . . . Moreover, the attitude of nurse administrators and staff is often not helpful to learners because of their lack of understanding of the goals held for students and the rationale underlying changes in nursing education. In addition, the modus operandi in nursing service has tended to engender rigidity; conformity; dependence on rules, regulations and superiors; and adherence to long-standing patterns which lacked established scientific bases. Nurse educators and nursing service administration were, and still are, hypercritical of each others' policies and practices to the detriment of both patients and students. (pp. 1–2)

From a more subtle vantage point, Ford (1981) quietly observed that "the immediacy of the service demands (is) an anathema to the studious and contemplative nature of . . . faculty (p. 4)."

In any case, it becomes reasonably clear that these models as we currently know and understand them arose from fairly common concerns: (1) the growing rift between nursing practice and nursing education; (2) lack of access and input into the practice setting by nurse educators in order to control the quality of student education; and (3) mutual lack of understanding of the characteristics and mission of either organization.

Undoubtedly, the earliest of these was developed at Case Western Reserve University (CWRU) Frances Payne Bolton School of Nursing in Cleveland. The model, described as "inter-institutional," was designed not to unify, as under one administration, but "to have nursing service and nursing education join forces in a common endeavor (Nayer, 1980, p. 1111)." Although service and education maintain their independent administrative structures, there are joint appointments between service and education and unification exists at the clinical department level, "where nursing service and nursing education meet in the care of patients (Nayer, p. 1111)." What can be noted here (*see* Fig. 2–1) is that the director or chair of a clinical specialty retains administrative responsibility

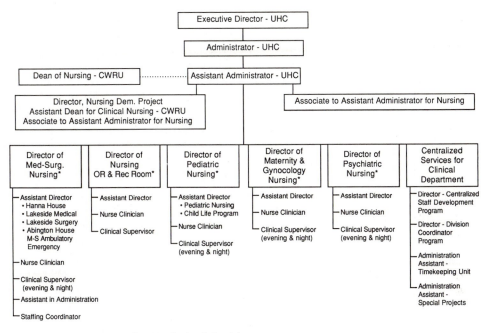

Figure 2-1. Nursing in the medical center.

both academically and clinically. Thus, the model reflects a combination of collaboration and unification.

The nursing model at the University of Rochester (New York), on the other hand, reflects a complete organizational merger of nursing education and nursing service under the directorship of a single dean and director of nursing (*see* Fig. 2–2). Unlike the CWRU model, which maintains two separate and distinct corporate administrations, the Rochester model—described as unification—is clearly under one governance structure, although as one moves through the model the similarities with CWRU emerge at the clinical point where the "clinical nursing chief" is accountable for research, education, and service, and where joint appointments (based on the level of educational preparation) exist among the various components of the nursing staff.

A totally different approach was taken at the Rush Presbyterian-St. Luke's Medical Center in Chicago. Although quality of patient care is certainly an ultimate issue in this model as in the others, the foundation of the Rush model rests with professional role synthesis and implementation (the professional practitioner as teacher), and thus in some respects could be categorized as a behavioral model. Yet, despite the matrix design (which is square as opposed to pyramidal—*see* Fig. 2–3), and in a practitioner-teacher model, the concepts of collaboration and even more unification are clearly there; it should be noted

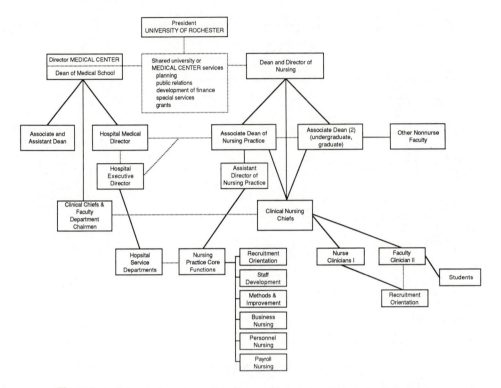

Figure 2–2. School of nursing within the medical center: University of Rochester.

that there are not dual or joint appointments. The CWRU and Rochester models follow more of a traditional organizational design as opposed to the Rush matrix, but the overall intent of promoting and facilitating integration and synthesis of the full professional nursing role encompassing education, practice, and research is present in all. In describing the matrix model, Christman (1979) points out that "matrix models . . . are useful because they permit the various major elements in the care structure to be arrayed so that appropriate loci of power, within and between professions can be arranged for the benefit of total organizational effectiveness (p. 10)."

It is Christman's posture that we in nursing make the mistake of fractioning student education by having students taught by the best prepared in nursing and then utilize staff nurses for role models, when as a rule the staff nurse is least prepared to carry out this function. Thus, the student is alienated, as it were, or deprived of highly educated behavioral models in the practice setting. For this reason, Christman claims, it is essential to have a critical mass of practitioners prepared at advanced educational levels "who could affectively change the clinical influence of nursing (pp. 8–9)." The matrix model, then, provides for more than unification of education and service; it provides for a fusion of the full professional role.

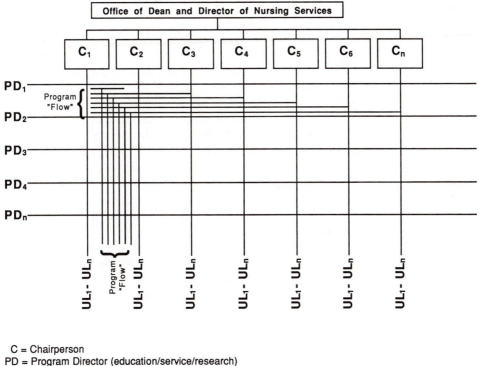

C = Chairperson
PD = Program Director (education/service/research)
UL = Unit Leader (each department has as many unit leaders as required to manage the workload)

Figure 2-3. Matrix model for unification of nursing effort.

The matrix configuration clearly illustrates the interdisciplinary collaborative process and focuses less on the hierarchy—which by its very nature of purpose exists to a greater or lesser degree in all organizations. Additionally, Christman posits that the matrix configuration arrays roles in such a manner that complementation and collaboration are encouraged and "decision-making power is lodged among equals (p. 11)."

By no means does the description of these three models complete the picture. These three, the most noted and most publicized, have in their own right become the paradigms for the rest of us. There are many other institutions, both service and academic, struggling with the challenge. Some have opted for contractural arrangements, others for joint appointments from one institution to another, and still others utilize adjunct appointments with shared salaries.

Whatever the case, there is every evidence that there is a strong movement either to replicate or develop other models to accomplish this highly desirable modus operandi.

EDUCATION AND SERVICE MERGER

There are multiple and varied opinions as to why education and service continue to struggle for a unified profession. Clearly, although we are the oldest of the defined groups of health care providers, and certainly the largest in terms of numbers, we continue to be divided in our efforts.

Service-oriented people are suspect of the "nonconforming" academicians and are reluctant to have institutional practices and practice modalities examined by scholars; academicians, on the other hand, tend to look askance at the rigid adherence to policies and procedures in the service setting. Additionally, service still longs for the days when the neophyte nurse required little orientation and was quite adept at practice skills immediately following graduation; service tends to overlook the increasing complexities of practice, changing modern technologies, and the fact that it is virtually impossible to prepare a beginning practitioner for every variation of the health care setting.

Interestingly enough, although we tend to view the medical model with a degree of envy because of the status it has wrought (as this relates to medicine's traditional "teacher-practitioner" model), it must be kept in mind that medical education functions largely as it did some 40 or more years ago. Although not referred to with such terminology, apprenticeship still prevails—as does rote learning of many thousands of scientific laws and facts—with little attention paid to curriculum development, teaching strategies, communication skills, interpersonal relationships between physicians and clients, or trends in health care delivery systems.

Despite its problems, and although some may say we have a long way to go, nursing in many respects is very advanced. There is absolutely no doubt that education should be done by those who are prepared to teach; at the same time there is absolutely no doubt that the product of that education—the nurse—must be prepared to practice—effectively, competently, and in a professional manner. Those involved in the models discussed in this chapter strive to do exactly that. Clearly, they are not without their problems. Sovie (1981), for example, in discussing the Rochester model points out that clinical chiefs carry a major responsibility for education and practice. The dearth of doctorally prepared nurses makes it extremely difficult to fill these positions.

Another problem is the fact that the decentralization of patient services during the weekdays must, by necessity, revert to a centralized model during evenings, nights, and weekends. A third concern is the huge workloads of the principle players who must meet all requirements for promotion and tenure academically while carrying practice and research responsibilities which, Sovie states, "cannot be carried out successfully without a strong career commitment and excellent support in one's personal life (p. 32)."

Baker (1981) points out that in addition to Sovie's first-hand information many of the problems associated with attempts at collaboration between education and service stem from a traditional commitment to either one or the other.

Baker asserts that many nursing service administrators see the process as a threat to their power base, yet economic realities are forcing the issue of interdependence. From a personal vantage point, it is one thing to hand-pick the principles involved where there is mutual understanding and agreement on common goals; it is quite another to deal with the defenses of individuals from a variety of backgrounds where there is little or no value placed on higher education and its potential impact on the quality of care provided within a particular facility. In addition, given the national economic mood and thrusts toward improved fiscal management, it is essential that the profession as a whole consider more expeditious utilization of scarce resources with benefits to be gained by both entities. As Styles (1984) put it, "the realization is inescapable that the two sectors—service and education—need each other, not just for strength but for survival (p. 23)." As it stands, the lack of effective communication strategies, sufficient planning, and built-in evaluation strategies—as well as the lack of clear, explicit expectations of either party and the lack of courage to risk isolation by colleagues and peers who may be less prepared in order to provide nursing at its best—has often resulted in aborted attempts toward collaboration, partnerships, or unification.

On the positive side, Christman (1979) views the matrix model as one that capitalizes on economy of effort, given all the right parameters of high accountability, high self-directedness, and a high degree of interdependence. He also notes—clearly through very valid experience—that "the fusing of the nursing effort in an organization can greatly enrich the resources of nurses (p. 11)." Sovie too points out that efforts at the University of Rochester have resulted in excellent patient care (based on evaluations of patients, families, physicians, and nursing staff). All faculty practice in areas of expertise, faculty and staff participate in interdisciplinary research, and the nursing model has become predominantly a professional one, with ancillary personnel reduced to a minimum and increasing numbers of licensed practical nurses enrolled in professional nursing programs. Perhaps more importantly, Sovie (1981) tells us that "nursing at Strong Memorial Hospital and the University of Rochester enjoys professional respect and recognition and occupies a position of influence and power in patient care (p. 31)."

Finally, for those of us interested in taking the step, Baker (1981) offers a model that has the potential for multiple variations on a theme (Fig. 2-4). Baker proposes that the three major components of nursing can be reflected through the use of overlapping circles to demonstrate areas of collaboration and joint efforts. As Baker explains, the model can

> illustrate different ways for the individual nurse to implement collaboration efforts. At different times and in different settings a nurse may choose to focus on different professional components. For example, within one year a nurse may be an educator for nine months and a practitioner for two months. Another nurse might practice three months, conduct research three months, and then combine the two functions on a weekly or monthly basis. And another nurse may wish to function in a professional academician position integrating

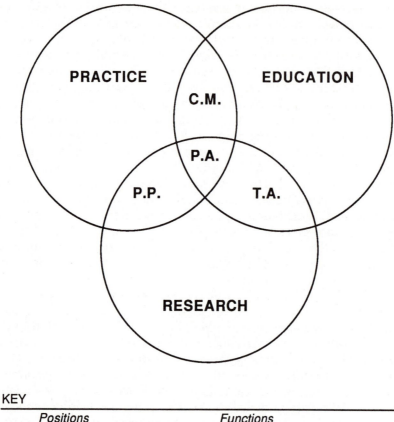

	Positions	Functions
T.A.	Tradional Academician	Research and Teaching
P.P.	Professional Practioner	Practice and Research
C.M.	Clinical Mentor	Practice and Teaching
P.A.	Professional Academician	Practice, Research and Teaching

Figure 2–4. The multiple functions of professional nursing.

a practice, research, and teaching on a full-time basis. Whatever approach the individual nurse selects, employment policies need to be flexible to foster such career choices and movement between components. (p. 29)

Educationally, Baker continues, a baccalaureate should be required for practice, a master's degree for teaching, and, of course, the doctorate for research. "The model suggests different educational emphasis for the other four positions," she asserts.

Master's preparation with emphasis on practice and teaching is required for clinical mentors. Doctoral preparation with emphasis on practice and research (the clinical doctorate) is required for the professional (research committed) practitioner. Doctoral preparation with emphasis on education and research (the research doctorate) is required for the traditional academician. If professional nursing's long-range goals is to blend practice, teaching, and research functions within a single nurse, the model suggests educational emphasis. (p. 29)

Clearly there are many unanswered questions and issues to be resolved: salary structures; standards for educational entry into practice; research "privileges" in clinical settings; mutual institutional benefits; the yet unaddressed issue of cost-effectiveness in a dollar-driven industry; the inevitable internal dissentions regarding the definitions of "professional" practice; and the issue of territoriality.

Nurses know what nursing can do; they know its potential and they certainly know its very positive contributions to the health care field.

In commenting on the two models (unification/collaboration) Styles (1984) poignantly stated that

just as joining rather than combining efforts seems to be the mode of the day, collaboration more than unification seems also to be the wave and hope of tomorrow. Collaboration, for its many purposes and in its many forms, can be a potent force to achieve our professional aims. (p. 23)

Lewis, editor emeritus of *Nursing Outlook,* once made an interesting observation. "Have the gulfs between our individual identities—the practitioner, the educator, the researcher, the administrator, the theorist, and others—become so deep and wide," she queried, "that it is no longer possible to bridge them in order to take collective action for the common good (1980, p. 159)?"

"If indeed," she went on to say, "we are agreed upon what the common good is (1980, p. 159)."

Lewis continued:

Possibly the root of our difficulties lies in the fact that so few of us see nursing whole; we just seem to see our own little piece of it and guard it zealously. I'm reminding [sic] of Kipling's line about "each in his separate star," which he seemed to think was a desirable state of affairs. But for stars to throw any real light, they have to be joined with others in a galaxy; otherwise, all they can do is twinkle. (p. 159)

REFERENCES

Baker, C. (1981). Moving toward inter-dependence: Strategies for collaboration. *Nurse Educator, 6*(6), 27–31.

Christman, L. (1979). The practitioner-teacher. *Nurse Educator, 4*(2), 8–11.

Fawcett, J. (1984). *Analysis and evaluation of conceptual models of nursing.* Philadelphia: Davis.

Ford, L. (1981, Fall). Unification model of nursing at the University of Rochester. *Nursing Administration Quarterly,* 1–9.

Hall, L. (1963). A center for nursing. *Nursing Outlook, 11,* 805–806.

Lambertson, E. (1953). *Nursing team organization and management.* New York: Columbia University Press.

Lewis, E. P. (1980). Downbeat. *Nursing Outlook, 28*(3), 159.

MacPhail, J. (1972). *An experiment in nursing: Planning, implementing, and assessing planned change.* Cleveland: Case Western Reserve University Press.

Nayer, D. (1980). Unification: Bringing nursing service and nursing education together. *American Journal of Nursing, 80*(6), 1110–1114.

Pannell, M. (1982, Feb. 1). Teaching hospitals build models for nursing organization. *Hospitals, 56,* 60–63.

Sovie, M. (1981). Unifying education and practice: One medical center's design. Part 2. *Journal of Nursing Administration, 12*(2), 30–32.

Styles, M. M. (1982). *On nursing: Toward a new endowment* (p. 212). St. Louis: Mosby.

Styles, M. M. (1984). Reflections on collaboration and unification. *Image: The Journal of Nursing Scholarship, 16*(1), 21–23.

Nursing Conceptual Frameworks
Content Analysis of Themes Related to Humans, Environment, Health, and Nursing Used in Nursing Education

Margaret Jopp

Today more than ever, the discipline of nursing, seeking to develop its scientific base, has a vital need for a theoretical body of knowledge to guide education and improve clinical practice. Historically, nursing education guided practice and influenced research. Today nursing education is being influenced by theorists and researchers who have developed conceptual models for nursing practice. In contemporary nursing education, conceptual frameworks have been designed, modified, and used as the foundation upon which curricula are built. Within the context of the conceptual framework approach in directing curricula structures and influencing course content, teaching methods, and clinical practice, many questions may be posed as to the outcome and future of such endeavors.

Conceptual framework development serves as a vehicle for labeling and classifying phenomena pertinent to the discipline of nursing. The process of using a conceptual framework as a guide in education, practice, and research provides a medium for theoretical growth, conceptual coherence, continuity, and unity within the profession. Educators' efforts to develop ideas and concepts into a nursing science are an indispensable requirement for professional nursing practice.

In nursing education, faculty have accumulated a body of knowledge and organized it through networks of conceptual ideas into a conceptual model for nursing practice or as a model for curricular design. The structures that have been developed convey basic assumptions, descriptions of concepts, and their interrelationships concerning the nature of human beings, the environment, health, and nursing.

PROBLEM AREA OF THIS STUDY

Kerlinger (1973) states that "education has suffered from a lack of analysis of
the educational information people absorb from the press and other media of
public communication (p. 533)." This point can be translated into the need for
analysis of conceptual framework documents used in curricula when knowledge is conveyed to students from educators in which the conceptual model
serves as the guiding tool. The development of conceptual frameworks has fos-
tered research based upon frameworks implemented in the clinical setting as
well as in some nursing educational programs (Lowry & Jopp, 1988). Over the
last several years, a number of textbooks have provided guidelines for analyzing
conceptual frameworks formulated by approximately 17 nurses (e.g., Johnson,
1980; Levine, 1971).

Since the National League of Nursing mandate of 1977 that all educational
programs organize nursing curricula on a designated conceptual framework,
curricular development has posed a tremendous challenge to educators in attempting to work out how to link the different and complex components of
knowledge into a unified conceptual scheme. Although faculty are still wres-
tling over issues surrounding the focus of a framework approach in curricula,
educators have moved forward to utilizing a conceptual model approach
within the curriculum. Thus, diploma, associate degree, and baccalaureate programs throughout the United States are still in the process of developing, expanding, and refining models within curricula. However, the general direction
in which conceptual frameworks have evolved within nursing curricula remains generally unexamined.

An earlier study by Riehl (1980) was selected to establish whether conceptual models were taught in the classroom and implemented in the clinical area
by students, and to determine what nursing model was employed by faculty
members who maintained a clinical practice. In this earlier study, all three
levels of education were included in the sample. From the 31 questionnaires
returned it was determined that 91 percent of these schools taught a conceptual
model and 89 percent used the models in the clinical areas.

PURPOSE OF THE STUDY

The purpose of this project was to examine conceptual framework documents
within the three levels of nursing educational curricula in Maryland and
Delaware to identify how the four major concepts of human beings, the environment, health, and nursing were described and used. This study was an off-
shoot from a preliminary investigation in which a sample of 12 documents was
examined. The data from the initial study were incorporated into the final data
of this research investigation, which conveyed information in written documents known as conceptual frameworks utilized in nursing education. The
following questions were explored:

1. What subconcepts are used to describe human beings, the environment, health, and nursing in the conceptual frameworks used in diploma, associate degree, and baccalaureate nursing programs in Maryland and Delaware?
2. How are these subconcepts described?
3. What subconcept similarities, central themes, and differences are found in the conceptual framework documents?

METHODOLOGY

Nursing administrators from 32 programs were asked to participate in this study. The philosophy and conceptual framework documents were requested in a letter explaining the project's purpose and summarizing the project. Follow-up telephone calls in 3 weeks were made to correspondents. If further clarification or input was requested in writing by the potential participant, a telephone call was made in order to clarify the intent of the project. This strategy was employed to obtain a higher participation response.

The sample included 32 programs that constituted all of the existing nursing educational institutions in Delaware and Maryland. Twenty-seven programs agreed to participate. The responses included an 80 percent rate from the diploma programs (4 out of 5), a 94 percent rate from the associate degree programs (15 out of 16), and a 73 percent rate from the baccalaureate programs (8 out of 11). The participants in the study included 2 associate degree programs and 1 baccalaureate program from Delaware; and 4 diploma, 13 associate degree, and 7 baccalaureate programs from Maryland.

A content analysis was employed for this study. Content analysis is a method of studying and analyzing communications to determine the emphasis or frequency of various communication phenomena. Content analysis is defined as any technique for making inferences by objectively and systematically identifying specified characteristics of messages (Holsti, 1969).

The history of content analysis as a research technique dates from the beginning of the twentieth century although scattered studies date back to the 1740s (Dovring, 1954). In the 1950s, applications of the technique appeared in such disciplines as folklore, biography, history, psychoanalysis, linguistics, propaganda, cognitive organization, and psychotherapy (Pool, 1959). This method has also been employed in nursing research.

This method is particularly useful where large bodies of data require analysis, as was the case in this study. The units of analysis were subconcepts and themes describing the nature of human beings, their environment, health, and nursing within conceptual framework documents used by diploma, associate degree, and baccalaureate nursing programs. The content analysis method allowed the researcher to formulate descriptive schemes that demonstrated coherent data as well as to cover all of the pertinent subconcepts and themes. According to Kerlinger (1973) "a theme is often a phrase or sentence; a proposition about something (p. 528)" and may be combined into sets of themes. Berelson (1954) states that if the themes are complex, content analysis is difficult and perhaps unreliable; however, the theme as a unit of analysis is important and useful because it is ordinarily realistic and close to the original content.

Content analysis serves as a multipurpose research method developed for investigating any problem in which the content of communication serves as the basis of inference (Holsti, 1969). It is acknowledged that any adequate account of written data must inevitably be in terms of complex and interrelated descriptions with a view to sharpening and clarifying them (Bliss, Monk, & Ogborn, 1983). Features that have something in common with each other need to be grouped together with structured summaries to more clearly describe the findings. It is vital to retain the characteristics and features described in the written data. The frequency with which certain themes occur does not necessarily indicate the weight or value of the specific themes. In addition, the data will provide information as to the existing features or themes that are presently being described in the data. However, this does not negate the value of data that is addressed to a lesser degree. There are potential factors that may influence the frequency of themes. These possible factors include philosophical biases of the faculty members who wrote the document; the knowledge development of a particular subconcept, theme or theoretical trend; research; and societal expectations.

It was suggested by Holsti (1969) that before constructing categories an investigator may want to read over a sample of his or her data to get a feeling for the types of relevant symbols of themes (p. 11). This was done in the pilot study of this investigation in order to familiarize this researcher with relevant subconcept descriptors and themes.

Another important factor in using content analysis relates to the requirement of objectivity—that only those symbols and combination of symbols actually appearing in the message be recorded (Holsti, 1969). In the coding stage of research—the stage at which specified words (subconcepts) and themes are located in the document and placed into categories—one is limited to recording only those items that actually appear in the document (Holsti, 1969). After the coding and data analysis have been completed, Holsti recommends that one may check the face validity of the results by rereading parts or all of one's documents. The investigator carried out this suggestion in the conduct of a preliminary study.

The preliminary investigation examined how the four major concepts of human beings, the environment, health, and nursing were described in the written philosophies and conceptual framework documents used by the baccalaureate degree, associate degree, and diploma programs in Delaware and Maryland. The rationale for initiating the preliminary study was to ascertain (1) if the four major concepts were addressed within the documents and (2) what type of subconcept descriptors and themes were used to describe the four major concepts. Familiarity with one's data is an important aspect for developing valid and reliable categories. Holsti states that "even the most knowledgeable investigator may want to test one's definitions on a small sample of data" in order "to judge whether the content units fall within its boundaries (p. 6)." This strategy proved to be a valuable and useful task in delineating groups of pertinent subconcepts.

Networking or grouping defined categories allows the researcher to elaborate on those categories to the point that enough of the individual essence of data is preserved and represented (Bliss, Monk, & Ogborn, 1983). Developing a network of category schemes was useful to visualize data that conveyed similar or different points of view.

Coding and categorizing processes were a central part of the methodological design. In carrying out the preliminary study, the investigator found that it provided an opportunity to refine the classification process through sorting and coding the documentary material from a representative small sample. The analysis had to be reshaped and attempts to recode were undertaken in order to produce effective formal summaries and at the same time retain the essential characteristics of the data.

FINDINGS AND DISCUSSION

Data used in this study were gathered from 21 conceptual framework documents as well as six program philosophy documents in instances where formal conceptual frameworks had not been developed or were limited. The documents varied in length ranging from a 1-page diagram to a 62-page document. Seven documents contained a glossary of terms, and 11 programs included diagrams of their conceptual framework. Only three programs incorporated written assumptions with their model.

Generally, the four major topics were addressed in the written philosophies. However, the approach used in addressing the concepts varied greatly within the conceptual framework documents. From them, two particular approaches to describing major concepts, subconcepts, constructs, and their interrelationships emerged. The first approach used was the Curricular Model, whereby unifying themes or major concepts and constructs were defined. In addition, these themes were described as to how they fit into the curricular design and content. The second approach was characterized as a Model for Nursing Practice, in which the nature of humans' internal and external environment, health, and nursing were described. The concepts, subconcepts, or constructs depicted in these various models depended on the program philosophy as well as the focus of the model. It was evident that faculty beliefs and knowledge regarding ideas, concepts, constructs, and their interrelationships were conveyed not only in the written philosophy but also in the conceptual framework document. The models formulated by educators demonstrated conceptual interrelationships through the selection and use of specific ideas that conveyed designated ideas with regard to the four concepts.

There were a total of 38 subconcept categories identified in the data that described the four major concepts of human beings, the environment, health, and nursing. Of these, there were 16 subconcept descriptors referring to human beings, 6 environment subconcept descriptors, 5 health subconcept descriptors, and 11 nursing subconcept descriptors (*see* Tables 3–1 through 3–4). The total number of subconcepts for each document ranged from 11 to 35 (*see* Tables 3–5 through 3–7). From these subconcepts, 15 themes were identified relating to the four major concepts. These included five themes of humans—holism, interaction, development or potential, needs, and adaptation. Three themes of the environment were identified—interaction between the internal and external environment; the external environment (such as events, conditions, society, and the health care system); and the internal response of humans. Three themes were found depicting health—internal and external environmental influences, the nature of health, and human adaptation and response. Four themes of nursing were found—nursing process, roles, recipient of care, and goal of nursing.

Person

Forty-two percent of the total number of subconcept categories described the concept of person. The terms mankind, human being, person, individual, mem-

TABLE 3–1. HUMAN BEING SUBCONCEPT CATEGORIES: PERCENT BY PROGRAM TYPE

Subconcepts*	Baccalaureate	Associate	Diploma	All
Holism	100	100	100	100
Interaction	100	93	100	96
Development/potential	100	93	100	96
Needs	75	87	100	85
Adaptation	100	60	50	70
Behavior: response/pattern	100	60	25	66
Unique	38	73	25	55
Active participant	50	47	100	55
System	88	20	50	44
Stress/stressors	25	60	25	44
Responsible to care for self/accountability	50	40	50	44
Freedom of choice/rights	75	20	50	41
Dignity/worth	38	33	50	37
Autonomy/self-determination	38	7	0	33
Energy	50	13	50	30
Change	38	7	0	15

*Subconcepts are presented in rank order as used in all programs.

TABLE 3-2. ENVIRONMENT SUBCONCEPT CATEGORIES: PERCENT BY PROGRAM TYPE

Subconcepts	Baccalaureate	Associate	Diploma	All
Interaction between internal/ external environment	100	100	100	100
External environment: events, conditions, society, health care system	100	73	100	85
Internal response	100	67	100	81
Factors, forces, elements, stimuli	63	40	25	44
Stress	25	60	0	41
Stressors	25	40	25	33

ber of a group, client, patient, family, small groups, and community were used to define the concept. Within the philosophy or conceptual framework document all programs depicted humans as holistic and interactive. The origin of the subconcepts addressed in the documents was speculative. References were cited within the documents reviewed. However, documentation that served as the original basis for the ideas conveyed in the documents (such as Gestalt theory or needs theory) was limited.

Many of the nursing theorists whose models were presented in the book *Conceptual Models for Nursing Practice* (Riehl & Roy, 1980) viewed person as a system in interaction with their environment. In the documents examined in this study, four nursing theorist models were cited as being the basis for the designated conceptual framework. The cited models that were identified in four documents included Roy's adaptation model, Orem's self-care nursing model, Neuman's Systems Model, and Orlando's meeting expressed needs model.

The baccalaureate programs in this study focused on person as having many different conceptual dimensions, which included a system, development and potential, needs, adaptation, behavioral response, and patterns. Based upon what terms were used in the baccalaureate models, it appears that system theory has been drawn upon heavily to describe people and their environment.

TABLE 3-3. HEALTH SUBCONCEPT CATEGORIES: PERCENT BY PROGRAM TYPE

Subconcepts	Baccalaureate	Associate	Diploma	All
Internal/external environmental influences	100	80	100	89
Nature of health	88	73	100	81
Adaptation	100	60	50	70
Continuum	38	67	75	59
Illness	50	53	75	56

TABLE 3-4. NURSING SUBCONCEPT CATEGORIES: PERCENT BY PROGRAM TYPE

Subconcepts	Baccalaureate	Associate	Diploma	All
Nursing process	100	100	100	100
Roles	100	100	100	100
Recipient of care	100	100	100	100
Goal of nursing	100	93	75	93
Role function	50	67	100	63
Knowledge base	50	67	25	55
Scientific/practice discipline	63	47	0	44
Action/intervention	63	40	25	41
Level of care	38	53	0	37
Skills/abilities	63	27	0	33
Accountability	50	27	25	33

At the same time developmental theory was evident throughout the documents. The concepts of direction, states, forces, form of progression, and potentiality were conveyed in the data that related human beings as a developing system. In addition, humans were described as a developing system that has needs. The terms *needs* or *basic needs* were depicted as an essential aspect of the developing system, whereas other programs used needs theory (Maslow) and developmental theory as the central themes of the conceptual framework with adaptation and behavioral responses or patterns as a consequence of human needs. Needs, developmental and adaptation descriptions were used in diploma models. Most associate degree programs also depicted a similar perspective; however, those models in the associate degree programs that did describe adaptation included stress or stressors as a central aspect within the model. In comparison, the baccalaureate degree programs depicted person as an adaptive system but did not emphasize stress or stressors, with the exception of one model.

Behavioral responses or patterns were depicted to a much greater degree in baccalaureate conceptual frameworks. These models describe person as a behavioral interactive adaptive system, whereas the associate degree models convey person as a developing interacting being with basic needs.

TABLE 3-5. RANGE OF SUBCONCEPT CATEGORIES FOR EACH MAJOR CONCEPT

Educational Level	Man	Environment	Health	Nursing
Baccalaureate	8–13	3–6	3–5	5–9
Associate degree	6–15	1–5	0–5	4–10
Diploma	6–13	2–6	3–5	4–7
All	6–15	1–6	0–5	4–10

TABLE 3-6. COMBINED RANGE OF ALL SUBCONCEPT CATEGORIES BY EDUCATIONAL LEVEL

Level of Education	Range
Baccalaureate	19–33
Associate degree	11–35
Diploma	15–31

In Riehl's (1980) study, it was found that systems theory, developmental theory, and adaptation theory were addressed by all three levels of education. However, need theory was not addressed at all. Therefore, one may speculate that need theory had not been the focus or even developed within conceptual models at that time. Thus, need theory has apparently developed quite extensively within nursing conceptual frameworks within curricula over the last 10 years in all three levels of nursing education, as evidenced by the term being used in this study.

Environment

For the major concept of environment, all documents in this study depicted in some manner an interaction between the internal and external environments. The external environment was described by depicting various aspects such as society; events, conditions, and elements that make up the client surroundings; and the health care system. Generally, the message communicated throughout the documents was that an internal response exists to human interaction with the external environment. The baccalaureate degree and diploma models employed a more in-depth description of the external environment, whereas the baccalaureate and associate degree documents focused on the internal response of person.

Health

The nature of health was described by 21 models in which health was related as a state of wellness or optimal functioning. Internal and external environmental influences were seen as primary determinants of the health state. To reflect the

TABLE 3-7. SUBCONCEPT CATEGORY MEANS FOR EACH MAJOR CONCEPT

Educational Level	Man	Environment	Health	Nursing
Baccalaureate	10.63	4.13	3.875	7.375
Associate Degree	8.60	3.80	3.27	7.13
Diploma	8.75	3.50	4.00	5.75

dynamic nature of health, the themes of adaptation and health continuum were used. The baccalaureate degree models used *adaptation* the most frequently, whereas the associate degree and diploma documents used the term *continuum* to depict the degree or measurement of health. The term *illness* appeared to be the least described in all three levels of education. It is interesting that the practice of nursing, which deals with the ill client, describes illness much less clearly or extensively than it does wellness. Another way of looking at this is that there may be a conscious choice by educators in the development of conceptual frameworks for nursing education to focus more on wellness than on illness. In contrast, a major focus on an illness perspective would be the main theme in the traditional medical model.

Nursing

The last major concept, nursing, was described the second most frequently following the major concept of person. Three major ideas were used by all of the reviewed documents: the nursing process, the recipient of care, and the roles in nursing. Also, the goal of nursing was addressed in most documents.

The purpose and components of the nursing process were quite clear throughout all documents examined. Generally, the nursing process was defined as a four-step problem-solving process that facilitated interaction and decision making as well as directing nursing action.

Even though all models reflected the individual as the recipient of care, only the baccalaureate programs included the community as the recipient of care. The diploma and baccalaureate models also focused upon the family.

The roles in nursing addressed in the documents examined included leader, researcher, teacher, counselor, collaborator, communicator, advocate, caring helper, provider of care, manager of care, member of the profession and change agent. All of the documents emphasized communication and interpersonal interactions as well as collaboration. However, there were differences among the three levels in what role(s) were emphasized. One difference noted was that the baccalaureate models addressed leadership and research. This finding is not surprising, because in higher education it would be expected that the graduates would assume a leadership and research role within the profession at an earlier stage in their career because of the curricular focus.

The goal of nursing intervention was clearly described by all three levels of education. Depending upon the theoretical construct(s) of each model, the nurse was said to assist, restore, maintain, enhance, or promote one of the following: system integrity, meeting human needs, achieving the optimal human health state, or adaptation by diminishing or eliminating stressors.

SUMMARY

As mentioned earlier, a content analysis was the method used for tabulation of the data. This method had its limitations. A goal of the researcher was to maintain objectivity and to diminish subjectivity in the structuring of the content. In addition, four major concepts were used as the methodological framework because these four areas were described within the nursing conceptual framework literature as the most influential determinants in nursing education, clinical practice, and research. Therefore, the analysis was limited only to those descriptors relating the four major concepts of person, the environment, health, and nursing. The content analysis of the nursing conceptual framework documents provided that appropriate statements be placed in one of the four designated categories. However, in reviewing the documents there were a few concepts and subconcepts that could not be suitably placed in one of the categories. Because this content was not included within the methodological framework, some areas were not addressed in this study.

An analysis of the nursing models examined indicated that there were more similarities than differences. Although details within the conceptual frameworks varied with major themes or theoretical emphases within the models—which may indicate the stage of development of the document itself—it is possible to sketch a broad outline of a universal metaparadigm. This sample conveys that within nursing curricula the conceptual framework relates four major concepts of person, the environment, health, and nursing. Within the global concepts of nursing's metaparadigm different dimensions and structures exist that affect the theoretical development of nursing as a science.

The subconcepts and themes identified in this study could be further examined to more clearly specify and define the essential attributes of each concept for theory development as well as for clinical practice. This study was conducted with nursing programs from a two-state region. A comparison of curricula documents in other geographical regions could add to the existing data. In using the design in this study, other work could further clarify to what extent and how specific subconcepts of conceptual frameworks are used within nursing curricula throughout the United States.

It is hoped that this study will promote in educators an interest to further examine the utility of conceptual frameworks within nursing curricula. Educators are challenged to determine which conceptual frameworks effectively guide curricula, influence teaching strategies, improve student and graduate clinical performance, influence knowledge expansion, and lead to theory development. In summary, at this stage of the development of the body of knowledge known as nursing science, the validation of concepts and themes within conceptual framework documents in nursing curricula remains an indispensable requirement.

REFERENCES

Berelson, B. (1954). *Content analysis.* In Linzey (Ed.), *Handbook of social psychology* (Vol. 1). Reading, MA: Addison-Wesley.

Bliss, E. O., Monk, M., & Ogborn, J. (1983). *Qualitative data analysis for educational research: A guide to use in systematic networking.* London: Croom Helm.

Dovring, K. (1954). Quantitative semantics in 18th century Sweden. *Public Opinion Quarterly, 18*, 389–394.

Holsti, O. R. (1969). *Content analysis for social sciences and humanities.* Reading, MA: Addison-Wesley.

Johnson, D. E. (1980). The behavioral system model for nursing. In J. P. Riehl & C. Roy (Eds.), *Conceptual models for nursing practice* (2nd ed.). New York: Appleton-Century-Crofts.

Kerlinger, F. N. (1973). *Foundations of behavioral research* (2nd ed.). New York: Holt, Rinehart, & Winston.

Levine, M. E. (1971). Holistic nursing. *Nursing Clinics of North America, 6*, 253–264.

Lowry, L. W., & Jopp, M. C. (1988). Strategies and development of an evaluation instrument for assessing associate degree nursing curricula based on the Neuman Systems Model. In J. Riehl-Sisca (Ed.), *Conceptual models for nursing practice* (3rd ed.). Norwalk, CT: Appleton & Lange.

Pool, I. (1959). *Symbols of internationalism.* Stanford: Stanford University Press.

Riehl, J. (1980). Nursing models in current use. In J. P. Riehl & C. Roy (eds.), *Conceptual models for nursing practice* (2nd ed.). New York: Appleton-Century-Crofts.

Riehl, J., & Roy, C. (1980). *Conceptual models for nursing practice* (2nd ed.). New York: Appleton-Century-Crofts.

Part 2

Systems Models for Nursing Practice

Of the models presented in this text, three are classified as systems models. The frameworks by Neuman and Roy have always been labeled as systems models by their authors. Historically, King's model, which is also included in this unit, has been thought of by some as an interaction model. However, King believes that her framework best fits in the systems model group. The rationale for this becomes clear in reading her description in Chapter 13.

In Chapter 4, a case study is presented using Neuman's framework. Because she has diagrammed and discussed her model in the second edition of this text and in her own book*, a review of it is not included. The reader is referred to the other sources for that information. Neuman's case study is followed by a critique by Campbell and Keller, who use the analysis criteria offered by Stevens.† In Chapter 6, Lowry and Jopp demonstrate the use of the Neuman model in the curriculum design of a community college where Lowry is the director. A follow-up study of their graduates is also included. Chapter 7 is by Mrkonich, Hessian, and Miller, who participate in a consortium that utilizes the Neuman Model. They illustrate its application in their setting. Finally, in Chapter 8 Louis reports on research she completed using Neuman's concepts as the theoretical framework.

---

*Neuman, B. (1989). *The Neuman Systems Model* (3rd ed.). East Norwalk, CT: Appleton & Lange.
† Stevens, B. J. (1984). *Nursing theory: Analysis, application, evaluation* (2nd ed.). Boston: Little, Brown.

Roy's adaptation model is presented in Chapter 9, followed by a critique by Pioli and Sandor. They, too, used Stevens' evaluation criteria. Mengel, Sherman, Nahigian, and Coleman are faculty members at a community college who share their experience in Chapter 11 in applying the Roy model in their curriculum. In Chapter 12, Andrews describes her experience working with this model in Canada.

King's model is described in the lead chapter (13) of the last set in this unit. A critique written by DiNardo, and an illustration by Daubenmire of the use of King's conceptual framework in a baccalaureate nursing program follows.

4

The Neuman Nursing Process Format
A Family Case Study

Betty Neuman

Because several books and articles are available on the Neuman model, it is assumed that the reader is knowledgeable about it. With this understanding, the Neuman Systems Model, per se, is not described here. What is addressed is the Neuman Nursing Process Format, which supplements the model. This format has been designed to complement and facilitate the use of the Neuman Systems Model. To illustrate the format and its application, a case study is presented. The steps of the nursing process employed include obtaining a history, analyzing the data, determining a nursing diagnosis, identifying nursing goals, and evaluating outcomes.

The Barry family is the case study presented. It is based upon an actual situation in a family caseload encountered by graduate nursing students supervised by Neuman. The approach taken in this chapter is primarily from the perspective of a nurse applying the Neuman Nursing Process Format (*see* Appendix 4–A). Use of the prevention as intervention modes as a typology for nursing intervention is also illustrated (*see* Appendix 4–B). Both of these tools were designed to implement the Neuman systems model.

A BRIEF HISTORY OF THE BARRY FAMILY

The Barry family consisted of Gregory and Marie, the parents, and their daughters Rose, age 16, and Angela, age 14. They had just moved to a small town where Gregory had accepted the position of local school superintendent. It was his first job since completing his hard-earned Ph.D. His wife Marie had made many personal and family sacrifices to help him complete his education.

Gregory and Marie were in their mid-30s. They were an attractive and personable couple. Marie had grown up in a deprived rural area and lacked the opportunity for higher education. However, she was very energetic and meticulously devoted her energies to her family. Like many teen-agers, Rose and Angela were both obese, shy, and somewhat unsociable. Neither of them had yet dated, as their parents were protective and selective concerning their associates. The Barry family was extremely proper with overt demonstrations of closeness such as shopping as a family, attending church every Sunday, and taking 300-mile trips every other weekend to visit grandparents and extended family members. Marie had not wanted to make this move because of her mother's failing health with terminal bone cancer. Their contact with the local townspeople was of a superficial nature. They projected an image of the "perfect" family.

The Barry family did become friends with their neighbors, Paula and Donald Storrs, a couple in their 20s. The Storrs prided themselves on physical accomplishments such as house and yard work, minor carpentry, and car repairing. They both worked. Don was a contractor and Paula was employed in a local dairy. When they were home, they seemed to fight a lot. Often their violent arguments were heard by nearby neighbors, including the Barrys.

During the second summer of their move to the small town, Marie decided to get a job. She obtained one at the same local dairy where Paula worked and was able to ride back and forth with Paula. This worked out fine at first, but soon after Marie's employment, Paula's behavior became erratic as her arguments with her husband increased. She threatened Marie's physical safety by near accidents in the dairy barn and by hazardous driving to and from work. Marie made several attempts to help Paula—for example, by inviting her to attend church with the family—but to no avail. Paula's behavior only continued to get worse.

Marie, fearing for her personal safety, finally quit her job. She thought it best to find other work and for her family to disengage themselves from their close friendship with the Storrs. Her daughter Rose and Paula were becoming best friends, and when Marie attempted to limit their growing friendship, Rose rebelled. Marie was concerned that the excessive time that Rose and Paula spent together could threaten Don and Paula's marriage.

During January, 2 weeks after Rose became 18 years of age, she told her mother that she and Paula were in love. Marie attempted to attack Paula physically but was intercepted by her husband. She became ill. In a state of hypoglycemic shock, she was hospitalized for a week. Soon after discharge, she attempted suicide by overdose because Rose had moved into Paula's home during her hospitalization and refused to return. Paula's husband was forced out of his bedroom to accommodate Rose.

For Gregory, business went on as usual; the school board decided not to retaliate or accept his offer of resignation when they heard about his family problems. Angela continued to attend school without any communication with her sister. Rose rejected attempts of her family and others at school and in the neighborhood to encourage her to return home. She continued to attend school, however, and completed her senior year. Following Marie's hospitalization for her suicide attempt, the family moved into another nearby town. With Rose living across the street with Paula, the stress was too great to handle, especially for Marie.

In the spring, Paula and Rose moved into a mobile home near the dairy where they both now worked. Don filed for a divorce. The Barry family decided when summer arrived that Gregory would resign his position so they could return to the area near both their parents from which they had come. Gregory had secured another position as school superintendent with the fear that he would be terminated if his family crises were known. Marie's mother died a few days before their return. Her father was recovering from a heart attack that occurred during his wife's last week of illness. The Barry family did not keep in contact with anyone in the town where they had lived for the past two years.

APPLICATION OF THE NEUMAN NURSING PROCESS FORMAT TO THE BARRY FAMILY CASE STUDY

The case study was analyzed in the following three-part format: nursing diagnosis, nursing goals, and nursing outcomes. Seven steps were used to gather relevant data for determining the nursing diagnosis and the variance from wellness.

In **step 1,** the predominate stressors for each Barry family member at the intra-, inter- and extrapersonal level were identified. These were as follows:

For Gregory
Intrapersonal   Self-image, values, and rules
Interpersonal   Maintenance of public or family image
Extrapersonal   Extended family

For Marie
Intrapersonal   Self-identity, values, mother role, physical health
Interpersonal   Paula and Gregory
Extrapersonal   Extended family and mother's health decline

For Rose
Intrapersonal   Identity, independence and growth, and development needs
Interpersonal   Rigid family expectations and rules
Extrapersonal   Don

For Angela
Intrapersonal   Identity
Interpersonal   Family status, rules, and expectations
Extrapersonal   School peers

In **step 2,** a general assessment of the condition and strength of basic structural factors and energy resources for the entire family revealed the following:

close intergenerational ties, family bonding, religious beliefs and values, and high moral standards that acted as "cohesive" forces prior to the family stress situation. From appearances, all variables would be considered above average in strength of the basic structure and energy resources to maintain it.

In **step 3,** an assessment was made of the characteristics of the flexible and normal lines of defense, lines of resistance, degree of potential reaction, and potential for reconstitution following a reaction. In the Barry family, the flexible line of defense was weak because of the family rigidity patterns. The normal line of defense was poorly developed because the energy resources of the family had long been focused on Gregory's professional development at the expense of the other family members. The lines of resistance were inadequate to provide the needed protection from major overt stresses occurring during the family crisis. In regard to the degree of potential reaction, there was a lack of previous experience with major family crises, and coping mechanisms were inadequate, as indicated by the following.

GREGORY: Became immobilized. He strengthened his denial defense mechanism.

MARIE: Developed physical health problems requiring hospitalization and later attempted suicide. However, she was open to support from external resources.

ROSE: Completely abandoned the family.

ANGELA: Increased her denial as a defense mechanism.

In the potential reaction category there was a complete family system disintegration, and the potential for reconstitution to the normal line of defense was low because even the basic structure was seriously threatened. That is, all family system variables were affected by the crises. For example, Marie's health and her mothering role, the father's social image and identity, the family's position, and the identity of both Rose and Angela were all areas for needed intervention toward reconstitution. Family beliefs and values were also seriously violated.

In **step 4,** an identification, classification, and evaluation of potential or actual intra-, inter-, and extrapersonal interactions between the family and their environment was considered. Four variables were used for the first interaction category and three were applied to the latter two. The intrafamily interactions (stressors) in the Barry family are indicated below.

Psychologically   Lack of individualization; communication problems between the parents and their educational differences; status differences and developmental needs of Rose and Angela; unidentified family member needs and threat of continued crises

Socioculturally   Rupture of the family system changed both private and public image of the family

Developmentally   Increased family rigidity as denial defense system strengthened

Physiologically   *Gregory*—increased physical stress due to recent gallbladder surgery with an incomplete recovery
Marie—overt hypoglycemia exacerbated requiring energy toward health maintenance

The interfamily interactions (stressors) for the Barry's were as follows:

Psychologically   Crisis conflict between families and violence potential
Sociologically   Social withdrawal of both families in conflict, image, and value changes
Physiologically   Hypoglycemic condition and suicide attempt of Marie

Finally, the extrafamily interactions (stressors) for the Barry's were also identified. They emerged as follows:

Psychologically   Adaptation to school, peer, and community reactions
Socioculturally   Potential and actual career and peer relationship damage
Developmentally   Community resources inadequate to meet family needs (church, mental health, children services, and police)

In **step 5**, an evaluation of the past, present, and possible future life-process and coping patterns on client system stability was made and revealed some interesting factors. In the past, the Barry family relationships were confused by rigid interaction patterns such as by rules and expectations. In the present, the family stability level was low due to long-term energy drain and family coping inadequacy in the recent family crises. In the future, past established interaction patterns are expected to generally continue, because Gregory and Angela received no intervention during the crises. Marie received only brief, inadequate counseling. Long-term or future family counseling seems unlikely. However, long-term goals for intervention can be determined by short-term outcomes (crisis counseling for Marie) and life events occurring since that time.

In **step 6**, an evaluation of actual and potential internal and external resources for optimal family wellness was made. For the internal resources, the family status position of Angela was altered because of Rose's absence. Her developmental needs could receive more consideration from her parents.

No external resources existed. The family crises were not shared with the extended family. The Barry family, including Marie, refused to acknowledge a need for long-term counseling. The fault of the crises was projected onto Paula. As a defense mechanism, denial by the entire family increased.

For potential resources, future employment, social and personal development activities are possible for Marie. Social, creative, and age-related activities will help Angela. Family counseling and school and community support for individuals and the family is needed.

Finally, in **step 7** the family perception was that Paula had unjustly invaded the family system that created the major crises that occurred. However, the perception of the caregiver was that Gregory and Marie had failed to effectively relate to their daughters' developmental needs and that rigid family interaction patterns were considered major causal factors in the family crises situation. Gregory also failed to recognize and support the needs of Marie. Community resources failed to resolve these perceptual differences and the family crises as well. These discrepancies could be resolved by helping the family gain an understanding of Rose's need for independence in light of her developmental needs and the deficits in the family interaction patterns.

NURSING DIAGNOSIS AND VARIANCES FROM WELLNESS

Variances from Wellness

In examining the variances from wellness, a synthesis of theory with the database allows for family problem definition and prioritization, determination of their level of wellness, family system stability needs, and total available resources to accomplish desired outcomes as follows.

- The accumulated energy drain weakened the flexible line of defense, allowing stressors to penetrate the solid line of defense, causing a series of near-fatal crises. A serious threat to the basic structure existed for which no previous coping mechanisms had been developed. This referred to the internal lines of resistance and to crisis, communications, and nursing process theory.
- Intervention for the family was grossly inadequate and uncoordinated. The family failed in proper resolution of their crises (Family, psychosocial, role, personality, and nursing process theory).
- Social role and function, as well as educational level, can influence family behavior. To integrate differing expectations (external stressors) into the intrafamily system is often difficult to accomplish while maintaining family system stability (Role and systems theory). Unless individual needs are identified and met, family integrity may be jeopardized, especially when new coping strategies are required (Family theory).
- Excessive energy was required to maintain the public image of Gregory, the father, while the growth and development needs of the two daughters and the mother were grossly compromised (Growth and development theory). The autocratic, rigid family interaction style failed to allow for free expression of emotions, differences, and ideas. The needs of one family part subsumed the needs of the other three parts, creating a dysfunction of the family system (Systems and interaction theories).

A serious threat to the family basic structure existed. Crisis intervention measures were necessary to prevent collapse of the basic structure. Although inadequate community resources were available, some degree of stability was accomplished through crisis counseling for Marie. Synthesis of client data with relevant theories substantiates the nursing diagnosis. Based upon the database and determined variances from wellness the following nursing diagnosis was made: Erosion of the family system due to the continuous stressor of rigid family rules to maintain Gregory's (the father) public image; bankruptcy of family emotions and energy negated sustaining communications.

Hypothetical Interventions

Hypothetical interventions are postulated to reach the desired client stability or wellness level—that is, to maintain the flexible and solid line of defense.

In this family situation first priority was given to crisis intervention strategies in order to strengthen the lines of resistance so that the basic structure could be protected. Unfortunately, family intervention did not materialize. Crisis intervention with Marie safeguarded the basic structure of the family.

The following interventions were considered.

1. Use crisis intervention strategies.
2. Identify and resolve individual family member needs.
3. Reduce family energy drain related to impacting stressors (physical, social, psychological, and developmental).
4. Clarify family role relationships and establish meaningful communication patterns for all family members, thus reducing the existing rigidity.
5. Facilitate age or stage-appropriate family member activities and behaviors.
6. Identify family spiritual needs and possible resources.

The above intervention strategies are those determined most appropriate for this particular family's crisis situation and long-term needs.

NURSING GOALS

Negotiate with the family for desired prescriptive change to correct variances from wellness, based on classified needs and resources identified in the nursing diagnosis.

Based on the family's previous (anticipated) resolution of perceptual differences, the caregivers will, at this point, explore and expand their understanding of both individual and family needs and possible resources for their resolution. The caregivers will, when appropriate, seek cooperative family involvement in an intervention plan to treat, reconstitute, and prevent further system disruption or instability. Some examples of possible nursing roles are offered, such as advocacy, coordination or acquisition of resources, and health education and counseling. It is valid for nursing to function within these roles.

Appropriate intervention strategies are postulated for retention, attainment, or maintenance of client system stability as desired outcome goals.

Intervention Strategies and Desired Outcome Goals

Immediate Goals
Action should be taken to attain family stability by reducing effects of the family crises by strengthening the internal lines of resistance.

The family will develop adequate coping behavior during the crises. Appropriate resources involvement will reduce guilt, shame, and effects of self-blame, anxiety, and stressor reactions, helping to stabilize the family and protect the basic structure.

Intermediate Goals
Action should be taken to maintain family stability by facilitating reconstitution toward a new solid and flexible line of defense.

Family stability will be reestablished and maintained by appropriate use of available community resources. Continued family counseling will further stabilize the family system. Hypoglycemia will be controlled through health education and improved nutrition. Clergy, school, and community will provide necessary support to the family.

Long-Range Goals
Action should be taken to retain family stability by developing the necessary coping to strengthen the flexible line of defense.

Recurrence of similar crises will be avoided by strengthening family coping strategies and changing patterns of family communication and interaction. A new life style will have emerged as a result of adaptations made during the crises, facilitating family stability. Health education will consolidate learning from past experiences and establish new approaches to family health. Previous outcome goals will be understood and integrated into the family system to enhance future stability.

NURSING OUTCOMES

Nursing intervention is accomplished through use of one or more of the following three prevention modes: (1) primary prevention (action to retain system stability); (2) secondary prevention (action to attain system stability); and (3) tertiary prevention (action to maintain system stability), usually following secondary prevention.

Evaluation of the outcome goals following intervention either confirms that the outcome goals were established or serves as a basis for reformulation of subsequent nursing goals. The caregivers will then review the nursing goals to confirm their degree of accomplishment. Based on this appraisal, subsequent reformulation of goals may be required.

Intermediate and long-range goals for subsequent nursing action are structured in relation to short-term goal outcomes. Short-term goal outcomes must be critically evaluated in terms of their relevance to family stability needs prior to reformulation of intermediate and long-range goals for subsequent nursing action.

Client outcome validates the nursing process.

NURSING DIAGNOSIS BASED ON THE NEUMAN NURSING PROCESS FORMAT

The logic for gathering comprehensive client data is that sufficient information is available for making an accurate diagnosis of problem areas for subsequent consideration or resolution.

Using the Neuman Nursing Process Format, the database acts as a foundation for determining variances from the usual state of wellness, which is one component of arriving at the nursing diagnosis. It is imperative in determining variances from wellness, based on client data obtained, that theoretical tie-ins be made in an explicit manner. The fact that theory is closely related to actual data gives assurance that a valid nursing diagnostic statement can be made. A nursing diagnosis must be a comprehensive statement that encompasses the client's general condition or circumstances. From this general diagnostic statement, prioritization of client needs, resources, and hypothetical interventions can be made.

It is assumed that the professional nurse operates from a theoretical perspective as client data are gathered. It is most often in the interpretation of client data that theory is either not explicitly used or improperly related to client data, resulting in confusing and often faulty diagnoses. It is more common for theory to be related to interventions than to diagnoses. Professional nurses should (to be considered truly professional) be able to justify their diagnostic statement based upon specific theoretical relationships with available client data. To substantiate and clarify this position further, data from the preceding case study analysis is summarized as follows:

- The Barry family diagnostic statement was "Erosion of the family system due to the continuous stressor of rigid family rules to maintain Gregory's (the father) public image; bankruptcy of family emotions and energy negated sustaining communications."
- It was determined that the Barry family system integrity was in a weakened state normally (normal line of defense). This fact was based on

both data gathered and theory as to healthy family system developmental needs and communication requirements.

• When the initial family crisis occurred (Rose's relationship was revealed) as well as their subsequent responses, the family reflected both a lack of coping skills and energy resources to protect the family system integrity (flexible line of defense and internal lines of resistance). Theoretical considerations such as crisis, family systems, role, psychosocial, physiological, and developmental theories, all confirmed the fact that family disintegration was imminent (basic structure jeopardized). Immediate use of external resources was required to develop and support family coping skills and energy conservation during and following the crisis period.

When client data are specifically related to social sciences theories in developing the nursing diagnosis, nurses can present themselves as professional in a knowledgeable manner. It is a responsibility to one's self, profession, clients, colleagues, and other health disciplines to be able to present a logical and rational justification for such decision making. Unless nurses can clearly articulate to others, particularly to the client, the *why* and *how* for arriving at a particular nursing diagnosis, they cannot claim the validity of their position; nor can they be certain of appropriate subsequent interventions.

CONCLUSION

The Barry family case study is presented without taking into consideration all possible factors inherent in the situation. Because it is retroactive in nature, hypotheses were made as to the most likely approach to the family crisis situation in order to best illustrate the use of all steps of the Neuman Nursing Process Format. This format was designed to follow the Neuman Systems Model and its terminology. The application of this process tool will act as a guide for future use of the Neuman Systems Model.

It is the author's purpose that this explication will provide guidelines to facilitate future student use of the Neuman Systems Model as a nursing practice model.

Appendix 4-A

The Neuman Nursing Process Format

Nursing Diagnosis

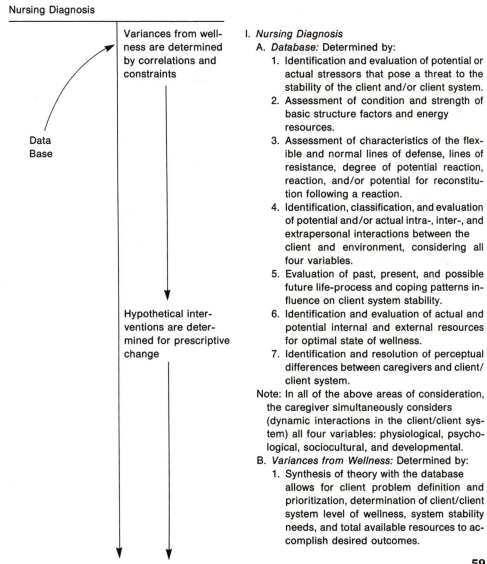

Variances from wellness are determined by correlations and constraints

Data Base

Hypothetical interventions are determined for prescriptive change

I. *Nursing Diagnosis*
   A. *Database:* Determined by:
      1. Identification and evaluation of potential or actual stressors that pose a threat to the stability of the client and/or client system.
      2. Assessment of condition and strength of basic structure factors and energy resources.
      3. Assessment of characteristics of the flexible and normal lines of defense, lines of resistance, degree of potential reaction, reaction, and/or potential for reconstitution following a reaction.
      4. Identification, classification, and evaluation of potential and/or actual intra-, inter-, and extrapersonal interactions between the client and environment, considering all four variables.
      5. Evaluation of past, present, and possible future life-process and coping patterns influence on client system stability.
      6. Identification and evaluation of actual and potential internal and external resources for optimal state of wellness.
      7. Identification and resolution of perceptual differences between caregivers and client/client system.
      Note: In all of the above areas of consideration, the caregiver simultaneously considers (dynamic interactions in the client/client system) all four variables: physiological, psychological, sociocultural, and developmental.
   B. *Variances from Wellness:* Determined by:
      1. Synthesis of theory with the database allows for client problem definition and prioritization, determination of client/client system level of wellness, system stability needs, and total available resources to accomplish desired outcomes.

59

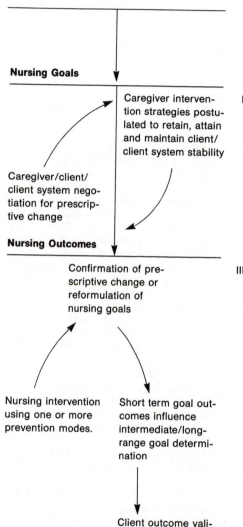

60

Nursing Diagnosis (cont.)

Nursing Goals

Caregiver intervention strategies postulated to retain, attain and maintain client/client system stability

Caregiver/client/client system negotiation for prescriptive change

Nursing Outcomes

Confirmation of prescriptive change or reformulation of nursing goals

Nursing intervention using one or more prevention modes.

Short term goal outcomes influence intermediate/long-range goal determination

Client outcome validates nursing process

2. Hypothetical interventions are postulated to reach the desired client stability or wellness level, i.e., to maintain the flexible and solid line of defense.

II. *Nursing Goals:* Determined by:
  1. Negotiation with the client for desired prescriptive change to correct variances from wellness, based on classified needs and resources identified in the nursing diagnosis.
  2. Appropriate intervention strategies are postulated for retention, attainment, and/or maintenance of client system stability as desired outcome goals.

III. *Nursing Outcomes:* Determined by:
  1. Nursing intervention accomplished through use of one or more of the following three prevention modes: (1) primary prevention (action to retain system stability), (2) secondary prevention (action to attain system stability), (3) tertiary prevention (action to maintain system stability), usually following secondary prevention/intervention.
  2. Evaluation of outcome goals following intervention either confirms outcome goals or serves as a basis for reformulation of subsequent nursing goals.
  3. Intermediate and long-range goals for subsequent nursing action are structured in relation to short-term goal outcomes.
  4. Client outcome validates the nursing process.

Appendix 4–B

Assessment Summary Guide

THE PREVENTION AS INTERVENTION MODES

Primary Prevention	Secondary Prevention	Tertiary Prevention
Nursing Action † to:	Nursing Action to:	Nursing Action to:
1. Classify stressors‡ as to client/client system threat to stability. Prevent stressor invasion.	1. Following stressor invasion, protect basic structure.	1. During reconstitution, attain/maintain maximum level of wellness and stability.
2. Provide information to maintain or strengthen existing client/client system strengths.	2. Mobilize and maximize internal/external resources toward stability and energy conservation.	2. Educate, reeducate, and/or reorient as needed.
3. Support positive coping and functioning.	3. Facilitate purposeful manipulation of stressors and reactions to stressors.	3. Support client/client system in appropriate goal directednes and change efforts.
4. Desensitize existing or possible noxious stressors.	4. Motivate, educate, and involve client and client system in health care goals.	4. Coordinate and integrate health service resources.
5. Motivate toward wellness.	5. Facilitate appropriate treatment/intervention measures.	5. Provide primary and/or secondary prevention/intervention as needed.
6. Coordinate/integrate interdisciplinary theories and epidemiologic input.	6. Support positive reaction toward illness.	
7. Educate/reeducate.	7. Promote advocacy by coordination/integration.	
8. Use stress as a positive intervention strategy.	8. Provide primary prevention/intervention as required.	

Reproduced with permission from Neuman, B. (1982). The Neuman Systems Model: Application to nursing education and practice. *Norwalk, CT: Appleton-Century-Crofts, p. 26. Copyright © 1980 by Betty Neuman.*

†Some nursing action examples are: intuition, planning, organization, monitoring, coordinating, implementing, integrating, supporting, and evaluating.

‡An example of a classification system is the following list of four basic categories of stressors: (1) deprivation, (2) excess, (3) change, and (4) intolerance.

PREVENTIONS AS INTERVENTIONS

Immediate Interventions

Secondary	*Primary*	*Tertiary*
Hospitalization crisis counseling (Marie)	Counseling crisis (Gregory and Angela) counseling (family)	—

Intermediate Interventions

Tertiary	*Primary*	*Secondary*
Clergy support (family) Continued counseling (Marie) School/community support (Gregory) School/recreational/social support (Angela) Support immediate goal outcomes (family)	Counseling (family)	Nutritional counseling (Marie)

Long-Range Interventions

Primary	*Tertiary*	*Secondary*
Continued family counseling (family) Nutritional counseling (family) Church support (family) Social/recreational support (family) Health education (family)	Support immediate and intermediate goal outcomes (family)	—

The Betty Neuman Health Care Systems Model
An Analysis

Vicki Campbell
Kathryn Buchanan Keller

The function of a theoretical framework is to guide the research process. Nursing has passed the point where it operates within the framework of functionalism—only relating one variable to another. A conceptual framework is needed to guide the research process and ultimately develop sound nursing theory. The theory must be both understandable and applicable to the real world of nursing. An analysis and evaluation of the Neuman Systems Model utilizing Stevens (1984) methodology is presented. The approach taken encompasses a description of the model, definitions of commonplaces, an internal evaluation, an external evaluation, and a summary.

DESCRIPTION OF THE NEUMAN MODEL

This health care systems model is called the "Total Person Approach to Patient Problems." The conceptual framework encompassing this model views people as unique individuals with a composite of characteristics within a normal given range of response. Each person in a state of wellness or illness is a dynamic composite of the interrelationship of physiological, psychological, sociocultural, and developmental variables. Although Neuman uses the term *composite*, the conceptual framework encompasses Gestalt theory, which holds that each of us is surrounded by a perceptual field that is in a dynamic equilibrium. A field theory approach such as this maintains that all parts are intimately related and interdependent. The total organization of the field and its impact upon the functional behavior of the individual is the primary focus. In this total person model, the organization of the field considers:

1. The effect of the stressors.
2. The reaction of the organism to the stressors.
3. The organism itself, while taking into consideration the simultaneous interaction of the physiological, psychological, sociocultural, and development variables.

This total person framework, then, is an open system model with two major components, stress and the reaction to stress. In Gestalt theory each stressor would affect the individual's reaction to any other stressor. The individual's behavior then would be a function of the dynamic interaction between stressors and the defenses against stressors supplied by the individual as well as the supporting environment.

COMMONPLACES

Commonplaces are topics commonly addressed by most theorists. These topics are usually vague, indicating locations rather than specific entities. The commonplaces in a theory may be used to organize a theory or as structures with which to evaluate and understand a theory. Definitions of the commonplaces utilized in the Neuman Systems Model are made by identifying the elements and relationships that have significance for Neuman.

Person

The conceptual framework encompassing this model views people as unique individuals who are a composite of characteristics within a normal given range of response. Each person in a state of wellness or illness is a dynamic composite of the interrelationship of physiological, psychological, sociocultural, and developmental variables. Person is an open system with interaction with the environment.

Nursing

Nursing is viewed as a unique profession in that it is concerned with all the variables affecting an individual's response to stressors. The nurse has an obligation to seek the highest potential level of stability for each individual.

Health

Wellness is considered the ability of an individual's flexible line of defense against any stressor to maintain equilibrium. Any variances of wellness occur when stressors are able to penetrate the flexible line of defense. Neuman views health on a continuum with levels of wellness and variances of wellness. If a person's total needs are met, he or she is in an optimal level of wellness. Hence, a reduced state of wellness is the result of needs not being met.

Person to Nurse

The nurse assesses and validates the individual's response to stressors. Response to some stressors are known whereas others are manifested depending on the meaning of the experience to the individual. The nurse has a knowledge of the relation of the environment and the person's reaction to stress and reconstitution.

Person to Health

People retain harmony and balance with the environment by a process of interaction and adjustment. Persons are viewed as a total person composed of physiological, psychological, sociocultural, and developmental variables. The interrelationship of these variables determines the degree of reaction an individual has to any stressor. Each individual is seen as unique, but containing a blend of common attributes within a normal range of response. This normal range of response is known as a normal line of defense—that which is necessary to maintain an individual's equilibrium.

Nursing to Health

The nurse assists individuals, families, and groups to attain or maintain a maximum level of wellness by appropriate interventions. Nursing actions are interventions at the primary, secondary, and tertiary prevention levels that will reduce stress factors, strengthen the line of defense, and maintain a reasonable degree of adaptation.

Environment

The environment consists of internal and external factors. Internal is the flexible line of defense against stressors, such as the body's immune response pattern or the mobilization of white blood cells. External consists of an individual's coping ability, life style, developmental stage, and so forth, and is known as the normal line of defense.

Stressors

Stressors may vary as to impact or reaction. There are three types of stressors:

1. Intrapersonal forces occurring within the individual.
2. Interpersonal forces occurring between one or more individuals.

3. Extrapersonal forces occurring outside the individual (Neuman, 1980, p. 50).

A stressor attempts to penetrate an individual's normal line of defense to cause disequilibrium.

INTERNAL EVALUATION

Clarity

The criterion of clarity is adequately met in that Neuman's theory is easily understood by this writer. However, in the analysis by Fawcett et al. (1982) it is felt that there is a need for further clarification with specific terms of environment, health, wellness, and reconstitution. This writer feels that Neuman adequately defines these terms. "Health or wellness is the condition in which all parts and subparts (variables) are in harmony with the whole man. Disharmony reduces the wellness state. Environment consists of the internal and external forces surrounding man at any point in time (Neuman, 1982, p. 9)." Neuman goes on to further explain internal and external environments and variables in greater detail. Neuman (1982) further defines reconstitution as a dynamic state of adaptation to all stressors in the environment, whether internal or external, synthesizing all factors to obtain the best use of all resources. Therefore, Neuman's model does meet the criterion of clarity.

Consistency

Fawcett et al. (1982) state in general that Neuman's Systems Model is logically consistent. Dunbar (1982) further supports this view in her statement that "Neuman's cyclical approach leads logically from tertiary prevention back to primary prevention," thus providing guidelines for nursing practice (p. 297). Neuman is consistent in her use of terms. However, Fawcett et al. (1982) point out that Neuman's definition of the person as an open system is not fully supported, and instead feel Neuman's discussion of the relation between person and environment presents a more closed system view. Fawcett et al. (1982) indicate that nowhere in the model is the output from the person to the environment described as is necessary for an open systems viewpoint (p. 39). On the contrary, Neuman's (1980) repeated statement that the person "interacts with this environment by adjusting himself to it or adjusting it to himself (p. 122)" supports the idea that the person does indeed have impact and therefore output in the environment.

Neuman has based her theory on a combination of two principles: comprehensive and simple. According to Stevens (1984) a comprehensive principle explains a phenomenon by reference to a larger whole. A simple principle explains a phenomenon by reference to its component parts. In Neuman's model she has incorporated both of these principles in her view of the person in a total person approach. Neuman's (1982) definition of person as an individual in a state of wellness or illness is a dynamic composite of the interrelationship of physiological, psychological, sociocultural, and developmental variables. This interrelationship determines the nature and degree of an individual's response to stress.

Stevens (1984) finds that Neuman is inconsistent in her interpretation, stating "the theorist defines adaptation as stimulus response patterning and later uses the same term to mean psychological adjustment to a complex environmental change conceptualized in a Gestalt framework (p. 56)." In the opinion of this author, Neuman has been consistent throughout her conceptual framework as it encompasses Gestalt theory, which holds that each of us is surrounded by a perceptual field that is in a dynamic equilibrium. A field theory approach such as this maintains that all parts are interrelated and interdependent. Neuman recognized the necessity of connecting a psychological model to the responses of a physiological substrate. To supplement Gestalt theory, Neuman incorporates Selye's (1950) work, which carries the effects of the environment directly to the physiological substrate and the response of the individual on this level. There is room for disagreement with Stevens' (1984) interpretation when Neuman's model is seen as encompassing the best of several theories in attaining a total person approach.

Stevens (1984) also views Neuman's model as an entitative approach to nursing theory. Stevens defines transcendental interpretations as being beyond human experience, with an entitative interpretation seeing reality as reductive (consisting of units that are microscopic or microcosmic). It is limiting to attempt to label Neuman's model as purely one approach over another as is done with most theories. Neuman's model, due to its ability to encompass already existing models, is therefore a combination of essential interpretation and entitative interpretation. Stevens' definition of essential interpretation is one of human experience or one in which the nursing phenomenon is explained by reference to the circumstances in which it occurs. Neuman does indeed describe people in their multicomponents, but she also relates people and their interaction with the environment—both internal and external. These are not mutually exclusive but are utilized simultaneously to ensure the total person approach.

Neuman has chosen to use the logistic mode of thought in constructing her systems model. In this method a system, event, or entity is organized by reference to its parts and their relationship to each other (Stevens, 1984). The construct of the Neuman model rests on its analysis of parts and their relationships. Neuman includes physiological, psychological, sociocultural, and developmental variables as influencing factors in determining an individual's interaction with a stressor. Further, she has organized these stressors into three categories: intrapersonal, interpersonal, and extrapersonal. Stevens states that she equates a systems approach with a logistic method of thought; Neuman meets this criteria consistently throughout her model.

Adequacy

Stevens (1984) defines a theory as being adequate "if it carefully accounts for the subject matter with which it deals, however broad or limited the subject matter may be (p. 60)." Fawcett et al. (1982) feel the Neuman model places less emphasis on the acutely ill person. This error lies in the choices of application. Although initially the focus of Neuman's model was the community health setting, Dunbar (1982) has successfully utilized this approach in the critical care setting and has developed a modified assessment tool. Morales and Richards (1985) also state that "the family systems approach has been successfully applied to Neuman's nursing model, and the concepts of a systems stress have been incorporated into an assessment tool for critical care nursing (p. 51)." Therefore, the Neuman model clearly meets the criterion for adequacy.

Logical Development

Stevens (1984) states "the criterion of logical development requires that a theory grow naturally from its premises, that any assertion or conclusion flows reasonably from the groundwork laid for the assertion (p. 64)." Neuman has based her model on the following nine assumptions:

1. Although each individual is viewed as unique, he or she is also a composite of common knowns or characteristics within a normal, given range of response.
2. There are many known stressors. Each stressor is different in its potential to disturb an individual's equilibrium or normal line of defense. Moreover, a particular relationship of the variables—physiological, psychological, sociocultural, and developmental—at any point can affect the degree to which an individual is able to use his or her flexible line of defense against possible reaction to a single stressor or combination of stressors.
3. Each individual over time has evolved a normal range of responses, which is referred to as a normal line of defense.
4. When the cushioning, accordionlike effect of the flexible line of defense is no longer capable of protecting the individual against a stressor, the stressor breaks through the normal line of defense. The interrelationship of variables (physiological, psychological, sociocultural, and developmental) determines the nature and degree of the organism's reaction to the stressor.
5. Each person has an internal set of resistance factors (lines of resistance) that attempt to stabilize and return the individual to the normal line of defense should a stressor break through it.
6. The person in a state of wellness or illness is a dynamic composite of the interrelationship of the four variables (physiological, psychological, sociocultural, and developmental) that are always present.

7. Primary prevention relates to general knowledge that is applied to individual patient assessment in an attempt to identify and allay the possible risk factors associated with stressors.
8. Secondary prevention relates to symptomatology, appropriate ranking of intervention priorities, and treatment.
9. Tertiary prevention relates to the adaptive process as reconstitution begins, and moves back in a circular manner toward primary prevention (Neuman, 1982, p. 12).

Logical deductive conclusions can be made from these nine premises. Because it is beyond the scope of this chapter to elaborate on this point, the reader is referred to publications written by Neuman which provide excellent examples.

Level of Theory Development

Neuman's Systems Model falls into the second level of sophistication in theory development. Explanatory theories attempt to tell why or how the given components of a theory relate to and with each other. They may deal with cause and effect, correlations, or with rules that regulate interactions among a theory's components (Stevens, 1984). Neuman's model utilizes a combination of both predictive theory and situation producing theory. Predictive theory is utilized in Neuman's assumption that people are a composite of common knowns or characteristics within a normal given range of response. Situation producing theories are those in which certain interventions into a phenomenon will alter the outcome (Stevens, 1984). Neuman's model is based on primary, secondary, and tertiary interventions in altering the outcome and attainment or maintainment of client system stabilization. Therefore, Neuman's model is at a higher level of sophistication in theory development than most nursing models today.

EXTERNAL CRITICISM

Reality Convergence

Neuman's model emphasizes the total person approach. The basic premises underlying the Neuman Systems Model are sound. These are expressed in the principles, interpretations, and methods of the Neuman model. Neuman has chosen to incorporate within her conceptual framework philosophies that emphasize the unity of the person, as well as the use of Gestalt and field theories, and her total approach is clearly applicable to the real world of nursing today.

Utility

A nursing theory that is useful in nursing practice, education, research, or administration is one that meets the criterion of utility. The Neuman model is universal in its applicability to various educational and nursing practice settings. Fawcett et al. (1982) state that the model is able to provide general yet comprehensive guidelines for application. Neuman's model is useful in many areas of nursing practice—from community health to critical care—with the inclusion of interventions through primary, secondary, and tertiary preventions. Neuman's writing clearly indicates the utility of her model by presenting the application of the model in nursing practice, education, research, and administration.

Significance

According to Stevens (1984), a theory is considered significant if it addresses the essential issues in nursing and contributes to the development of nursing knowledge. As health care continues to evolve with an expanded focus on primary prevention, the Neuman Systems Model will be of major significance. The focus of traditional nursing roles in the acute hospital setting has expanded to include primary and tertiary prevention. This model indeed addresses a very up-to-date issue in the realm of nursing today and provides clear guidelines for nursing management. The Neuman Systems Model focuses on the wellness and variances of wellness along with environmental influences on health, and reflects nursing's interest in a total person or holistic approach.

The Neuman Systems Model research potential is clearly demonstrated by Dunbar (1982) in her study of transfer stress of patients in a surgical intensive care unit. Dunbar modified Neuman's original assessment intervention tool. This tool was found to be useful in developing nursing diagnoses and care plans to include interventions in areas of primary, secondary, and tertiary prevention. Although the sample was small, Dunbar's results indicate the importance and value to nursing practice of investigation into the nature of stressors affecting patients. This research is a step toward the development of an assessment tool that is guided by theoretical requirements of the Neuman model.

Discrimination

The criterion for the capacity to discriminate is whether the theory differentiates nursing from other health professions on one hand, and other caring and tending acts on the other (Stevens, 1984). Although Neuman (1982) defines nursing as a unique profession concerned with all the variances affecting an individual's response to stressors, the nurse is not assigned a unique function or role. On the contrary, the Neuman Systems Model is an attempt to provide a conceptual framework appropriate for health care providers in areas other than nursing. Therefore, the Neuman model does not meet the criterion for discrimination. However, Venable (1980) notes that "since the total person approach is so useful, the lack of a unique role for nursing is not seen as a detriment but rather as a call for reexamination of traditionally defined roles assigned to health care workers in general (p. 141)."

Scope

There are conflicting views in nursing as to whether nursing theories should be of broad or limited scope. Recognition must be given to the validity of a need for both types of constructs. The Neuman Systems Model is of broad scope and addresses the total domain of nursing. The multidimensional nature of the model and its recognition of the multivariable nature of humans and interactions with human and physical environments is of great import in the world of nursing theories.

Complexity

The criterion for complexity is when a theory is able to achieve a balance between parsimony and complexity. Parsimony is seen as too simple—the fewest possible variables within a theory's components. Complexity allows for explanation and interrelationships of many more variables (Stevens, 1984). On a scale from one to ten, with parsimony being one and complexity being ten, this writer rates the Neuman Systems Model as a six. The model is based on the interaction and interrelationship of many variables. In its comprehensive approach to the total person, the multiple terms used in the model are familiar and therefore do not require learning an extensive new vocabulary. Hence, this writer believes Neuman has achieved an appropriate balance between parsimony and complexity.

SUMMARY

Neuman has successfully combined the theoretical construct of Gestalt theory with that of Selye's (1950) theory on stress and adaptation. This integration of theory is in the tradition of scientific advance and is perhaps one of Neuman's most significant contributions at the present for the development of an experimental model compatible with nursing theory and clinical data. Frankly, exploratory experimentation is in order, because theoretical development in nursing has not yet reached the level of sophistication where theory requiring rigorous hypothesis testing would be appropriate.

REFERENCES

Dunbar, S. B. (1982). Critical care and the Neuman model. In B. Neuman (Ed.), *The Neuman Systems Model*. East Norwalk, CT: Appleton-Century-Crofts.

Fawcett, J., Carpenito, L. V., Efinger, J., et al. (1982). A framework for analysis and evaluation of conceptual models of nursing with an analysis and evaluation of the Neuman Systems Model. In B. Neuman (Ed.), *The Neuman Systems Model.* East Norwalk, CT: Appleton-Century-Crofts.

Morales, M., & Richards, E. (1985). Family centered critical care nursing. *Focus on Critical Care, 12*(4), 45–51.

Neuman, B. (1980). The Betty Neuman health-care systems model: A total person approach to patient problems. In J. P. Riehl & C. Roy (Eds.), *Conceptual models for nursing practice* (2nd ed.). New York: Appleton-Century-Crofts.

Neuman, B. (1982). *The Neuman Systems Model.* East Norwalk, CT: Appleton-Century-Crofts.

Selye, H. (1956). *The stress of life.* New York: McGraw-Hill.

Stevens, B. J. (1984). *Nursing theory: Analysis, application, evaluation.* Boston: Little, Brown.

Venable, J. F. (1980). The Neuman health-care systems model: An analysis. In J. P. Riehl & C. Roy (Eds.), *Conceptual models for nursing practice* (2nd ed.). New York: Appleton-Century-Crofts.

An Evaluation Instrument for Assessing an Associate Degree Nursing Curriculum Based on the Neuman Systems Model

Lois W. Lowry
Margaret C. Jopp

Many nurse educators attest to the effectiveness of models for curriculum development, claiming that students learn and practice more effectively from a conceptually based curriculum (Fawcett, 1984; Lindeman, 1980; Neuman, 1982; Riehl & Roy, 1980). The Neuman Systems Model has been adopted as a curricular framework by more than two dozen baccalaureate and higher degree nursing programs in the United States and Europe because of its holistic, interdisciplinary, systems approach to client care. Yet associate degree nursing programs that emphasize the preparation of nurses for direct patient care have been slower than professional programs to design curricula from nursing models.

The purpose of this article is to share the strategies of developing a curriculum and evaluation instrument from the Neuman Systems Model for a newly established associate degree nursing program. The faculty of the nursing program at Cecil Community College (in North East, Maryland) believe that nursing models provide a logical framework for nursing curricula, based on several assumptions:

1. Models provide a structure for organizing curricular content for students.
2. Models introduce relevant nursing concepts and help illustrate the relationships among them.
3. If broad in scope, models remain adaptable as future changes occur in the health care system.

4. Models provide a guide for nursing practice—that is, concepts taught in the classroom apply equally well to clinical practice settings.

The Neuman Systems Model was selected as the framework for this new associate degree program because it was consistent with the assumptions and philosophy of the faculty. The Neuman model provides a systems approach for organizing curricular content and describes the interrelationships among person, environment, health, and nursing. It particularly focuses on the relationship between nurse and client and the client's response to stressors. These concepts are critical to nurses prepared at an associate's level, and the model is therefore appropriate for an associate degree curriculum. The nursing program at Cecil Community College is the first associate degree program in the United States to use the Neuman Systems Model as a conceptual framework.

STRATEGIES AND EXPERIENCES

The processes of curriculum development and evaluation occurred in two phases: (1) internalization of the model by the faculty and (2) development and testing of the evaluation instrument.

Faculty Internalization of the Model

Several tasks needed to be accomplished before the faculty was ready to work creatively with the model. All faculty members participated in an intensive review of the literature, defined model terms, and identified subconcepts. The concepts and subconcepts became the curricular threads that formed the outline of each nursing course. The depth, breadth, and complexity of the courses increased throughout the curriculum but the outline remained consistent. For example, the developmental variable was introduced in the beginning of each course in relation to the clients who were the focus of care in that course. Stressors that affected the health status of these clients were then presented with the appropriate nursing interventions.

Concomitantly, the faculty planned clinical learning experiences that applied model constructs to clinical practice. For example, client assessment was designed in a logical sequence based upon the five variables of person—psychological, physiological, sociocultural, developmental and spiritual. Clients' responses to stressors and perceptions of their illness were noted. Nursing diagnoses, care plans, and charted notes followed a logical pattern derived from the model concepts.

The faculty determined which aspects of the model should receive greater or lesser emphasis within an associate degree nursing program. Because the primary aim of associate graduates is to provide care for clients in acute and chronic care settings, the faculty agreed that secondary prevention as intervention must be emphasized in all theory and practice courses. Primary and tertiary prevention as intervention concepts would be introduced in some theory courses, with special emphasis on health teaching and illness prevention, and on referrals and discharge planning, although fewer clinical experiences were provided. The concept of a holistic person impacted by stressors received major emphasis in all nursing courses; first, the person as a unique being, and then in the second year, the person as a member of a family and community.

Working with the constructs enabled the faculty to gain ownership of the model and to begin to use it creatively. However, not all faculty members chose to become as involved with this new way of thinking and developing a curriculum. In other words, they were resisting change. Variations existed among faculty members as to their acceptance and utilization of the model both in the classroom and in clinical practice. Some were enthusiastic role models for integration of the model concepts into their teaching, and students were able to observe the usefulness of a nursing model in practice. Others persisted in using traditional approaches. Thus there was inconsistency in the use of the model throughout the total curriculum. As this became evident, a comprehensive strategy for change was effected so that commonalities could be identified and differences resolved.

With an emphasis on cooperation and communication, team building was instituted. Specific times were set aside for faculty discussions and the sharing of perceptions and values in the use of the model. The group goals were to develop trust, mutuality, and group cohesion. Achievement of these goals was a vital step in team building that when achieved became a major factor in enabling faculty members to effectively work together toward the common goal of internalizing the model.

The group discussions were relaxed and supportive; trust was maintained and fear of expressing differing ideas decreased with time. Faculty members shared many innovative ideas, took risks, thought in unique ways about familiar concepts, and were willing to experiment with new approaches— resulting in the emergence of creative ways to use the model. One creative innovation was to consider the student as the center of the system in the educational process just as the client is the center of the system in the caretaking process. This model adaptation depicts the faculty member, student, and client as interacting and responding to stressors during the teaching and learning process. An atmosphere of excitement and enthusiasm continued to permeate the faculty discussions. Curriculum development became a creative experience!

As the model began to give shape and form to the curriculum, the faculty proposed the following: development of a format for a client care plan based upon the Neuman model. It was anticipated that such a care plan would provide consistency and continuity throughout the curriculum and would be used in all clinical courses. The format was general enough to contain the major model constructs, while specific enough to allow for the inclusion of curricular subconcepts necessary for client assessments in specialty areas, such as maternal–child and psychiatric nursing. The more the faculty worked with the model, the more creative they became in adapting it to their own use.

Throughout this faculty internalization phase (a period of 2 years), the faculty became aware that curriculum development evolved within the concept of change and implied a long-term commitment. Their commitment was to an open system process involving information input, interpretation, information output, and a feedback loop. This process necessitated adaptation and change within the system. It required time, effort, energy, perseverence, and continual support and acceptance of new ideas. Creativity continued, resulting in a curriculum that was both internally consistent and unified by the model constructs themselves. Table 6–1 lists the strategies that enable successful curriculum development and evaluation.

Instrument Development

The experiences shared in phase one were requisites for phase two, the actual development of the evaluation instrument of the Neuman Systems Model.

Early in phase one, the faculty realized the necessity of networking with other professionals who were utilizing the model. They began to communicate

TABLE 6–1. STRATEGIES LEADING TO SUCCESSFUL EVALUATION OF A CONCEPTUAL MODEL

1. Review the literature about the model.
2. Define the constructs of the model.
3. Define the scope of the model for your program.
4. Encourage faculty to choose areas of exploration and development in which they are most interested.
5. Share agreeably the responsibilities among the members.
6. Provide opportunities for team building and values clarification.
7. Set specific times for faculty work sessions.
8. Select locations conducive to productivity and free from interruptions.
9. Maintain an informal atmosphere at work sessions.
10. Encourage creativity, risk-taking, and innovation.
11. Eliminate "tunnel-vision" and criticism.
12. Establish a written timetable for short- and long-term goals.
13. Appoint one member to keep group interaction notes to review from session to session to provide continuity.
14. Encourage members to keep idea logs to record creative thoughts, strategies, and ideas.
15. Establish a network with faculties from other institutions that utilize the model.
16. Identify and contact resource-persons assisting with research design and statistical analyses.
17. Plan the research design.
18. Plan for reliability and validity tests appropriate to the design.
19. Plan the method of data collection.
20. Analyze data and draw conclusions.

with other nursing programs and exchange ideas for curriculum development. Most of these were at the baccalaureate level. This not only provided opportunities to discuss the commonalities and differences in the use of the model at specific levels of education but also to explore the possibilities of articulation between programs. Further, it was necessary to begin networking as well as to identify necessary resources for assistance with the design and testing of the evaluation instrument.

Three steps were involved in the development of the evaluation instrument: (1) selection of constructs to be measured; (2) formulation of test items for each construct; and (3) testing the instrument for validity and reliability. Brainstorming was the process that faculty members engaged in to list all the aspects of the model that required evaluation. Two major sections were identified from this exercise. The first section focused on graduates' perceptions of the four major concepts of the model—person, stress or adaptation, health or illness, and nursing. The second section focused on graduates' use of the model in clinical practice. The five interrelated roles of associate degree graduates as identified by the National League for Nursing (1979) and defined by the Western Interstate Commission on Higher Education (WICHE, 1985) were the subconcepts for section two of the instrument; that is, provider of care, communicator, teacher, coordinator of care, and member of the discipline of nursing.

The second step was to formulate test items for each section of the instrument that reflected the perceptions of that concept as interpreted by the Neuman model. For example, an item under the subconcept *person* read, "I assess person as composites of five variables: physiological, psychological, sociocultural, developmental, and spiritual." An item from *stress/stressors* read, "I categorize stressors as: intrapersonal, extrapersonal, and interpersonal forces". Each item reflected an important concept of the Neuman Systems Model. The number of items for each concept varied between 8 and 20 depending on the emphasis placed on that concept by Neuman. The concepts *person* and *nursing* were described more fully by the model than *stress/adaptation* and *health*, and thus required more evaluative items. The intent was to include a sufficient number of items for each concept so that all aspects of the concepts were addressed. Table 6–2 includes several examples for each concept in section one of the instrument.

In section two, application of the model in practice, test items were written for the following roles: provider of care, communicator, teacher, coordinator, and member. Each item referred to a behavior related to that role. The number of items per role varied between 8 and 25, depending on the emphasis on a specific role for an associate degree graduate. For example, the provider of care role contained the greatest number of items, whereas the coordinator and member roles contained the least. Further, the communicator and teacher roles were subdivided into sections related to client and related to self. Table 6–3 contains several examples of items for the practice roles.

Initially, the evaluation instrument, comprised of seven categories (four in

TABLE 6-2. SECTION ONE: CONCEPTS OF THE NEUMAN MODEL

Concepts	Focus	Sample Evaluation Items
Person	Perception of clients	1. I view persons as holistic beings.
		2. I assess person as a composite of the five variables (physiological, psychological, sociocultural, developmental, and spiritual).
		3. I relate to persons as open systems in dynamic interaction with the environment.
Stress or stressors	Perception of environment	1. I evaluate the stressors that affect a client's normal line of defense.
		2. I identify the stressors that affect my client's condition. . . .
		3. I attempt to reduce the effect of stressors on the client.
Wellness or illness	Perception of health	1. I view wellness and illness as a continuum between which individuals fluctuate.
		2. I assist clients to reconstitute from illness.
Nursing	Perception of nursing	1. I function to assist individuals to obtain and maintain maximum wellness.
		2. In my experience to date, I have utilized: 　　Primary intervention 　　Secondary intervention 　　Tertiary intervention
		3. I attempt to involve families and significant others in planning client care.

section one and three in section two), had a total of 95 items (about half in each section). Subjects were asked to evaluate each item according to how well they had internalized the concepts in section one and how much they implemented the behaviors of section two in clinical practice. A Likert scale was used, with five choices of responses (never, rarely, sometimes, mostly, and always). At the end of the questionnaire one open-ended question was included to elicit data about unique applications of the model in practice.

Validity and Reliability

The third step was to test the instrument for reliability and validity so that it could be used with confidence. Content validity was determined by submitting

TABLE 6–3. SECTION TWO: APPLICATION OF MODEL TO CLINICAL PRACTICE

Concepts	Focus	Sample Evaluation Items
Provider of care	Role as caregiver	The Neuman Systems Model . . . 1. Provides me a consistent way of interpreting clinical situations. 2. Provides me a basis for thinking ahead proactively rather than reactively. 3. Increases the probability that I will select care modalities from a wider range of relevant behaviors.
Communicator and teacher	Roles as communicator and teacher Related to client	The Neuman Systems Model enables me to . . . 1. Provide the structure for client teaching and learning activities. 2. Promote a positive client response to my nursing care.
	Related to self	The Neuman Systems Model . . . 1. Increases my understanding of new information. 2. Makes a difference in my communication.
Coordinator and member of discipline of nursing	Role in coordinating client care	1. I feel comfortable sharing the Neuman Systems Model with my colleagues at work. 2. Nursing administration encourages the use of the Neuman model.

the instrument to two groups: faculty members in a baccalaureate program who used the Neuman Systems Model for their curriculum framework and senior nursing students in the same baccalaureate program.

The questions asked were:

1. Did the items represent the essential content for each model concept?
2. Were the items in the application section appropriate for nursing graduates?
3. Were statements clear and unambiguous?
4. Were there sufficient reverse-score items?

5. Were the statements written in an unbiased way?

6. Was there consistency in person and tense?

7. Did the respondents have any comments on the response format?

Faculty evaluated the first six criteria positively. Several suggestions were made about the format by both faculty and students, and these were implemented to enhance clarity and facility in answering the questionnaire.

Reliability of the instrument was demonstrated by a test-retest procedure to measure stability over time and the Spearman-Brown split-half formula to measure internal consistency. The Pearson product-moment correlation statistic was used to analyze the results. The method of conducting the reliability procedures was to administer the instrument to a group of 24 senior nursing students in a classroom setting allowing 20 minutes for test administration. Each instrument was coded to identify each student. One week later the same instrument was readministered by matching code numbers to the same group of students under the same testing conditions.

The first step in analysis was to examine the matching pairs of questions for the 24 students to note changes in responses from the first administration to the second. It was noted that 25% to 35% of the students (between six and nine students) had changed their first response by one point at the second testing. Sometimes the response change was from "mostly" to "all the time" and vice versa, or from "never" to "rarely" and the reverse. Seldom was change noted from the midpoint on the Likert scale "sometimes" to "mostly" or from "sometimes" to "rarely," even though these were one-point changes as well. The literature indicates that minor changes in response categories is quite common in tests that measure attitudes and behaviors because of differences in human perceptions at any given point in time. This phenomenon is referred to as trait instability, and accounts for some error in reliability testing (Mehrens & Lehmann, 1980).

The faculty decided that a one-point change between the two upper categories (mostly and all the time) and the two lower categories (rarely and never) was not enough to be considered a statistical gain or loss. Therefore, one point changes in either direction at the two ends of the scale would be counted as the same and not be considered different responses.

The next step was to calculate a total score for the questionnaire. The Pearson r was calculated to be 0.50. Because of this low correlation, a closer examination of the individual pairs of tests was necessary. Scatter plots were run for each matched pair of questions to visualize the pattern of responses and to identify outliers. The result was that five questions which had a Pearson r of less than 0.30 were eliminated from the final instrument. Each questionnaire was again carefully scrutinized and it was discovered that seven questionnaires were incomplete (either whole pages were missing or individual questions were skipped), and two were invalid. That is, two individuals had selected one group of responses (all the time) on the first administration and the opposite set (never or rarely) on the second administration. Thus, these 9 pairs of questionnaires were eliminated from the sample and another correlation was calculated on the remaining 15 sets. The resulting Pearson product-moment correlation was found to be 0.920, an excellent correlation that indicated stability of the instrument.

The procedure used for measuring internal consistency was the Spearman-Brown split-half formula. To accomplish this, 18 questionnaire items were written in reverse order that matched up with 18 items asking the same question in a different way. For example, the following two statements are matched: "I relate to persons as open systems in dynamic interaction with the environment" and "I consider persons as closed systems." The purpose of this procedure was to validate that two questions stated in different ways would be answered in a consistent manner. The result of the procedure yielded an alpha level of 0.922, indicating that there was internal consistency in the instrument.

Having completed validity and reliability tests and the subsequent revisions, the final instrument was ready for use in the longitudinal study. The final instrument consisted of 90 items, 44 in section one and 46 in section two. Figure 6–1 shows a portion of the final evaluation instrument.

Pilot Testing

The instrument was pilot tested with the first two classes of graduates who had been introduced to the model during their first nursing course in the program. The first group (A) consisted of 23 members from the first graduating class; the second group (B) consisted of 22 members from the second graduating class. Both groups were similar in age and sex. The instrument was mailed to group A 5 months after their graduation and resulted in a 50% return rate. Group B completed the instrument in a classroom setting 3 weeks prior to their graduation, with a 100% completion rate. The two groups simulate a pre- and postgraduate comparison, which is the intent of the study, to note changes over time. Each group was directed to answer each item in section one according to what extent they had internalized the concepts and in section two to what extent they had applied them in practice.

Respondents from both groups tended to cluster their answers in the two highest categories ("most of the time" and "always") for the test items about person and stress or adaptation. When answering the items concerning health or illness, there was more diversity. One sixth of the postgraduates (group A) selected the category "sometimes" for six of the seven items, indicating that their perceptions of health and illness changed over time after exposure to the real world of sick clients. In contrast, the pregraduates (group B) selected the categories "mostly" and "all the time" to rate their internalization of the health or illness concepts.

Both groups tended to internalize the concept of nursing "mostly" and "all the time," reporting that they perceived the practice of nursing as collaborative care with primary, secondary, and tertiary interventions. One third of the post graduates were less apt to involve families in interventions and did not interpret

This questionnaire is for all graduates of the associate degree nursing program of Cecil Community College. Your responses to the statements will assist the faculty in evaluating the Neuman Systems Model as a basis for curriculum development. Please answer all of the questions. If you wish to comment on any of the questions or qualify your answers, please feel free to do so.

Thank you for your help.

ID NUMBER _____

Section I: Concepts of the Neuman Model

A. PERCEPTION OF PERSON (Circle the adverb which best describes your understanding of the concept.)

1. I consider persons as closed systems	Never	Rarely	Sometimes	Mostly	Always
2. I consider persons as unique individuals, all of whom have a normal range of responses ...	Never	Rarely	Sometimes	Mostly	Always
3. I think of person's normal range of responses as the normal line of defense	Never	Rarely	Sometimes	Mostly	Always

B. PERCEPTION OF STRESS/STRESSORS

1. I assess stressors as internal and external stimuli which have the potential to cause disequilibrium or crises	Never	Rarely	Sometimes	Mostly	Always
2. I categorize stressors as: intrapersonal, extrapersonal, and interpersonal forces	Never	Rarely	Sometimes	Mostly	Always
3. I evaluate the client's flexible line of defense which acts as a protective buffer from stress	Never	Rarely	Sometimes	Mostly	Always

Section II: Application of Model to Practice/Education

IIA. PROVIDER OF CARE (Circle the adverb which best describes your utilization of the model.)

The Neuman Systems Model:

1. Serves as a checklist to encourage thoroughness in providing client care	Never	Rarely	Sometimes	Mostly	Always
2. Enables me to improve my: diagnostic skills	Never	Rarely	Sometimes	Mostly	Always
3. observation skills	Never	Rarely	Sometimes	Mostly	Always
4. writing skills	Never	Rarely	Sometimes	Mostly	Always

Figure 6-1. Portion of evaluation instrument of the Neuman systems model.

5.   performance skills ....   Never   Rarely   Sometimes   Mostly Always
6. Makes no difference in my
    client care ....   Never   Rarely   Sometimes   Mostly Always

IIB. COORDINATOR/MEMBER OF PROFESSION (Circle the adverb which best describes *your experience* in the work setting.)

1. I am able to articulate the Neu-
    man concepts ....   Never   Rarely   Sometimes   Mostly Always
2. I feel comfortable sharing the
    Neuman Systems Model with
    my colleagues at work ......   Never   Rarely   Sometimes   Mostly Always
3. Is there anything else about the Neuman model you would like to share? (Please describe any unique opportunities you have had to use the model.)

_____

_____

_____

Thank you very much for your contribution to this effort. If you would like a summary of the results, please print your name and address and we will see that you get it.

Name _____

Address _____

_____

Figure 6-1. (continued).

the meaning of stress to their clients; the pregraduates selected responses that involved families in care. These group differences may be due to the influence of time constraints and pressures in the real work setting that impeded family involvement.

More differences in responses between the pre- and postgraduate groups were noted in the second section, "application to clinical practice." As care providers, 45% of the respondents in group B (pregraduates) stated they "always" utilized the model through all steps of the nursing process when providing care. In group A (postgraduates), 40% of the graduates responded that they utilized the model "most of the time." Five percent of this group indicated that they rarely used the model when providing care. Respondents from both groups affirmed that they "always" or "most of the time" used the model when recording on nurses notes, Kardex, nursing care plans, and nursing histories. One third or less of the group A graduates used the terms "flexible and normal lines of defense" when writing client care plans, but all the respondents in the group considered the five variables of person when assessing clients. The responses in group B were similar to those in group A regarding the use of Neuman terminology. Responses to the roles of communicator and teacher were similar for both groups in that 90% selected "most of the time" and "always" for statements relating to these roles.

The greatest difference in responses between the two groups was found in items associated with the coordinator and member roles. Two thirds of the respondents in group A indicated that their colleagues and administrators did not encourage them to use the model in their practice although half of this group claimed that their administrators were aware that they were using the model. On the other hand, half of those in group B expressed that they used the model. The other half of this group selected "never," "rarely," and "sometimes" as their responses to questions about their use of the model. These findings indicate that more communication about the utility of nursing models is necessary between nurse-educators and nursing service personnel, so that new graduates can actually practice in the way they have been taught.

Research Currently Being Conducted

The longitudinal evaluation study of the graduating classes of the Cecil Community College nursing program began in May 1985 and will conclude with the class of 1989.

A recurrent institutional cycle design was selected for the evaluation study because it combines longitudinal and cross-sectional approaches resulting in four comparisons. The combined approaches permit controls for history, instrumentation, test-retest, regression, and maturation.

Data collected from the class of 1985 tend to indicate that there is no change in the internalization of concepts over time; that is, model concepts are well internalized by time of graduation, and remain part of the graduates understanding and modus operandi of nursing 6 months later.

The degree to which the model is used in practice settings appears to vary according to the encouragement and recognition of model usage by the graduates' supervisors in agencies where they are employed. If graduates are encouraged to write comprehensive, systematic care plans, they are more likely to use the model. One graduate reported that she was asked to present an in-service program on the use of the model in assessing clients. Another graduate was asked to serve on a committee to redesign the hospital care plan format according to the Neuman variables. Thus, early evidence from the evaluation study seems to indicate that a curriculum based on a nursing model is effective. Not only is the curriculum internally consistent but the product of the program is able to provide comprehensive care to well and ill human beings.

CONCLUSION

This article was intended to share effective faculty strategies applied in the development of an associate degree nursing curriculum based on the Neuman Systems Model and an evaluation instrument to test the model. The future of conceptual models and their impact on nursing curricula will require in-depth evaluation studies. The effectiveness of these studies is dependent upon conscientious, dedicated faculty members willing to assume the arduous task of an effective evaluation system. Nurse-educators badly need information that can be used to improve the process of curriculum development. The sharing of innovative program evaluation data based on nursing models can be a vital force in facilitating significant change toward responsible nursing education.

REFERENCES

Fawcett, J. (1984). *Analyses and evaluation of conceptual models of nursing*. Philadelphia: Davis.

Lindeman, C. A. (1980). Putting theory to work: A changing approach to practice. Recorded at JONA's fourth national conference, Chicago: Teach-em, Inc.

Mehrens, W. A., & Lehmann, I. J. (1980). *Measurement and evaluation* (2nd ed.). New York: Holt, Rinehart & Winston.

National League for Nursing. (1979). *Current statement of competencies and ability*. New York: Author.

Neuman, B. (1982). *The Neuman Systems Model*. East Norwalk, CT: Appleton-Century-Crofts.

Riehl, J. P., & Roy, C. (1980). *Conceptual models for nursing practice* (2nd ed.). New York: Appleton-Century-Crofts.

Western Interstate Commission on Higher Education. (1985). *Model hospital job descriptions for the new associate degree and baccalaureate degree graduates. Table 2*. Author.

A Cooperative Process in Curriculum Development Using the Neuman Health-Care Systems Model

Dorothy Evanson Mrkonich
Marguerite Hessian
Marilee Woehning Miller

How does a faculty begin to create an innovative curriculum designed to prepare graduates for the complex system of health care delivery today and for future practice? The Neuman Health-Care Systems Model provided the framework for the development of a new curriculum for the Minnesota Intercollegiate Nursing Consortium (MINC).[1] The focus of this chapter is to describe how three accredited baccalaureate nursing programs in private, religious, and liberal arts colleges accomplished this task.

Multiple factors provided an incentive for cooperation throughout the entire process of development. Political, economic, and demographic forces necessitated a fresh look at how educational systems are dependent on each other for a more efficient use of resources and for growth. With a desire to maintain high-quality nursing education at a time of decreasing student numbers, it was decided to pool resources to maintain and increase the quality and marketability of a baccalaureate nursing program. Another of the many factors providing an incentive for cooperation among one Catholic and two Lutheran colleges was the openness and desire of people to work together in the belief that what unified them was greater than what separated and divided them. The Minnesota Intercollegiate Nursing Consortium has become both a symbolic and substantive effort in ecumenicity.

In beginning to work together, three nursing representatives from each of the colleges were named to a steering committee to explore the feasibility of creating one program from three. As in any new group approaching a common task, it was essential to take time for members of the group to become acquainted and to learn about each other. As hopes and fears for the consortium were shared and roles were clarified, the trust level increased. Individuals became willing to let go of personal attachments to current programs and free themselves for creative, innovative thinking.

The further the steering committee moved into creative thinking the more it became apparent that this group had a life of its own and was comfortable with the trustee representative role. The process of differentiating the trustee from the delegate representative role necessitated an understanding of each role and a personal acceptance of the responsibility for decison making. The person in the trustee role follows his or her own convictions and makes judgments based on an assessment of the facts, understanding of the problems involved, and a thoughtful appraisal of the sides of the issue. The delegate role, in contrast, commits the person to follow the majority opinion of the group represented (Eulau, 1969). As members of the steering committee assumed the trustee role, they continued to value information sharing among faculty.

One of the expected short-term goals of this steering committee was to take a position on whether or not to continue planning for the implementation of the nursing consortium. In order to make that decision the group began to work on developing a common philosophy. The components of the philosophy were determined and small groups were used to generate and share beliefs about nursing, society, health, and learning. In the process of writing the philosophy, the members came to the realization that beliefs were shared and that they could work together to develop a common curriculum. After that realization the group decided to continue planning toward implementaton of the consortium.

At a day long retreat, the nursing faculties of all three colleges had an opportunity to share reactions and ask questions about the position paper. Following almost unanimous support in favor of the position, the faculties became actively involved in sharing ideas for a future-oriented program. The philosophy was reviewed, suggestions for change were considered, and a working document was accepted.

The combined faculties then examined the work of major nursing theorists in relation to their beliefs about nursing. They agreed to use an existing nursing model as an organizing framework to give structure to the curriculum and as a guide for selecting content. Data were gathered by reading, discussing, making comparisons, and meeting with experts in theory building and curriculum development. Five questions guided the discussion in selecting a nursing model:

1. Is the model congruent with the MINC philosophy?
2. Does the model provide direction for nursing practice?
3. Can the model be applied to the client as individual, family, and community?

4. Does the model allow for the use and development of a common structure and language for nursing diagnosis?

5. Is the model future oriented?

Neuman's Health-Care Systems Model was chosen because the answers to the five questions were affirmative. This reinforced the belief that a nursing model could provide a useful framework for curriculum development. The model, coupled with a strong liberal arts preparation, provides the education needed to carry out traditional nursing roles as well as a variety of innovative, futuristic roles.

A newly established consortium curriculum committee consisting of four nursing representatives from each college began to write the organizing framework for the new curriculum. Strategies used in expressing an understanding of this framework included assigning one group to write and one to depict artistically the integration of key elements into an articulated structure based on the Neuman model. Pictorial and narrative conceptualizations of the organization were a result of this effort.

The pictorial conceptualizations shown in Figures 7–1 and 7–2 reflect Neuman's model from a three-dimensional and top view. They depict the client (person, family, or community) as an open, holistic, autonomous system adapting to and interacting with other systems through an exchange of energy. Wellness is a dynamic self-perceived, multidimensional state that is influenced by the interrelationship of five client variables: physiological, psychological, sociocultural, spiritual, and developmental. Variances of wellness occur when stressors act as disruptive forces that mobilize the lines of defense. When the flexible lines of defense are no longer able to protect the normal lines of defense, the internal lines of resistance are called into play to protect the core. At this point, reconstitution or death results. Reconstitution of the lines of defense stabilizes the client system and may occur above, below, or at the previous level of adaptation. Reconstitution occurs with the mobilization of all internal and external resources and is facilitated by the purposeful, collaborative intervention of the professional nurse with the client system.

The professional nurse uses the nursing process in a variety of roles and settings to intervene at the various levels of prevention. This assists the client system to retain, attain, and maintain stability with growth as a potential outcome at any time. The nursing process is a complex skill implemented within an interpersonal relationship and requires self-awareness, critical thinking, creativity, and application of ethical principles.

Nursing is an open system and has a reciprocal relationship with the environment, which includes the health care system as well as the larger social system. Nursing is accountable to society for responding to its health needs and for creating change.

The pictorial and narrative conceptualizations guided the selection of prerequisite and supporting courses for the major in nursing. These selected

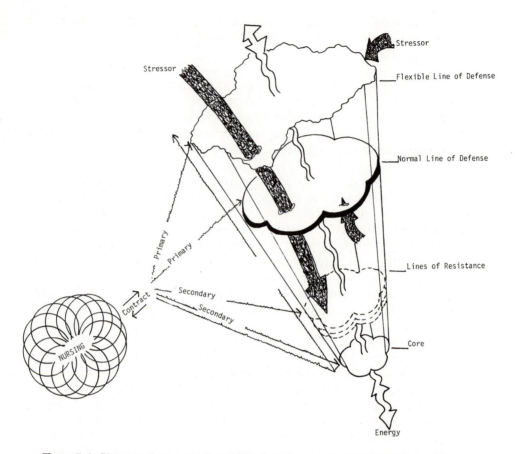

Figure 7-1. Diagram of conceptual model for the Minnesota Intercollegiate Nursing Consortium. (*Diagram by Mary Ellen Kitundu, Gustavus Adolphus College. Copyright © 1985 Minnesota Intercollegiate Nursing Consortium.*)

courses provided a balance of emphasis among the five variables. The overall educational schema makes it possible for students to have choices among other general education and elective courses, thus insuring the integration of the liberal arts and nursing.

A further step in development of the curriculum was to establish program goals, definitions of terms, and characteristics of the graduates. Major concepts were traced from the philosophy through all these documents and were placed in levels congruent with four semesters of nursing. Table 7-1 explains how two major concepts, client system and nursing process, can be taught at these levels with increasing complexity. This in turn dictates course content including the selection of clinical experiences. *Client system* is defined as person, family, or community and *nursing process* is defined as nursing diagnoses, nursing goals, and nursing outcomes, in keeping with Neuman's model (1982). At the first

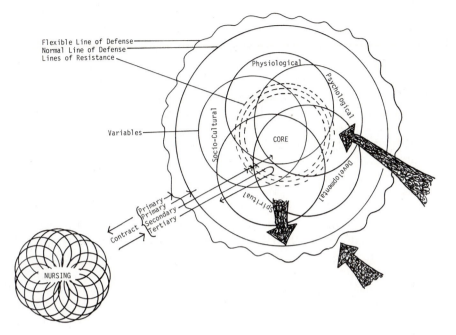

Figure 7–2. Diagram of conceptual model for the Minnesota Intercollegiate Nursing Consortium. (*Diagram by Mary Ellen Kitundu, Gustavus Adolphus College. Copyright © 1985 Minnesota Intercollegiate Nursing Consortium.*)

TABLE 7-1. THE NURSING PROCESS AS APPLIED TO CLIENT SYSTEMS AT FOUR LEVELS OF COMPLEXITY

Nursing Process	Levels of Complexity			
	I	II	III	IV
Nursing diagnosis	Well persons	Persons with variances of wellness	Persons and families with variances of wellness	Communities
		Well families		
Nursing goals		Persons with variances of wellness	Persons and families with variances of wellness	Communities
Nursing outcomes		Persons with variances of wellness	Persons and families with variances of wellness	

level the student assesses well persons. At the second level the student also assesses well families as client systems, and in addition carries out all three steps of the nursing process with persons having variances of wellness. Families, as well as persons with variances of wellness, are added at the third level, and the student is expected to use all steps of the nursing process. Continuing to build the complexity, communities as client systems are added at the fourth level and students apply the first two steps of the nursing process in working with communities.

Determination of objectives at each of the four levels was the next step in curriculum design and set the stage for future course development. Examples of two of the ten expected characteristics of the graduates and level of objectives are shown in Table 7-2.

In using the Neuman Health-Care Systems Model, the steering committee discovered that certain aspects of the model needed further development because of beliefs stated in the MINC philosophy. For instance, Neuman (1982) views the holistic person as a dynamic composite of interrelationship among physiological, psychological, sociocultural, and developmental variables. The sociocultural variable could be interpreted to include the spiritual but the choice was made to identify it as a separate fifth variable. This was in keeping

TABLE 7-2. CHARACTERISTICS OF GRADUATES AND LEVEL OBJECTIVES

Characteristics of the Graduate	Level Objectives			
	I	II	III	IV
Incorporate ethical principles into nursing practice	Identify principles of ethical behavior related to self and society	Explain ethical responsibilities inherent in professional nursing	Apply ethical principles in the use of the nursing process with persons and families	Analyze ethical dilemmas in nursing based on the principles of ethical decision making
			Justify the importance of having an ethical framework for decision making in nursing	Demonstrate ethical decision making within the nursing profession
Combine creativity with a realistic, futuristic view of professional nursing	Explore own creative potential in problem solving	Consider a variety of alternatives in nursing practice	Apply creative approaches in nursing practice	Formulate creative strategies for change within nursing and the health care system based on an analysis of trends

with the mission statement of the three Christian liberal arts colleges and the commitment to viewing the client system as holistic.

Another illustration of how the model was individualized is reflected in the characterization of the role of the nurse. Neuman (1982) provides the framework for the description of the nurse as actor or intervenor who works in collaboration with the client to reduce the system's encounter with stressors or to strengthen the system's flexible line of defense. According to the MINC philosophy, the intervenor was further delineated as practicing in the roles of caregiver, collaborator, coordinator, consultant, advocate, educator, counselor, researcher, manager, and leader. In these and many other ways the Neuman Health-Care Systems Model allowed for the expansion of thinking and for the personalization of the framework without limiting creativity.

Throughout this entire endeavor, support for the development of the consortium and for curriculum planning was provided by the three colleges as well as private foundations. Teams comprised of one nursing chairperson with an academic dean of one of the other two colleges approached the executive officers of foundations, determined their interest in funding the project, and submitted grant proposals. The uniqueness of the plan, the cooperative approach, and the promise for the future prompted several foundations to support this effort. Monies obtained were used primarily for total faculty workshops, small group summer curriculum planning, and consultants.

Additional curriculum work that challenges the consortium faculty includes content mapping, course structure, and the formulation of an assessment tool. The recent experience of working cooperatively to build an undergraduate program gives assurance that these tasks will be accomplished. Options for creative ventures in education for the consortium remain an exciting possibility for the future.

The Neuman Health-Care Systems Model provided the organizational framework in the development of a future-oriented curriculum for the Minnesota Intercollegiate Nursing Consortium. It is a model for education as well as for professional nursing practice. The model provides a common language that facilitates understanding among health care professionals, stimulates research, and invites further development of theory.

REFERENCES

Eulau, H. (1969). *Micro-macro political analysis.* Chicago: Aldine.
Neuman, B. (1982). *The Neuman systems model.* East Norwalk, CT: Appleton-Century-Crofts.

ENDNOTES

Minnesota Intercollegiate Nursing Consortium: The College of St. Catherine, St. Paul; Gustavus Adolphus College, St. Peter; St. Olaf College, Northfield.

Steering committee members, Minnesota Intercollegiate Nursing Consortium: Marguerite Hessian, Chairperson, Department of Nursing, The College of St. Catherine; Mary Louise Krall, Gustavus Adolphus College; Jean Marie Martinson, The College of St. Catherine; Marilee Miller, Chairperson, Department of Nursing, Gustavus Adolphus College; Dorothy Mrkonich, Chairperson, Department of Nursing, St. Olaf College; Helen Schmitz, The College of St. Catherine; Valborg Tollefsrud, St. Olaf College; Devra Westover, St. Olaf College; Kay Wold, Gustavus Adolphus College.

Curriculum committee members, Minnesota Intercollegiate Nursing Consortium: Sally Harding, Gustavus Adolphus College; Marguerite Hessian, Chairperson, Department of Nursing, The College of St. Catherine; Carol Hocking, St. Olaf College; Jean Marie Martinson, The College of St. Catherine; Marilee Miller, Chairperson, Department of Nursing, Gustavus Adolphus College; Dorothy Mrkonich, Chairperson, Department of Nursing, St. Olaf College; Dee Reedy, The College of St. Catherine; Judi Sateren, St. Olaf College; Devra Westover, St. Olaf College; Kay Wold, Gustavus Adolphus College.

An Intervention to Reduce Anxiety Levels for Nurses Working with Long-Term Care Clients Using Neuman's Model

Margaret Louis

It is widely accepted that nurses working with clients requiring intensive care are under high stress and have resultant high anxiety levels. Experience and observation suggest that this is also true for nurses working with clients with long-term health problems particularly clients seen in rehabilitation units and those with chronic diseases.

The purpose of this study was to test the effect of short-term group meetings to reduce anxiety levels of the nurses working with clients with chronic or long-term health problems.

Conceptual Model

Neuman's Systems Model (1980, 1982) provided the framework for the intervention and hypotheses tested. Neuman describes three levels of nursing intervention: primary (preventative), secondary (acute response to stress), and tertiary (stabilized or rehabilitative). The intervention in this study was identified as primary or preventative, because all of the study's participants were registered nurses working full time who did not have any preidentified line-of-resistance responses.

Neuman's Systems Model (1980, 1982) proposes that individuals have lines of defense to resist stressors. These lines are further delimited as follows:

1. The flexible line of defense, which is dynamic rather than stable, can be altered over a relatively short period of time (for example, daily), and

can be controlled by the individual through such things as sufficient rest, balanced diet, and expression of feelings.

2. The normal line of defense, amounting to what a person has become over time, or his or her normal or steady state (life style, coping patterns).

These lines of defense are used to resist or repel stressors. However, if the stressor(s) penetrates the individual's lines of defense, a reaction occurs— symptoms of illness or disease. The flexible lines of resistance are identified as factors that attempt to stabilize and return the individual to the normal line of defense (as with body immobilization of white blood cells or activation of the immune response mechanism). The model provides guides to measuring response to stressors through assessment of the lines of defense and resistance. In this study, the lines were measured in the response to the intervention (mutual help group) to the stressor of work in clients with long-term health problems. The goal of the intervention in this study was to strengthen the flexible line of defense.

Intervention

Use of groups to deal with stress is not new. Self-help groups have been reported to be successful in dealing with many types of stressors. Studies reported since the early 1900s (Cartwright & Zander, 1968; Shaw, 1971) show group experiences have been used by people to deal with all sorts of stressors, including chronic illness, cancer, rape, work problems, divorce, and depression (Baker & McCoy, 1979; Campbell, 1986; Gallese & Treuting, 1981; Marram van Servellan & Dull, 1981; Trainor, 1981; Waller & Griffin, 1984). In addition, the use of group experiences has been demonstrated as being helpful in many situations including the work setting (Gaumont & Dworak, 1980; Oda, 1974).

The effect of a group on its members has been identified as (1) letting its members know they are cared for; (2) giving a place where members can feel they belong; (3) allowing members to express themselves without fear; and (4) receiving honest feedback in a safe environment (Marram, 1973). Through the group experience the individual can learn that his or her problems and concerns are not unique but shared, and a shared load is easier to carry.

Group membership is a natural phenomenon and with minimal intervention can become a successful therapeutic tool. A self-help group is a form of preventative intervention that attempts to reduce the possibilities of further emotional distress that may lead to pathology and necessary treatment (Newton, 1984). Because help is both received and given in these groups, "mutual help" group would be a more appropriate term to use.

With the substantiation of information from the literature, it was decided to implement a planned mutual help group experience and to assess its effect in reducing the anxiety level of the caregivers in response to the stresses of working with clients with chronic, long-term problems. For this study, *group* was defined as associations between two or more persons who were in some kind of interdependent relationship concerning behavior or perceptions. When people interact and communicate together, taking one another into account and modifying their own behavior in light of the behaviors of others, they belong to a group (Sampson & Marthas, 1981).

The intervention provided for an uninterrupted exchange, sharing of problems, and resolutions or support from the group. Problems of a personal nature, not related to the work situation, were purposefully not identified as a topic for discussion. However, in both groups personal problems were discussed by the participants.

Instruments

A problem with most conceptual frameworks is determining measures to use for empirical testing. For this study, using Neuman's model, a comparison of the definitions of the lines of defense to the definitions of the concepts measured by state-trait anxiety scales (SAS and TAS) (Spielberger, Gorsuch, & Luchene, 1970) and the self-rated anxiety status inventory (ASI) (Zung, 1971) suggests a direct relationship between the concepts measured by these instruments and the lines of defense and resistance of Neuman's model. A comparison of the definition of a flexible line of defense (factors that change on a short-term basis) to the SAS (reflection of how an individual feels at a particular moment in time) showed a very close relationship. A similar relationship was demonstrated between the normal line of defense (factors that are characteristic of the individual and are changeable over time) and TAS (indicator of how the individual feels in general). Zung identified the variable measured on the ASI as anxiety concerned specifically with a clinical disorder. It was determined that this score provided a measure of the line of resistance (the individual's attempt to stabilize and return to his or her normal line of defense). These relationships supported the use of the SAS, TAS, and ASI to measure the lines of defense and resistance.

Whenever signs or symptoms of disease or disruption could be observed, the model suggested that the lines of defense had been penetrated, with the line of resistance coming into action to protect the core of the individual. It was judged that the ASI scores would be within the normal range (score less than 45) when the subjects were identified as being in a primary prevention state, or having their lines of defense intact. It was determined that a decrease in the ASI score with the study group population could be interpreted as being a reflection of the strengthening of the lines of defense. If the intervention was seen as long-term, a change in the normal line of defense could be expected, resulting in a decrease in the TAS score. If, however, the intervention was seen as short-term, a decrease in the TAS score would not necessarily occur. If the intervention was working, a change in the flexible line of defense and an SAS score decrease could be expected. The model further suggested that a change in the flexible and normal lines of defense could be obtained without a similar change in the line of resistance if the stressor had not penetrated the lines of defense.

Research Hypotheses

Based on the model, the following research hypotheses were proposed:

1. Nurses participating in the mutual help group will have lower SAS scores after participating in the mutual help group experience.
2. TAS scores will not be different after participating in the mutual help group experience (intervention not strong enough to produce change).
3. For nurses participating in the mutual help group, a decrease in the ASI scores will be accompanied by a decrease in the SAS scores as compared to control group scores.
4. The nurses participating in the self-help group will have lower ASI scores than the nurses not participating in the group experience.

RESEARCH METHODOLOGY

Design

A nonrandomized, two-group pretest-posttest design was used in this study. The design provided control for most of the components of internal validity, but control of external validity was, of course, weak. To compensate for this, the study was repeated using two different groups of nurses working with long-term care clients.

Sample

One group of participants consisted of ten public health nurses whose client load included many individuals with long-term illnesses. The second group of participants had ten nurses who were working in a rehabilitation unit of a general hospital. Both groups had similarities in clients, with the exception that the public health group had hospice patients and the rehabilitation group had infrequent deaths of clients. Five nurses from each agency group were identified for the mutual help group experience and the other five nurses were identified to act as controls at each agency. This gave a total of ten nurses in one of the two group process intervention situations and ten different nurses acting as controls. It should be noted that Shaw's (1971) review of group research concluded that five is the ideal number for a group. He concluded that this size is large enough to allow participation by all and still provide variety of the participants.

Procedure

The intervention consisted of four 1-hour group meetings for the nurses in the public health department and another four 1-hour sessions for the nurses in the rehabilitation unit. The groups met once a week in a conference room at the respective agencies. One group attended on the agency's time and the other after regular work hours.

The groups were co-led by two registered nurses not employed by either agency. These nurses had taken a three-credit-hour course in group process and had studied and done work in change theory related to group leadership as part of their basic nursing education.

Meeting Format

The first 5 to 10 minutes of each meeting consisted of orientation of the participants to what they would be doing at that meeting. The next 35 to 45 minutes was used for discussion by the participants of their experiences and feelings in relation to the discussion area for that session. The last 10 to 15 minutes were used by the leader to summarize. Topics identified for discussion at the sessions were:

Week 1 Things I handle well; things I do not handle well.
Week 2 My most stressful experience in the recent past (the last week or so).
Week 3 Things about my work that make me feel good (positive attitude and feelings about my job).
Week 4 Discussion of the group sessions—likes, dislikes, benefits, feelings, and suggestions for future group sessions.

The pre- and postmeasures were administered at the beginning of the first session and at the end of the last session. Data for the control groups were collected during the first and last weeks of the group meetings at that agency.

FINDINGS

Analysis of the data indicated the reliability of the instruments with this population was of an acceptable level. The split-half *r* values ranges from 0.86 to 0.92 for the three instruments with this sample. Internal consistency (alpha) was identified as $r = 0.92$ or greater for the three scales.

The prescores for the two mutual help groups were not significantly different as analyzed by the independent t-test. This was also found for the two control groups of nurses. Therefore, the scores for the two intervention and two control groups were combined for the remaining analysis.

Hypothesis 1

Nurses participating in the mutual help group will have lower SAS scores after participating in the mutual help group experience.

The mean SAS score for the intervention group decreased significantly (Table 8-1). However, the mean post-SAS scores for the intervention group were not significantly different from the control group, which did not change significantly during the study period. An analysis of covariance (ANCOVA) controlling for the preintervention score differences did not elicit a significant difference between the two groups' postscores even though the intervention group did show a significant decrease in SAS scores. Consequently, the rejection of the null hypothesis should be accepted with caution.

Hypothesis 2

Trait Anxiety Scale scores will not be different after participating in the mutual help group experience (intervention not strong enough to produce change).

This hypothesis was supported because the mean TAS scores did not change significantly pre to post for either group of nurses (*see* Table 8-1).

Hypothesis 3

For nurses participating in the mutual help group, a decrease in the ASI scores will be accompanied by a decrease in the SAS scores as compared to control group scores.

The data did show a significant difference in both ASI and SAS scores for the intervention group (SAS, $t = 3.84$, $df = 7$, $p < 0.05$; ASI, $t = 3.89$, $df = 7$, $p < 0.05$). The control group did not reflect such a change. These findings support rejection of the null hypothesis.

Hypothesis 4

The nurses participating in the mutual help group will have lower ASI scores than nurses not participating in the group experience.

This hypothesis is supported, with the ANCOVA results of $F = 7.08$, 1, 1, 12, $p < 0.05$ when controlling for the pre-ASI scores (Table 8-2). The multiple R^2

TABLE 8–1. SUMMARY OF MEANS, SD, AND T-VALUES PRE-TO-POST-SCORES OF BOTH GROUPS

	Prescore			Postscore			
	Mean	*SD*	*N*	*Mean*	*SD*	*N*	*t Score*
Intervention Group							
State (SAS)	46.00	13.31	8	35.50	7.96	8	3.84*
Trait (TAS)	41.50	10.58	8	38.00	8.03	8	1.74
Anxiety status (ASI)	38.62	7.98	8	33.12	4.70	8	3.89*
Control Group							
State (SAS)	39.14	14.71	7	36.42	13.89	7	1.51
Trait (TAS)	34.00	9.64	7	36.57	6.80	7	−0.92
Anxiety status (ASI)	33.85	4.41	7	35.85	8.35	7	−1.08

*$p < 0.05$.

TABLE 8-2. SUMMARY TABLE OF ANCOVA FOR ANXIETY STATUS INVENTORY

	SS	df	MS	F	Prob
Covariate (preanxiety status)	236.79	1	236.79	12.39	0.004
Main effect (group sessions)	135.46	1	135.46	7.08	0.021
Explained	372.26	2	186.13	9.74	0.003
Residual	229.33	12	19.11		
Total	601.60	14	42.97		

Multiple R^2 = 0.619

was 0.619, supporting the appropriateness of the use of the covariate (*see* Table 8–2).

DISCUSSION

The data suggest that short-term low-intensity nurse lead group process experience is a tool nurses can use to improve their lines of defense and lines of resistance to stressors encountered while working with long-term care clients. This intervention is low in cost and relatively easy to institute. It does seem to be a viable way to help nurses deal with the stress they encounter while working with clients with long-term health problems. Additional support for the use of the intervention of mutual help group was supplied by the participants in their comments about the overall experience: "It helped me to increase my self-awareness," "I am more aware of the thoughts and feelings of other nurses," "I believe I am more responsive to my co-workers," "Overall, the experience was worthwhile, and I would recommend future groups to others." The comments are similar to other reported findings (Gaumont & Dworak, 1980; Knight, Waller, & Levy, 1980). These comments are supportive evidence that a group cohesion was formed during the study (Sampson & Marthas, 1977).

An informal follow-up was made of the participants after a 9-month period. The information obtained indicated the group intervention did work for the rehabilitation nurses during and for a period of time following the sessions. However, 9 months after the end of the group meetings, the conditions were identified as being much as they were prior to the group intervention. The public health group identified the group sessions as worthwhile and their work conditions as being much as they were at the end of the group intervention. A factor that must be considered with this group of nurses is that they also participated in a similar group experience for hospice work shortly after this study was completed. This information suggests a longer intervention may be needed to maintain a more lasting impact, or that nurses willing to continue the self-awareness process are better able to manage their work-related anxiety.

Limitations for this study include the small sample size and lack of random selection. Consequently, further study with other nurses in similar situations is recommended to validate these findings. Other recommendations for future study include longer follow-up of participants to determine if the change in lines of defense lasts beyond the group meeting and to determine if group sessions lasting longer than 4 weeks will impact differently on lines of defense.

The findings in this study support the predictions made based upon the Neuman Systems Model and the use of mutual help groups to aid nurses in dealing with stress related to working with clients with long-term problems. This support of Neuman's model is contrary to Ziemer's (1983) finding that the "model may be faulty and primary prevention may not increase resistance to stressors or lines of defense may not be important in reducing the penetration of stressors and development of symptoms (p. 286)." Comparison of these two studies shows stronger reliability for the instruments used in this study, which may have affected the findings. This study should be considered a test of only one area of a complex system (Neuman's model). More testing is needed to assess the validity of the Neuman model, because it is only through systematic planned testing of the models that data can be compiled to support or refute the validity of models for nursing assessment and intervention.

Acknowledgements to Nell Jacobs, BSN, RN, and Nona Schnieder, BSN, RN, for their assistance with the study.

REFERENCES

Baker, C. G., & McCoy, P. L. (1979). Group sessions as a method of reducing anxiety in patients with coronary disease. *Heart and Lung, 8*(3), 525–529.

Campbell, J. (1986). A survivor group for battered women. *Advances in Nursing Science, 8*(2), 13–20.

Cartwright, D., & Zander, A. (1968). *Group dynamics: Research and theory* (3rd ed.). New York: Harper & Row.

Gallese, L. E., & Treuting, E. G. (1981). Help for rape victims through group therapy. *Journal of Psychosocial Nursing and Mental Health Services, 19*(8), 20–21.

Gaumont, B., & Dworak, M. H. (1980). Group work with nurses. *Social Work Research, 5* (3), 76–77.

Knight, B., Wollert, R. W., Levy, L. H., et al. (1980). Self-help groups: The members' perspectives. *American Journal of Community Psychology, 8*(1), 53–56.

Marram, G. (1973). *The group approach in nursing practice* (2nd ed.). St. Louis: Mosby.

Marram, G., & Dull, L. V. (1981). Group therapy for depressed women: A model. *Journal of Psychosocial Nursing and Mental Health Services, 19*(8), 25–31.

Neuman, B. (1980). The Betty Neuman health-care systems model: A total person approach to patient problems. In J. P. Riehl & C. Roy (Eds.), *Conceptual models for nursing practice* (2nd ed.). East Norwalk, CT: Appleton-Century-Crofts.

Neuman, B. (1982). *Neuman Systems Model.* East Norwalk, CT: Appleton-Century-Crofts.

Newton, G. (1984). Self-help groups. *Journal of Psychosocial Nursing, 22*(7), 27–31.

Oda, D. S. (1974). Increasing role effectiveness of school nurses. *American Journal of Public Health, 64*(6), 591–595.

Sampson, E. E., & Marthas, M. (1981). *Group process for the health professions* (2nd ed.). New York: Wiley.

Shaw, M. E. (1971). *Group dynamics: The psychology of small group behaviors.* New York: McGraw-Hill.

Spielberger, C. D., Gorsuch, R. L., & Luchene, R. E. (1970). *STAI manual for the state-trait anxiety inventory.* Palo Alto: Consulting Psychologists Press.

Trainor, M. A. (1981). Acceptance of ostomy and the visitor role in a self-help group for ostomy patients. *Nursing Research, 31*(2), 102–106.

Waller, M., & Griffin, M. (1984). Group therapy for depressed elders. *Geriatric Nursing, 10,* 309–311.

Ziemer, M. M. (1983). Effects of information on postsurgical coping. *Nursing Research, 32,* 282–287.

Zung, W. K. (1971). A rating instrument for anxiety disorders. *Psychosomatics, 12,* 371–379.

The Roy Adaptation Model

Sister Callista Roy

The Roy Adaptation Model can be viewed primarily as a systems model, although it also contains interactionist levels of analysis. The person as patient is viewed as having parts or elements linked together in such a way that force on the linkages can be increased or decreased. Increased force, or tension, comes from strains within the system or from the environment that impinges on the system. The system of the person and his or her interaction with the environment are thus the units of analysis of nursing assessment, while manipulation of parts of the system or the environment is the mode of nursing intervention. The person has four subsystems: physiological needs, self-concept, role function, and interdependence. The self-concept and role function subsystems are seen as developing in an interactionist framework. Thus the interaction process is one of the elements to be assessed within the system. Likewise, one of the nurse's primary tools in manipulating elements of the system or the environment is his or her own or others' interaction with the patient. Within a systems model, therefore, interactionist concepts are relevant. They can be used in the explication of the Roy Adaptation Model.

The Roy model had its beginning in 1964, when the author was challenged to develop a conceptual model for nursing in a seminar with Dorothy E. Johnson at the University of California, Los Angeles. The adaptation concept, presented in a psychology class, had impressed the author as an appropriate conceptual framework for nursing. The work on adaptation by the physiological psychologist, Harry Helson, was added to the beginning concept and the model's present form began to take shape. In subsequent years the model was developed as a framework for nursing practice, research, and education. In 1968 work began on operationalizing the model in the baccalaureate nursing curriculum at Mount Saint Mary's College in Los Angeles. The first class of students to study with the model began their nursing major in the spring of 1970 and were graduated in June of 1972. Use of the model in nursing practice led to further clarification and refinement. In the summer of 1971 a pilot research study was conducted and in 1976 to 1977 a survey research study was done that led to some tentative confirmations of the model. Thus the Roy model

105

has been more fully developed and operationalized than some other models in spite of its relatively recent origin.

BASIC ASSUMPTIONS OF THE ROY ADAPTATION MODEL

An *assumption* is a statement accepted as true without proof. All models of nursing have certain underlying basic assumptions. Assumptions may be explicitly stated or they may be implied within the discussion of the model. The assumptions behind the Roy adaptation model are based on the model's approach to the concept of the person and to the process of adaptation. These assumptions are outlined and discussed in the following section.

Assumption One **The person is a bio-psycho-social being.**
This assumption states that the nature of the person includes a biologic component, such as anatomy and physiology. At the same time, the person consists of psychological and social components. Furthermore, the behavior of the individual is related to the behavior of others on a group level. Hence, methods of analysis of the person must come from the biological, psychological, and social sciences, and the person as a unified whole must be viewed from these perspectives.

Assumption Two **The person is in constant interaction with a changing environment.**
Daily experience supports this assumption. One need only cite the vicissitudes of the weather, or of traffic conditions, as examples. The person confronts constant physical, social, and psychological changes in the environment and is continually interacting with these.

Assumption Three **To cope with a changing world, the person uses both innate and acquired mechanisms, which are biological, psychological, and social in origin.**
At times learned or acquired mechanisms are used to cope with the changing world. For example, on a cool day one might wear a sweater, then remove it as the temperature warmed. Other mechanisms are innate. An example is the natural reaction of thirst in response to water loss through perspiration. Reiner (1968) discusses the chemical control systems of the organism as an adaptive device.

Assumption Four **Health and illness are one inevitable dimension of the person's life.**
This assumption states that each person is subject to the laws of health and illness. This dimension is therefore one aspect of the total life experience. The familiar greeting "How are you?" attests to the validity of this assumption.

Assumption Five **To respond positively to environmental changes, the person must adapt.**

Levine (1969) states that "a truly integrating system within the organism must be one that responds to environmental change (pp. 93–98)." She describes this process as adaptation. Thus a changing environment demands a positive response which, hopefully, is adaptive.

Assumption Six **Adaptation is a function of the stimulus a person is exposed to and his or her adaptation level.**

The person's adaptation level is determined by the combined effect of three classes of stimuli: (1) focal stimuli, or stimuli immediately confronting the person; (2) contextual stimuli, or all other stimuli present; and (3) residual stimuli, such as beliefs, attitudes, or traits, which have an indeterminate effect on the present situation.

   This assumption relies on the work of Helson (1964), whose systematic approach to behavior is assumed to be valid. Helson states that adaptation results from the response to a stimulus that stands in relation to the adaptation level. The strength of the confronting stimulus, the contextual or environmental stimuli, and other residual or nonspecific stimuli, go together to form an adaptation level. Thus, for example, the temperature outside, the humidity, and a person's previous experience with extreme temperatures all influence adaptation to changing temperatures.

Assumption Seven **The person's adaptation level is such that it comprises a zone indicating the range of stimulation that will lead to a positive response.**

If the stimulus is within the zone the person responds positively. However, if the stimulus is outside the zone, the person cannot make a positive response.

   This assumption, again based on Helson's theory, is illustrated in Figure 9–1. As noted in the example of assumption six, adaptation to environmental temperature depends on the temperature outside, the humidity, and a person's

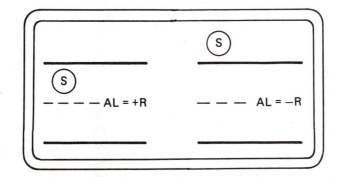

Figure 9–1. Process of adaptation.

previous experience with extreme temperatures. Thus a person raised in south-
ern California has a narrow range of adaptability to extreme temperatures
whereas someone raised in a high desert in New Mexico might have a much
wider range of adaptability. If both persons were exposed to the same high temperatures with the same humidity, the New Mexican might respond positively,
or adapt, whereas the Californian would respond negatively, or fail to adapt.

Assumption Eight **The person is conceptualized as having four
modes of adaptation: physiological needs, self-concept, role
function, and interdependence relations.**
Roy defines a mode as a way or method of doing or acting. Thus a mode of
adaptation is a way of adapting. Further, Roy assumes that the person has
various ways of adapting. Based on an initial survey of 500 samples of patient
behavior, Roy (1971) has tentatively identified four ways in which the person
adapts in health and illness.

First, the person adapts according to his or her physiological needs. The
previous examples about adaptation to temperature changes illustrate this
phenomenon.

Second, the person's self-concept is determined by interactions with
others. Outside stimuli cause the person to adapt according to his or her self-
concept. For example, when I switch from teaching to administration, my
concept of myself adjusts; I may no longer think of myself as a mild, unper-
turbed individual, but rather as someone who can respond quickly and even
vehemently.

Third, role function is the performance of duties based on given positions
within society. The way one performs these duties is constantly responsive to
outside stimulation. For example, the mother of a family constantly adapts her
mothering activity to the changing developmental needs of her children.

Finally, in relations with others, the person adapts according to a system of
interdependence. This system involves ways of seeking help, attention, and affection. Changes both inside and outside the person cause changes in this subsystem. As an example, when a person is separated from a loved one, his or her
mode of obtaining attention and affection is changed.

These eight assumptions about the person and the process of adapting are
basic to the Roy adaptation model of nursing.

ELEMENTS OF THE MODEL

Values

The elements of a practice-oriented model imply values and include goal,
patiency, source of difficulty, and intervention. To begin with, Dickoff and
James say that a model must specify values that indicate that its goal is desir-

able of attainment. Like assumptions, the worth of values is not proved but is believed to be true.

The Roy adaptation model implies four basic values which, taken together, point to the desirability of the model's goal content. The goal of the model will be discussed later. The basic values behind the goal can be summarized as follows:

1. Nursing's concern with the person as a total being in the areas of health and illness is a socially significant activity.
2. The nursing goal of supporting and promoting patient adaptation is important for patient welfare.
3. Promoting the process of adaptation is assumed to conserve patient energy; thus nursing makes an important contribution to the overall goal of the health team by making energy available for the healing process.
4. Nursing is unique because it focuses on the patient as a person adapting to those stimuli present as a result of his or her position on the health-illness continuum.

These values are not proven within the model, but are assumed to be truths that make the overall goal of nursing worthwhile.

Goal of Action

Perhaps the most important distinguishing characteristic of a specific nursing model is the way the specific model describes the goal of nursing activity. The Roy adaptation model describes the goal of nursing as the person's adaptation in the four adaptive modes.

All nursing activity will be aimed at promoting the person's adaptation in physiological needs, self-concept, role function, and relations of interdependence during health and illness. The criterion for judging when the goal has been reached is generally any positive response made by the recipient to the stimuli present that frees energy for responses to other stimuli. This criterion must be applied to each specific instance of nursing intervention for which a specific goal of adaptation has been set. For example, the patient may be confronted with the general stimulus of illness, and one necessary mode of adaptation is the role function. The relevant literature reveals particular behavior cues indicating when there has been positive assumption of the sick role (e.g., Martin & Prange, 1962). When patients are no longer fixated on the restrictions imposed on them but are able to take these in stride and to free their energies for other things, then adaptation regarding the sick role has occurred.

Patiency

A practice-oriented model must clearly describe who or what is the recipient of the activity. According to the Roy Adaptation Model, the patiency of nursing is described as the person as an adaptive system receiving stimuli from the environment inside and outside his or her zone of adaptation.

The person as a bio-psycho-social being in constant interaction with a changing environment has been discussed in conjunction with the assumptions of this model. Also, the process of adaptation and the person's four modes for adapting have been explored. At this time it should be pointed out that the recipient of nursing is the person in the dimension of his or her life related to health and illness. Thus the patient may be ill, or may be potentially ill and require preventive services. Also the patient may be adapting positively or not. If the patient is adapting, the nursing goal is to maintain that response. For example, when a public health nurse makes a postpartum visit and finds a new mother adapting positively to her changing role, the nurse aims to maintain this positive response. The person adapting in health and illness is the patiency of nursing care.

Source of Difficulty

The source of difficulty, the next element of the model, is described as the originating point of deviations from the desired state or condition. The current view of this deviation is implied in Figure 9–2. A need is a requirement in the individual that stimulates a response to maintain integrity. As internal and external environments change, the level of satiety for any need changes. When satiety changes, then a deficit or excess is created. This deficit or excess triggers off the appropriate adaptive mode. Within the modes are coping mechanisms whose activity is aimed at integrity. The manifestations of this activity are the

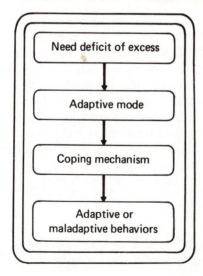

Figure 9-2. Source of difficulty.

adaptive or ineffective behaviors. The source of difficulty, then, is coping activity that is inadequate to maintain integrity in the face of a need deficit or excess.

Intervention

Intervention, as described earlier, includes both focus and mode. The intervention focus is the kind of problems found when deviations from the desired state occur. It describes the kinds of disturbances in the patiency that are to be prevented or treated. Roy has identified some commonly occurring adaptation problems in each of the adaptive modes. These can be thought of as a failure of coping mechanisms when excesses or deficits are present in the modes. Those currently identified are the following.

A. Basic physiological needs
  1. Exercise and rest
     Immobility
     Hyperactivity
     Fatigue and insomnia
  2. Nutrition
     Malnutrition
     Nausea and vomiting
  3. Elimination
     Retention and hyperexcretion
     Constipation and diarrhea
     Incontinence
  4. Fluid and electrolytes
     Dehydration
     Edema
     Electrolyte imbalance
  5. Oxygen
     Oxygen deficit
     Oxygen excess
  6. Circulation
     Shock
     Overload
  7. Regulation
     a. Temperature
        Fever
        Hypothermia
     b. Senses
        Sensory deprivation
        Sensory overload (pain)
     c. Endocrine system
        Endocrine imbalance

B. Self-concept
  1. Physical self
     Loss (e.g., depression following mastectomy)
  2. Personal self
     a. Moral-ethical-guilt (e.g., child with rheumatic fever blames illness on disobeying his mother)
     b. Self-consistency-anxiety (e.g., patient pacing the floor the night before surgery)
     c. Self-ideal and expectancy-powerlessness (e.g., teenager in traction unable to try out for varsity)
  3. Interpersonal self
     a. Social disengagement (e.g., elderly woman refuses to communicate with staff)
     b. Aggression (e.g., cardiac patient yells at nurse)
C. Role mastery
   Role failure—perceived inability to perform behaviors related to role (e.g., amputee: former truck driver concerned about supporting family)
   Role conflict—perceived expectations of others regarding role behavior differs from own expectations (e.g., wife with threatened abortion whose husband expects sexual relations)
D. Interdependence
   Alienation, rejection, aggression, rivalry, competitiveness, hostility, loneliness, disengagement, dominance, exhibition

The intervention mode is the major means of preventing or treating the problems identified in the intervention focus. It is the action that can be used to change the course of events toward the desired end product. In this model, it is what the nurse can do to promote patient adaptation. According to the Roy Adaptation Model, the nurse acts as an external regulatory force to modify stimuli affecting adaptation. The nurse's mode of intervention is to increase, decrease, or maintain stimulation. This mode of intervention takes place within the nursing process, a problem-solving approach to diagnosing patient problems and to planning, carrying out, and evaluating patient care.

Roy has developed a two-level assessment process. The first level includes the identification of patient behaviors in each of the adaptive modes and the recognition of the person's position on a health-illness continuum. This assessment can be carried out rapidly and utilizes both objective data and subjective reports from the patient. The nurse may read on the chart that the postoperative patient refused his breakfast tray, and the nurse may also hear the patient state that he is not hungry. For any behavior that the nurse is concerned about, either for purposes of reinforcement or modification, he or she begins a second level of assessment. In this the nurse looks for the focal, contextual, and residual factors influencing the behavior. For example, the nurse may question the patient further about his statement that he is not hungry and learn that the immediate cause for refusing the tray is that the patient is afraid of gas pains. But the nurse may also learn that the patient dislikes to eat in bed, a contextual factor. In addition, the patient lacks knowledge about return of peristalsis and about the effects of nutrition on healing. Finally, the diet may not be as well seasoned as the patient prefers. These conditions all would enter into a nursing assessment for possible intervention.

Based on the information from the assessment the nurse makes a diagnosis. This is either a summary label that connotes the nature of the problem (for example, one of the adaptation problems) or a statement of the relationship between the behavior and the impinging stimuli. Thus in our example the diagnosis might read, "Refused breakfast tray related to fear of gas pains."

At present, the Roy Adaptation Model is not sufficiently developed to include a typology of nursing interventions. Generally interventions are devised by the selection of influencing factors that can be manipulated. If possible, the focal stimulus is manipulated first, since it is the primary cause of the behavior. If this stimulus cannot be manipulated—as, for example, when the focal stimulus is a necessary but painful treatment— then the appropriate contextual or residual stimuli are manipulated. An example is the support given during treatment. In the situation we have been discussing the nurse might try to help the patient resolve his fear of gas pains by exploring this fear, and the basis for it, with the patient. The intervention focus thus is adaptation problems and the mode is the changing of stimuli through the process of assessment, diagnosis, planning, effecting, and evaluating nursing care.

SUMMARY

The Roy Adaptation Model has been developed as a nursing model and can thus be more easily analyzed according to the characteristics of models. However, this brief explanation of the model already points to the need for continuing development of many of its aspects. Some assumptions about the model should be validated—for example, the assumption that the person has four modes of adaptation. Assumed values, particularly the value concerning the uniqueness of nursing, need to be made more explicit, and perhaps should also be supported. The model's goal, patiency, source of difficulty, and intervention in terms of focus and mode are all replete with possibilities for further clarification. A particularly fruitful field for study is the patient's use of adaptive mechanisms and the nurse's support of these in each of the adaptive modes.

REFERENCES

Dickoff, J. & James, P. (1968). A theory of theories: A position paper. *Nursing Research*, *17*(3), 197.

Helson, H. (1964). *Adaptation level theory.* New York: Harper & Row.

Levine, M. E. (1969, January). The pursuit of wholeness. *American Journal of Nursing, 69*, 93–98.

Martin, H. W., & Prange, A. (1962). The stages of illness—psychological approach. *Nursing Outlook, 10*(30), 168.

Reiner, J. M. (1968). *The organism as an adaptive control system.* Englewood Cliffs, NJ: Prentice-Hall.

Roy, C. (1970). Adaptation: A conceptual framework for nursing. *Nursing Outlook, 18*(3), 42.

Roy, C. (1971). Adaptation: A basis for nursing practice. *Nursing Outlook, 19*(4), 254.

Roy, C. (1973). Adaptation: Implications for curriculum change. *Nursing Outlook, 21*(3), 163.

The Roy Adaptation Model
An Analysis

Cynthia Deibert Pioli
Janet Kwarta Sandor

Roy's model emerged when she was a graduate student in nursing and she was challenged by Dorothy E. Johnson to define nursing (Roy, 1980). Her response was that nursing promotes adaptation. This led to Roy's research of Helson's (1964) theory of adaptation level and the beginning of her conceptualization of the person as an adaptive system.

The Theory

An overview of Roy's model indicates that it is based upon Helson's (1964) concept of adaptation or the positive response to a continually changing environment. The three essential elements are the recipient of nursing care, the goal of nursing, and the nursing intervention. The recipient of nursing care, a patient or client, is synonymous with *person*, which is defined as a bio-psycho-social being with innate and acquired coping mechanisms. Nursing's goal is to promote adaptation or a positive response to changes within the internal and external environment. This can be accomplished when the nurse intervenes to assist the person in coping effectively with these changes (Duldt & Giffin, 1985; Roy, 1976a, 1984; Roy & Roberts, 1981).

These essentials will be further elaborated on as this chapter examines Roy's theory using Stevens' (1984) framework for internal and external evaluation.

Underlying Assumptions

Roy classifies her assumptions as scientific and philosophical. The scientific assumptions are those that relate to the systems theory and include the following:

115

1. The person is a bio-psycho-social being in constant interaction with a changing environment.
2. The person uses both innate and acquired mechanisms, which are biological, psychological, and sociological in origin, to cope with a changing world.
3. Health and illness are inevitable dimensions of the person's life.

A system is a set of parts connected to function as a whole for some purpose. Roy views the person as a system whose purpose is survival, growth, reproduction, and mastery—which are the goals of adaptation. The achievement of these goals promotes the integrity of the individual and thereby contributes to health.

The remaining scientific assumptions are those derived from Helson's Adaptation Level Theory (1964):

1. To respond positively to environmental changes, the person must adapt.
2. The person's adaptation is a function of the stimulus he or she is exposed to and his or her adaptation level.
3. The person's adaptation level is such that it comprises a zone indicating the range of stimulation that will lead to a positive response.
4. The person is conceptualized as having four modes of adaptation, which are physiological, self-concept, role function, and interdependence (Roy, 1980).

In 1984, Roy cited additional assumptions that were philosophical in nature and derived from humanism. As humanistic nurses, we believe in the person's own creative power and value their opinions and viewpoints, recognize the significance of interpersonal relationships, and see behavior as being purposeful and not as a mere chain of cause and effect.

Roy's scientific assumptions are explicit and provide the base from which her theory grows. Her philosophical assumptions have been added to enhance the holistic view of the person and to make the person more visible in the care process (Meleis, 1985).

INTERNAL EVALUATION

Commonplaces

Stevens (1984) identifies the commonplaces in Roy's theory as being values, goals of action, patiency of the recipient, and intervention. Using Stevens' own description of commonplaces, however, we see them as person, health, environment, nursing, and their interrelationships.

Person is defined as an adaptive system. He or she is a bio-psycho-social being in constant interaction with a changing environment. As a system, the person receives input from the environment, and along with feedback processes this information and responds as indicated by output. This outcome or output may consist of adaptive or ineffective responses (Fig. 10–1).

Roy has identified six subsystems within the person. The two internal processor mechanisms are the regulator and the cognator subsystems. The four effector subsystems or modes of adapting are physiological, self-concept, role function, and interdependence. The regulator is related primarily to the physiological mode and is the automatic response of the neural-chemical-endocrine systems within the body. The cognator is the mechanism of perception, information processing, learning, judgment, and emotion. Both the regulator and the cognator subsystems affect behavior in each of the four adaptive modes.

The concept of person can be expanded to include family, social organizations, and community.

Health is the state and the process of becoming integrated and whole. This concept is derived from person and environment. As an adaptive system each person is constantly growing and developing in a changing environment. Each person has the potential for becoming integrated and whole.

Environment is the most broadly defined concept, and includes all the conditions, circumstances, and influences surrounding and affecting the development and behavior of persons or groups. The environment may be internal or external, and is composed of all stimuli impinging upon the person at any given time. These factors which affect the person's ability to adapt are taken from Helson (1964) and consist of the focal or the immediate stimulus to which the person must respond, contextual or all other stimuli present, and residual stimuli or those that have an indeterminate effect on the situation.

Nursing is defined by Roy as being a science and a practice discipline. In either situation, it is the body of knowledge used to positively effect a person's health status. This is achieved through specific nursing activities, which distinguish nursing from other disciplines and are termed the nursing process. According to Roy, this process has six steps (Fig. 10–2). First, the nurse assesses the person receiving care in the four adaptive modes. This is a dual level assessment, which looks at behaviors and the factors or stimuli affecting these behaviors. A nursing diagnosis is formulated and goals set to promote a positive response or adaptation. The nurse then selects and carries out specific interventions that manipulate the stimuli to achieve these goals. Lastly, the nurse evaluates the effectiveness of the care given in relation to whether or not the goals have been attained (Andrews & Roy, 1986).

Nursing Domain

According to Stevens (1984), one of the domains used to classify a theory is that of intervention. In intervention theory, the nurse actively selects variables for manipulation in order to bring about a change in the present state of the individual. It is the nurse who decides which interventions apply in a particular

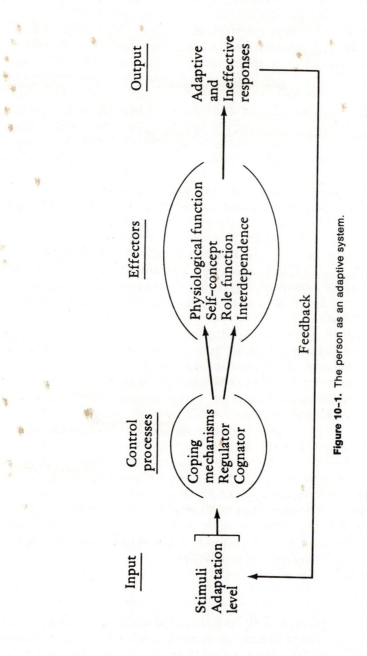

Figure 10-1. The person as an adaptive system.

Input

Stimuli
Adaptation
level

Control
processes

Coping
mechanisms
Regulator
Cognator

Effectors

Physiological function
Self-concept
Role function
Interdependence

Output

Adaptive
and
Ineffective
responses

Feedback

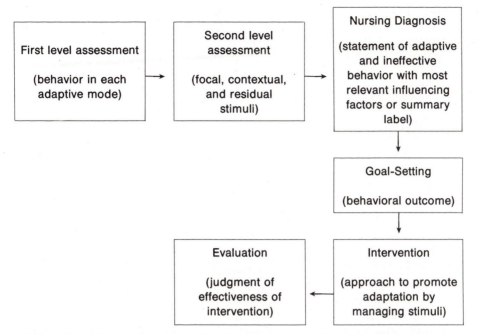

Figure 10-2. Roy's nursing process flowchart. (*Reproduced with permission from Roy, C.* [*1976a*]. Introduction to nursing: An Adaptation Model. *Englewood Cliffs, NJ: Prentice-Hall.*)

situation and who implements these interventions. Thus, action and decision making reside within the nurse. Once again, it is the nurse who manipulates the stimuli to promote an effective response. Therefore, Roy's model clearly falls within the domain of intervention theory.

Clarity

The underlying principles are identified and are clearly presented. The use of systems and adaptation theories are explained. The confusion lies within the interrelationships of the subsystems. For example, it is not made clear how the regulator and cognator mechanisms affect each other to bring about behavior in the four adaptive modes. Perception, as the key, has not been operationally defined. Roy's psychosocial modes of self-concept, role function, and interdependence do not have clear boundaries and tend to overlap. The concept of environment relative to internal and external stimuli is abstract and needs further clarification.

Consistency

Overall, Roy defines her terms consistently throughout her theory. There are a few exceptions. In her earliest writings, health is viewed as a position on a health-illness continuum (Roy, 1970, 1976a). Currently, health is defined as a state and a process of becoming integrated and whole (Andrews & Roy, 1986; Roy, 1984). The adaptive mode of role function was initially identified in the literature as role mastery (Roy, 1973). Mastery is now identified as one of the goals of adaptation with the others being survival, growth, and reproduction (Roy, 1984). The literature does not reflect the rationale for these changes.

Another inconsistency relates to patient participation in the care. Roy advocates that the person is the doer: "It is the client who does the adapting and his resources must therefore be used to cope with the situation (1976, p. 691)." In other words, it is the patient who ultimately must change. However, in the Roy model, this change would not take place without the nurse's assessment and intervention. It is the nurse who effects this change by identifying the problem and manipulating the stimuli. In reality, the patient remains the object of care with the nurse in control (Meleis, 1985).

The model is consistent with respect to principle interpretation and method. According to Stevens (1984), Roy uses a simple principle explaining person on the basis of stimulus, adaptation level, and response.

According to Stevens, interpretation is how the theorist perceives the world of nursing. Roy's theory is phenomenal in nature because it falls within the realm of human experience. More specifically, it would be considered essential in interpretation because the nursing phenomenon relates to the circumstances in which it occurs. The underlying reality is the patient's response to his or her environment at any given time. A person's behavior in the adaptive modes is influenced by the stimuli affecting the situation. Nursing is concerned with assessing behavior and stimuli and intervening to promote adaptation.

One of the limitations is the lack of a spiritual dimension to the definitions of Roy's person. The literature reflects person as being a bio-psycho-social being (Duldt & Giffin, 1985; Meleis, 1985; Roy, 1976a; Roy & Roberts, 1981). Humanistic assumptions have been added that could be considered transcendental. (Andrews & Roy, 1986; Roy, 1984). Generally speaking, these assumptions are philosophic in nature and have not been operationalized.

In evaluating Roy's model with respect to method, it is noted that Roy uses a logistic approach. Parts are used to organize the whole; relationship is added to relationship. Roy's view of person is logistic; she explains the person on the basis of four adaptive modes (physiological, self-concept, role function, and interdependence). These are further broken down into the subsystems of stimulus, adaptation level, and response.

When describing nursing, Roy switches to problematic language while continuing to use the logistic method. The inconsistency lies in what the nurse actually does and in what Roy says the nurse does. In Roy's model, the nurse is motivated by a clearly defined logistic method. She utilizes the nursing process—that is, she first assesses, identifies the problem, sets the goals, and then proceeds. In the true problem-solving approach, the problem is identified initially and then the nurse, as the problem solver, formulates and tests hypotheses until the problem is resolved. The major aim of problem solving is to eliminate the problem. On the other hand, nursing is goal directed with the aim being the achievement of one or more of the goals identified (Stevens, 1984).

Adequacy

The criterion of adequacy is met if the theory accounts for the subject matter with which it deals. The essential elements of Roy's theory, as previously discussed, are accounted for. The model is realistic and practical for nursing and is continually evolving in its development.

Logical Development

Roy's theory is logically developed and includes both deductive and inductive modes of reasoning (Blue et al., 1986). The deductive mode is predominate in that her scientific and philosophical assumptions are deduced from other disciplines, namely biology, psychology, and sociology.

Her conceptualization of person as having four adaptive modes is inductive and is derived from 500 samples of patient behaviors identified by Roy (1976a), her colleagues, and students in various practice settings.

Level of Theory Development

The level of Roy's theory development is explanatory and more specifically situation-producing—that is, it explains how the nurse can promote adaptation through the manipulation of stimuli. By reinforcing, reducing, or removing stimuli that affect a person's behavior, the nurse can change the person's adaptation level and elicit a positive response. This type of theory has the potential for being predictive based upon further development and testing.

EXTERNAL EVALUATION

Reality Convergence

For Stevens (1984), the criterion of reality convergence relates to the acceptance or rejection of a theory based upon the principle, interpretation, and method used. Although there are some inconsistencies, Roy's theory is generally acceptable in each of these areas.

Utility

The Roy Adaptation Model has been widely utilized in nursing practice, education, and administration, as documented in the literature (Blue et al., 1986; Meleis, 1985; Roy, 1973; Schmitz, 1980; Tiedeman, 1983). Practice areas include surgical, community, obstetric, pediatric, and geriatric settings. The intensive care setting proved to be the most difficult in which to implement the model due to the rapid changes in the patients' conditions. Roy's theory serves as the discipline model in many nursing programs in the United States, Canada, and abroad (Meleis, 1985). It has been operationalized successfully in nursing adminstration (Mastal, Hammond, & Roberts, 1982).

Roy's model evolved from her image of what nursing is; it was not developed from a research strategy. Much research has been done relative to the application of the model in various settings. However, with regard to the validation of the theory propositions and concepts, little research has been documented. Meleis (1985) notes that one of the reasons for this is the complexity of the propositions and their physiological perspective.

Significance

Essential issues in nursing are addressed. Roy's theory has contributed much nursing knowledge in the functional areas of practice, education, and administration (Blue et al., 1986; Meleis, 1985; Roy, 1973; Schmitz, 1980; Tiedeman, 1983). However, the theoretical propositions need to be further validated through empirical testing. The model does have research potential. More information is needed in regard to the regulator and cognator coping mechanisms and their relationship to each other. Roy's four adaptive modes tend to overlap and have not been supported with empirical evidence.

Capacity for Discrimination

Generally speaking, in Roy's model boundaries unique to nursing are not delineated. There is nothing identified that differentiates the nursing process, other than the terminology, from any similar problem-solving method used in other disciplines; that is, the steps of assessment, planning, intervention, and evaluation are not restricted to nursing. "The nursing process is no different than the medical process, the social work process, the school teaching process, and so forth (Stevens, 1984, p. 77)." Roy has attempted to differentiate her process by identifying six steps, which include the dual level assessment, nursing diagnosis, goal setting, intervention, and evaluation. However, Stevens' criteria for capacity for discrimination have not been met.

Scope

In reviewing the literature, Roy's theory has been cited as being both broad and limited in scope. Blue et al. (1986) state that Roy's theory is limited in scope because it primarily addresses the concept of person-environment adaptation. Schmidt (1981) agrees with this position. We find the theory to be broad in scope because it addresses numerous concepts from other disciplines as well as nursing. The theory has been applied in each of the functional areas of nursing and in a variety of settings. This view is similar to that expressed by Tiedeman (1983) and Meleis (1985).

Complexity

Roy's model is complex in that it deals with many concepts and the interrelationships between them. These relationships are not always clear, which adds to the complexity of the model. The nurse may find it difficult to integrate all the related concepts in each of the adaptive modes simultaneously in order to view the person as a unified whole.

SUMMARY

The Roy Adaptation Model has contributed to the science and practice of nursing as evidenced by its use in the functional areas of practice, education, and administration. The basic assumptions are clear and the concepts do generally reflect this. For Roy, nursing is concerned with the person's behavioral responses, which are affected by the internal and external environment. The nurse plays an active role in promoting effective responses or adaptation.

The inconsistencies noted lie mainly within the terminology and the definitions employed and do not alter the overall theory. The expanded views of person as an adaptive being with creative power, and of health as a state and a process of becoming whole and integrated, represent a few of the changes in Roy's model from its beginning approximately 20 years ago. The model is evolving theoretically and through practical application further development has occurred. With continued group and individual interpretation we believe that this theory can generate knowledge for nursing.

REFERENCES

Andrews, H., & Roy, C. (1986). *Essentials of the Roy Adaptation Model.* East Norwalk, CT: Appleton-Century-Crofts.

Blue, C., Brubaker, K., Papazian, K., & Riester, C. (1986). Sister Callistra Roy Adaptation Model. In A. Marriner (Ed.), *Nursing theorists and their work.* St. Louis: Mosby.

Duldt, B., & Giffin, K. (1985). *Theoretical perspectives for nursing.* Boston: Little, Brown.

Helson, H. (1964). *Adaptation-Level theory.* New York: Harper & Row.

Mastal, M., Hammond, H., & Roberts, M. (1982). Theory into hospital practice: A pilot implementation. *Journal of Nursing Administration, 12*(6), 9–15.

Meleis, A. (1985). *Theoretical nursing: Development and progress.* Philadelphia: Lippincott.

Roy, C. (1970). Adaptation: A conceptual framework for nursing. *Nursing Outlook, 18*(3), 42–45.

Roy, C. (1973). Adaptation: Implications for curriculum change. *Nursing Outlook, 21*(3), 163–168.

Roy, C. (1976a). *Introduction to nursing: An adaptation model.* Englewood Cliffs, NJ: Prentice-Hall.

Roy, C. (1976b). The Roy Adaptation Model: Comment. *Nursing Outlook, 24*(11), 690–691.

Roy, C. (1980). The Roy Adaptation Model. In J. P. Riehl & C. Roy (Eds.), *Conceptual models for nursing practice* (2nd ed.). East Norwalk, CT: Appleton-Century-Crofts.

Roy, C., & Roberts, S. (1981). *Theory construction in nursing: An adaptation model.* Englewood Cliffs, NJ: Prentice-Hall.

Roy, C. (1984). *Introduction to nursing: An adaptation model* (2nd ed.). Englewood Cliffs, NJ: Prentice-Hall.

Schmidt, C. (1981). Withdrawal behavior of schizophrenics: Application of Roy's model. *Journal of Psychosocial Nursing and Mental Health Services, 19*(11), 26–33.

Schmitz, M. (1980). The Roy Adaptation Model: Application in a community setting. In J.P. Riehl & C. Roy (Eds.), *Conceptual models for nursing practice* (2nd ed.). East Norwalk, CT: Appleton-Century-Crofts.

Stevens, B. (1984). *Nursing theory: Analysis, application, evaluation* (2nd ed.). Boston: Little, Brown.

Tiedeman, M. (1983). The Roy adaptation model. In J. Fitzpatrick & A. Whall, *Conceptual models of nursing—Analysis and application.* Bowie, MD: Brady.

11

Adaptation of the Roy Model in an Educational Setting

Andrea Mengel
Susan Sherman
Eileen Nahigian
Ivory Coleman

As is the case in many curriculum revisions, the impetus for curricular change at Community College of Philadelphia was an impending National League for Nursing (NLN) accreditation visit in 1978. All faculty members agreed that the existing curriculum lacked consistency and cohesiveness. Content was repeated in several courses and students had clinical laboratory experiences for two different nursing courses in each week. In addition, minimal coordination of content and student learning activities occurred among the faculty. Likewise, the total program of learning was not subject to rigorous faculty examination. One faculty member remarked that instead of a department of nursing with team teaching, we had a series of cottage industries where each teacher developed and taught her or his own course.

As a faculty, we agreed that a major curriculum revision was in order. After a year of development, the revised curriculum was implemented in the fall of 1978. In the ensuing years, we have experienced three periods: the period of excitement, the period of reorganization, and the period of acceptance. In the period of excitement we were naively overconfident that the revised curriculum would work. "Why doesn't it work?" was the theme of the reorganization period. During reorganization we began to make changes to meet our needs. Finally, in the period of acceptance, we discovered that with further adaptations, a curriculum based on the Roy (1970, 1973, 1976) model does meet our needs.

THE PERIOD OF EXCITEMENT

After deciding that a curriculum change was in order, the faculty discussed various options. Two faculty members were beginning their doctoral work in nursing and were interested in nursing conceptual models. Further, we had support from the administration to engage an NLN consultant for two days. After a mini-inservice by the two faculty members and discussions with the NLN consultant, the faculty selected the Roy model as a base for curriculum development. The Roy model was viewed as the most concrete, developed model and seemingly required only minor readjustments in our thinking. The philosophy, conceptual framework, goals, level objectives, and all course outlines were rewritten. The resulting curriculum was a thing of beauty: it was logical, clear, nursing-process oriented, and comprehensive. Each course outline adhered strictly to the Roy model. The curriculum was implemented only weeks before our NLN accreditation visit. The visitors commented on how easily the students had adapted to the model. Privately, we agreed that this was true but that the faculty was struggling. Our naive excitement was already being tempered by the realities of the major changes we had made.

This curriculum required alterations in the thinking of the faculty. Faculty members had learned nursing primarily by the disease-oriented medical model and had applied that model during prior teaching. We all believed we knew which content should be taught. Yet adaptation theory and a nursing process format required that we place less emphasis on medical diagnosis as we strengthened our presentation of nursing as a distinct entity. The faculty realized that in the prior curriculum, disproportionate hours had been allocated to content more aptly called "pathophysiology," but letting go of this content was difficult.

The initial solution was to develop two separate courses in each semester. The first course was a two-credit nursing science class dealing with behaviors (signs and symptoms exhibited by clients) of maladaptive states and the influencing factors (anatomy and physiology; pathophysiology; nutrition; and sociocultural, developmental, and pharmacological factors) that could be manipulated to promote adaptation. For some faculty members, identification of a nursing problem was pivotal in discussing behaviors and influencing factors. Other faculty members presented sets of behaviors and conceptual categories of influencing factors, arriving at a nursing problem identification secondarily.

The second course was a nursing theory course, which included a two-hour lecture, one-hour seminar, two-hour skills laboratory, and two consecutive six-hour clinical laboratory days each week. In the theory course, the nursing process was discussed for each of the problems identified in the nursing science course. This format was followed in the classroom and in the clinical laboratory. Some faculty members adapted to this format with relative ease because their graduate studies were organized in this manner. Others found it difficult to abandon the medical model.

The second, third, and fourth semesters had a nursing theory and a nursing science course. The first semester had only a nursing theory course. A nursing science course was not included in the first semester because the semester focused on health. Adaptive behaviors and influencing factors for each component of each mode were presented using the World Health Organization's (WHO) definition of health. Gradually, a philosophical shift in our definition of health occurred, which has resulted in the inclusion of a few health problems related to hospitalization, such as alteration in sleep patterns.

Specialty content such as maternity, pediatrics, and psychiatric nursing was integrated. This eliminated repetition of concepts applicable in many situations and enhanced team teaching by maximizing the contributions of specialty faculty in each classroom. Once concepts were presented by medical-surgical faculty, specialty faculty explained variations in application of the concepts within specialty settings.

Pediatric content was easily integrated into all components of Roy's modes. Maternity content was less easily integrated. Initially, maternity was taught in the first semester, which was the health semester. Logically, most maternity content fits well in a health semester. However, given the lack of nursing skills of beginning students and the need for a strong emphasis on nursing process in the first semester, we realized that maternity content was more than we could teach in this semester. We moved most of the maternity content to the second and third semesters, which deal with disruptions, but we continue to consider what maternity content is essential in an associate degree program. Responding to our marketplace and our graduates' needs, we eliminated an inpatient psychiatric nursing clinical laboratory experience and focused on the psychiatric and mental health needs of the patient in an acute care setting.

In the classroom and clinical laboratory, we used Roy's nursing care plan format. Students identified behaviors and labeled them as adaptive or maladaptive. Focal, contextual, and residual influencing stimuli were manipulated through nursing interventions to achieve goals. Nursing problems were categorized by Roy's components and modes.

As we implemented the curriculum, we encountered several disruptive factors, which precipitated modifications. The problems of faculty experiencing change was primary. Faculty interpretation of the conceptual model is essential to its effectiveness. Although change requires time, we were expecting faculty members to quickly alter their teaching styles. And although teaching styles are individual, we were requiring the faculty to use the nursing process to provide consistency throughout the curriculum.

Our revised curriculum was well-designed. As one of the first schools in our region to use Roy's conceptual model as a curriculum base, we were proud of our innovative spirit and open minds. Something was wrong, however, and evidence of discontentment began to grow.

THE PERIOD OF REORGANIZATION

Instead of representing a minor readjustment of our thinking, the revised curriculum required a major change in how we thought and what we did. Some of the faculty accepted that, as innovators, we would have to find our own way. Others found it frustrating to have few if any of the answers. Adding to this confusion and frustration was the model. Some parts of Roy's model were highly specified, especially the parts derived from sociological theory such as the role function mode; whereas some components of the physiological mode were underdeveloped. The interdependence mode was vague and the role of the nurse was unclear.

Recognizing our sincere struggle and good intentions, the administration funded 6 days of inservice training with nursing consultants who worked in the same educational setting as Roy. Yet we continued to have confusion, frustration, and discord. Why?

As a faculty, we were committed to a curriculum change which was still incomplete in 1980. We had designed an innovative curriculum which we expected a traditional faculty to implement. Some faculty members were excited, pleased, and adapting, while others were cautious, wary, and isolated. The curriculum change required restructuring the thinking of all 18 faculty members but after 2 years, only one half of the faculty was comfortable with the Roy model. The faculty reacted with puzzlement and a search for order. Discussions about whether an influencing factor was contextual or residual went on for what seemed like months. Philosophical debates over labeling client's behaviors as maladaptive ensued. Role function partitions were cumbersome.

Unplanned changes were also occurring. The head of the department of nursing resigned and a new department head who was familiar with Roger's conceptual framework was hired. Simultaneously a faculty member who had been one of the key leaders in curriculum development became ill and was unable to return to work. Four new faculty members were employed in the fall of 1980. Loyalties were disrupted and students, sensing disorder, expressed frustration and confusion.

Students complained that textbooks were not reflecting the terminology and framework of our curriculum. They could not use their textbooks to validate the approach to nursing required by the faculty. They complained about some of the faculty who were not using the model concisely and comfortably. Confusion about differences between medical and nursing diagnoses was endemic. Students had to use an idiosyncratic language and unfamiliar nursing process but were not receiving the support that they needed.

Moreover, affiliating agencies were not familiar with our language or model. Sometimes we felt that we were preparing students for tomorrow's world in a world of yesterday. During the clinical laboratory experience, students recognized this time lag and questioned whether the faculty were imposing a superfluous structure that hampered their ability to function.

Reactions from the staff at our affiliating agencies paralleled the reactions of some of our faculty, but staff resistance was manifested primarily by objection to the language of the model. During the period of reorganization, we developed a compromise language. *Influencing stimuli* became *influencing factors*, whereas *health* and *adaptation* were used interchangeably. When we agreed to use either the term *patient* or *client* depending on the agency's needs or wishes, staff resistance diminished and the staff began to compliment our students on their good nursing care plans.

When nursing diagnosis categories were well-developed at the national level, we substituted them for Roy's list of problems. This change facilitated the student's transition to employment and resulted in our students being viewed by themselves and others, as masters of the nursing process. Employer and graduate follow-up studies confirm this strength. For example, alumni report that they are being recruited to serve on nursing care planning committees at their places of employment.

Issues about content were not solved so easily. Although content was organized by mode and component in the curriculum revision, the faculty needed more direction and specificity to plan learning activities. Faculty members had to agree about what content would be taught in which semesters. We wrestled with these content questions endlessly. At lengthy curriculum committee meetings, the faculty debated how and what to teach. A circular process developed. What seemed to be understood and accepted at the end of one meeting stood for debate at a subsequent meeting. The nemesis of how to organize content remained. Should we follow a conceptual approach based on nursing diagnosis? Should we use common, well-defined health problems? The curriculum committee realized that all the faculty members needed to be involved in this decision.

After a full-day meeting of the entire faculty, we decided that we would use Roy's modes and components as an organizing framework for common well-defined health problems. For example, a unit of study is termed "The Client with Disruptions of Self-Concept." The unit outline lists common, well-defined health problems associated with self-concept disruptions. Lecture is presented in a nursing process format. For a diagnosis of "Alteration in Self-Concept Related to Ineffective Coping/Chemical Dependence," the faculty presents content related to ineffective coping and chemical dependence. The client's medical diagnosis is briefly discussed as an influencing factor. Nursing goals and interventions are developed based on current knowledge about ineffective coping and chemical dependence.

Changes in Roy's structure were made to meet our needs. The four modes were reduced to two: physiological and psychosocial. In our revision, the psychosocial mode has two components: self-concept and role function or interdependence. Collapsing the psychosocial modes simplified the structure and minimized the vague, artificial boundaries between role function and interdependence. Unquestionably, this has clarified the thinking of both faculty and students.

We found that faculty and students had difficulty labeling a client's behavior as *maladaptive.* Primarily for philosophical reasons, we now use the term *disrupted behavior,* which conveys fewer negative connotations and value judgments. Also, we found that categorizing stimuli as focal, contextual, or residual had little clinical significance, so we eliminated these categories. Students list all influencing factors, but do not use Roy's categories to sort them. Because of the nature of our clinical settings, we manipulate the influencing factors needing immediate attention and, when dealing with the role function or interdependence mode, focus only on the sick role.

During the period of reorganization, we learned that analysis and synthesis of content is facilitated by faculty members who explain relationships to students, who help them organize content, and who translate the medical model found in clinical practice to Roy's conceptual model. Our growth during this period culminated in abandonment of the view that nursing process functioned to compartmentalize information and acceptance of nursing process as a way to describe relationships among pieces of information.

THE PERIOD OF ACCEPTANCE

By 1983, content was stabilized and most of the faculty was comfortable. Faculty members were able to direct their energies to other important parts of the curriculum, such as strengthening the skills laboratory. When asked to identify inservice needs, the faculty named test construction and clinical teaching rather than further development of the Roy model. The curriculum committee was empowered to review and make recommendations on all content changes, and their meetings have become the hub of the program. Students commented positively on faculty expertise in content areas and on the collegial nature of faculty interactions. Students, graduates, and employers commended the program for its nursing process orientation.

Several factors external to our adaptation of the Roy model facilitated our movement through the first two stages to the period of acceptance. Increasingly, textbooks are organized by a nursing process format. *Nursing diagnosis* and other once-idiosyncratic language is now common terminology, so students find reinforcement in textbooks and in health care agencies. Further, the head of the department of nursing and other college administrators provided quiet, patient support for the faculty. Because few faculty members have resigned in recent years, we have established group cohesion and met individual development needs such as an extended orientation and mentoring program for new faculty members. All of these factors have contributed to our success.

CONCLUSION

Curriculum innovation is a trial and error process. Curriculum change can occur as a slow, evolutionary process or as a "big bang" transformation. We experienced both. The "big bang" transformation in 1978 was well-developed, logical, and a very pure implementation of Roy's conceptual model. But it did not work. It was met with resistance by faculty, students, and staff in our affiliating agencies. We persisted and as we used the Roy model we realized that we needed to adapt the model to meet our needs. A period of defining our needs and adjusting the model resulted in a successful reorganization. Movement through the reorganization process was slow, tedious, and disorienting. However, the curriculum that resulted from this evolutionary process responds to the requirements of practice settings, capitalizes on the strengths of our program, and provides students with an excellent knowledge base for clinical practice.

The primary goal of a curriculum or a conceptual model is facilitation of nursing practice. Each is useful only if it contributes to this goal. Neither should be adhered to because of tradition, principle, or loyalty. After a period of use, both evolve to meet the needs of those served. Our evolution was influenced by observations in practice settings, structured surveys of alumni, and discussions among faculty and students. We feel that we are firmly grounded in the period of acceptance because an NLN accreditation visit is scheduled for the near future and the faculty is not suggesting further curriculum revision!

REFERENCES

Roy, C. (1970). Adaptation: A conceptual framework for nursing. *Nursing Outlook, 18*(3), 42–45.

Roy, C. (1973). Adaptation: Implications for curriculum change. *Nursing Outlook, 21*(3), 163–168.

Roy, C. (Ed.). (1976). Introduction to nursing: An adaptation model. Englewood Cliffs, NJ: Prentice-Hall.

12

Implementation of the Roy Adaptation Model
An Application of Educational Change Research

Heather A. Andrews

Although there has been an increasing commitment on the part of nurse educators to base nursing education programs on one conceptual description of nursing, problems have been encountered. In some educational situations where the application of a nursing model has been attempted, the full potential of implementation has not been fully realized: difficulty in the isolation of major concepts and their relationships has occurred; there has been dwindling application of the model at subsequent levels of the program, especially if the course development has taken place over a number of years; and some faculty members, although initially committed to the use of the model, have had difficulty in applying it in their clinical settings. In addition, the significance of and support for the use of the model may not be recognized or understood by new faculty members. Thus, the commitment to the use of the model as a conceptual basis for the program is eroded.

Introducing a change into an educational setting always poses special problems and those just identified are not peculiar to nursing education. The literature pertaining to educational change in settings other than nursing attests to the fact that, wherever change occurs, problems must be overcome.

Arising from the literature on educational change, and of particular applicability for the situation just described, are a number of factors that have been identified as affecting the implementation of a change in an educational setting. The purpose of this chapter is to explore the applicability of these selected factors to a nursing situation—in particular, to the implementation of a nursing model as the conceptual framework for a nursing program. Initial discussion will focus on the implications of curricular use of a nursing model. Secondly, following a brief reference to one perspective on the change process, selected factors affecting educational change will be explored and applied to the process of implementing a nursing model as the conceptual basis for an educational program. Illustration will be provided of the manner in which one educational program proceeded with the implementation of the Roy Adaptation Model.

CONCEPTUAL MODELS AND THE NURSING CURRICULUM

Historically, nursing education programs have been plagued by such problems as lack of direction, unnecessary repetition of content, diversity of approaches to the study of nursing, and seeming irrelevance of support courses. In an effort to irradicate these concerns, there has been an increasing commitment by nurse educators to base educational curricula on one nursing model.

Nursing models, as conceptual descriptions of nursing, provide clear statements of what nursing is and the service it renders. The major parts of nursing (the person, the environment, health, and nursing activities) are described and their relationships to one another are specified (Roy, 1984).

The use of a nursing model as an organizing framework for a nursing curriculum accomplishes several goals. It facilitates the delineation of nursing knowledge and helps differentiate important and inconsequential material (Bevis, 1982); functions unique to professional nursing practice can be isolated. Core concepts can be identified and their presentation to students made progressive. This provides clear direction to each curricular level through the formulation of specific and progressive objectives. In addition, direction is provided for the selection of support courses through such aspects of the model as its theoretical basis and the skills inherent in its application. Thus, continuity and consistency within and among curricular levels are achieved and evaluation of student progress is facilitated.

According to Chater's (1975) conceptual framework for curriculum development, it is the nursing model that provides direction for the "subject component" of the curriculum framework. Each aspect of the curriculum must align with and reflect the nursing model if the full potential of implementation is to be realized. The nursing model must reflect the philosophy of the nursing program and the beliefs of faculty. It may either be developed by the faculty members or selected from models available in the nursing literature; however, the advantages associated with the choice of a published model relate to the degree of sophistication achieved by public application of that nursing model and the resulting human and literary resources.

Implementation of a nursing model as the conceptual basis for a nursing program represents a significant commitment and change for the nursing faculty; the complexity of such an undertaking must not be underestimated. Any factors that may facilitate the process should be considered. The theory and research pertaining to educational change offers some suggestions that may assist nurses in overcoming the problems associated with the process of implementing a nursing model in the curriculum. Before exploration of some of these factors is undertaken, however, a brief overview of one perspective of change will help to anchor the discussion in a body of theory and research.

OVERVIEW OF THE CHANGE PROCESS

Although detailed analysis of the stages involved in change is beyond the scope of this chapter, some background regarding conceptualizations of the process facilitates understanding of the factors affecting it.

Descriptions of the change process evident in the literature pertaining to educational and organizational change vary in specificity. Arising from the Rand Corporation Change Agent studies[1] as reported by Berman and McLaughlin (1976) was the identification of a three-stage change process that has become commonly accepted in the literature relating to educational change. The stages are (1) the initiation phase, consisting of processes leading up to and including the decision to proceed with a change; (2) the implementation phase, defined as the point at which the change is incorporated into practice; and (3) the incorporation phase, representing the extent to which the different practice becomes part of the ongoing activities and is thus maintained. Selected literature originating from the Rand Corporation Change Agent studies has been the major source of the factors influencing change as discussed here.

FACTORS INFLUENCING THE CHANGE PROCESS

Approaches to discussion of the factors affecting change in education vary in focus. Some authors, such as Berman and McLaughlin (1976), highlight categories of factors, whereas others focus on the phases and stages of change and the factors viewed as peculiar to each. However the factors are segregated, it is obvious that there is much overlap and interrelation; it appears that any division is arbitrary and aimed at ease of presentation.

The approach for discussion of factors influencing change assumed in this chapter contends that, although a few factors may influence one stage of the change process exclusively, most ultimately affect the process and the resulting innovation as a whole. Therefore, the factors will not be designated as applying to one particular phase unless the research cited has focused on a specific segment of the process.

Five major categories of factors influencing change in education have been identified for description and illustration: institutional motivation, project implementation strategies, institutional leadership, teacher characteristics, and staff and administrative turnover. As each factor is addressed, the findings of relevant educational research will be reported. To illustrate the relevance of each factor to a nursing education situation, the experience of one nursing program and its implementation of the Roy Adaptation Model as the conceptual basis for the program will be explored.

Institutional Motivation

Institutional motivation constitutes the receptivity of the institutional setting in terms of interest, commitment, and support (McLaughlin & Marsh, 1978). The change agent studies suggested that a major element of motivation, teacher commitment, was influenced by the motivation of upper-level managers, project planning strategies, and the scope of the proposed project.

Motivation of Managers

The motivation and commitment of upper-level managers, a factor identified by McLaughlin and Marsh (1978) relating to institutional motivation, provided signals to teachers in the change agent studies as to how seriously the project should be taken. Teachers then gauged their behavior accordingly. Administrative personnel provide indications of their commitment to change initiatives in a number of ways. Attendance and involvement in planning activities, the energy invested in obtaining additional resources for the project, and the priority given to the project were but a few indications of this commitment.

It was evident at the outset of the curriculum revision project that the administrative personnel at the school of nursing were supportive of and enthusiastic about the implementation of a nursing model as the conceptual basis for the program. In fact, it was at the director's initiative that the project was undertaken. Through ingenious planning, it was possible for the director to appoint a steering committee with two full-time members to oversee the process of the curricular revision and to release faculty members from their instructional responsibilities to participate for periods of time in course development activities. In addition, funds were made available for special educational initiatives related to the curriculum revision. Each of these actions, in addition to many more, provided an indication to faculty members that the project was of utmost importance.

Project Planning Strategies

As was demonstrated in the change projects studied by McLaughlin and Marsh (1978), collaborative planning was necessary for both short- and long-term success of a change initiative. Active engagement of faculty and administrators in all phases of the project was an important ingredient.

Collaborative planning was a significant aspect of the change initiative in the school of nursing. Faculty members were consistently and deeply involved with decision making throughout the project. For example, all faculty members participated in the identification and exploration of the nursing models that represented feasible conceptual options. By exploring various models and arriving at a consensus, all faculty members experienced the process involved in identifying the most appropriate model for their specific program. Through a democratic process, commitment to the implementation of the Roy Adaptation Model as the conceptual basis for the nursing program was obtained.

Scope of the Proposed Project

Contrary to early thinking regarding factors affecting success of an innovative project, the change agent studies demonstrated that the more effort required by teachers, and the greater the overall change in teaching style, the higher the proportion of commitment to the project (McLaughlin & Marsh, 1978).

The implementation of a nursing model in an educational program serves not only as an organizing framework for the nursing curriculum; there must also be evidence that faculty members are committed to the use of the nursing model in their instruction situations. This constitutes a great challenge and change for most faculty members.

Faculty members, as project planning progressed, began to recognize the implications of the implementation of the Roy model in their instructional situations. No longer would it be appropriate to present the steps of the nursing process as they had traditionally understood them; the six-step nursing process as described by Roy (1984) would become the framework for nursing care plans, clinical conferences, and classroom instruction. Through such major adjustments, the members of the faculty believed that consistency and continuity in the presentation of nursing concepts would facilitate and enhance the educational experience for the students. They were convinced that, although the changes were extensive, the product would be worthwhile.

Although factors associated with institutional motivation such as those presented above were identified in the change agent studies as a necessary condition for success of an educational change project, McLaughlin (1976) cautioned that they were not a sufficient condition. The next category of factors to be explored introduces a second category for consideration—project implementation strategies.

Project Implementation Strategies

Project implementation strategies are defined as those activities fostering staff learning and change. McLaughlin and Marsh (1978) reported that two variables—staff-training activities and training-support activities—accounted for a substantial portion of the variation in project success and continuation in the change agent studies. Other project implementation factors demonstrating a major impact on implementation were goal specificity, conceptual clarity, and local materials development.

Staff-Training Activities

Staff-training activities involve skill-specific activities—that is, instruction in how to carry out the innovation. Alone, these activities influenced outcomes only in the short run.

Staff-training activities in the curriculum revision project varied as the implementation project progressed. Initially, it was important to access information on the implications of using a nursing model as a conceptual basis for the program and how this task could be accomplished. Secondly, it was necessary to obtain input about the nursing models that represented potential choices as conceptual bases for an educational program of the type being offered. Once the choice of the Roy model had been made, it was necessary to receive specific instruction on the use of the Roy model and its implementation. On a number of occasions, individuals viewed as nursing experts were brought in to provide input and instruction relative to the topics described earlier to the faculty as a whole and to the nursing practice personnel who were part of the revision project. Each of these activities assisted faculty members in the curriculum development processes involved in the change initiative.

Throughout the implementation of the Roy model, staff-training activities focused on application of the concepts inherent in the model in the provision of nursing care. In addition to exploration of the basic concepts, the opportunity to apply the information in a patient care situation was provided. Frequently, this activity would focus on one of the four adaptive modes. As skill in the use of the model was achieved, more complex situations involving problems in two or more modes would be introduced.

Involvement of each faculty member in course development also assisted with skill development. The process of relating the Roy model to various content areas facilitated personal incorporation of model-specific concepts into nursing practice.

Training-Support Activities

Training-support activities such as classroom assistance by resource personnel, project meetings, and participative decision making, demonstrated a major positive effect on longer-term project outcomes.

Throughout the curriculum revision project, regular meetings involving all faculty members served to communicate the progress being made. Participative decision making was viewed as an important factor in achieving faculty commitment to the new program, and regular curriculum development meetings provided the means by which this could be achieved. Input from the faculty was consistently sought while the steering committee took the responsibility and leadership for generating specific plans of action for faculty consideration and decisions and for maintaining the momentum of the curricular revision activities. For example, it was the faculty as a whole that generated design features for the new program, after which the steering committee developed design options. The final selection as to which option provided the most appropriate sequencing of courses for the new program was made by faculty members. It was the faculty that identified the advantages of presenting the psychosocial mode to the students at the outset of their program. McLaughlin and Marsh (1978) explained the importance of teacher participation in decision making; not only were teachers in a better position to identify problems and make recommendations, but participative decision making enhanced the development of a "sense of ownership" of the innovation.

Once the revised program was operating, curriculum coordinators and experienced instructors were available to provide assistance for less experienced faculty members in their particular instructional areas. A number of faculty members found that they needed assistance in the application of the Roy model in their instructional situation. More experienced faculty members could relate readily to the problem and their assistance facilitated the process of achieving competence in the application of the model.

Goal Specificity

Two particular facets of goal specificity are relevant to an implementation project such as that being described. The first pertains to the goals related to the project itself: What will the new program look like? What is to be accomplished at what point in time? What elements must each course contain? Questions such as these can be addressed by meticulous planning activities. In the curriculum revision project, as each course development team began the task of design and research involved in the designated content area, specific goals related to the content of course outlines, application of the Roy model, and the time lines associated with the task were presented.

A strategic time line also assisted in achieving goal specificity. Target dates were established for each segment of the curriculum development process and deadline dates were adhered to. Throughout the process, the faculty was aware of the progress being made towards the final curricular product.

The second facet relates to the competencies expected of a graduate of the program. In this respect, terminal objectives were developed by faculty members to describe specific behaviors that would be necessary for successful completion of the nursing program. Reflected in these terminal objectives were the concepts inherent in the Roy model. Consider the following terminal objective:

> The graduate will be able to assess patient behavior and all relevant influencing factors by utilizing observational, interviewing, and measurement skills.

The fact that assessment of behavior and influencing factors is specifically addressed identified the first two steps of Roy's six-step nursing process. The subsequent objectives address the remaining four steps: nursing diagnosis, goal setting, intervention, and evaluation. Thus, each participant in the change process was provided with a clear perception of the competencies of a graduate from the program.

Conceptual Clarity

Conceptual clarity relative to the understanding of the essential elements of a nursing model is a particular challenge and of great importance if the conceptualization is to be effective in its application. Any nursing model represents complex conceptual interrelationships related to the practice of nursing. It was recognized that conceptual clarity was imperative if a successful implementation of the Roy model was to be achieved.

Initially, it was recognized that the members of the steering committee required thorough familiarization and working knowledge of the model before they could knowledgeably and effectively guide faculty members in the curriculum process. To accomplish this understanding, detailed study was undertaken by the four committee members.

Roy's (1976) definitive work was studied as was all accessible published material related to the model. Division of tasks among committee members permitted one person to gain a thorough understanding of one aspect of the model and subsequently share this knowledge with the other committee members. Study of the four adaptive modes was accomplished in this manner. Throughout the process, committee members began to identify the utility of diagrams to demonstrate relationships in the model, thereby facilitating its conceptual understanding.

Bloom (1956) has suggested that the achievement of understanding of such concepts may be facilitated by their translation into briefer terms or symbols. Although it was not the initial intent of the steering committee, in their achievement of personal competence in the use of the Roy model a diagrammatic conceptualization (a simplification) of the model was developed (Fig. 12–1).

Roy's conceptualization of the person as an adaptive system could be simplified as illustrated by the central circle in Figure 12–1. Stimuli from the internal and external environment and adaptation level act as inputs to this system, activating coping mechanisms (the controls of the system), and resulting in behavior as output of the system. By adding peripheral circles representing adaption to this diagram, it was possible to designate adaptive and ineffective behaviors as arrows remaining within the adaptation circle and arrows extending beyond the circle. Four overlapping circles designating the physiological, self-concept, role function, and interdependence modes were introduced within the adaptation circles to indicate that behaviors could be observed relative to each of the modes.

It was also possible to illustrate the six steps of Roy's nursing process (the outer circle). By aligning the stimuli and behavior arrows appropriately, it became possible to demonstrate how each step in the nursing process relates to specific aspects of the person. For example, the first step of the nursing process involves assessment of the person's behavior. According to the diagram, this step is next to a behavior arrow.

Clarity and utility of this diagrammatic conceptualization has been ratified in a number of respects. When the diagram was initially presented to faculty members, all felt that it clearly portrayed the Roy model. The conceptualization is one tool that has achieved interest from nurses outside the organization: it has been used by other nursing programs and has been implemented by Andrews and Roy (1986) in a text addressing the essential elements of the Roy Adaptation Model.

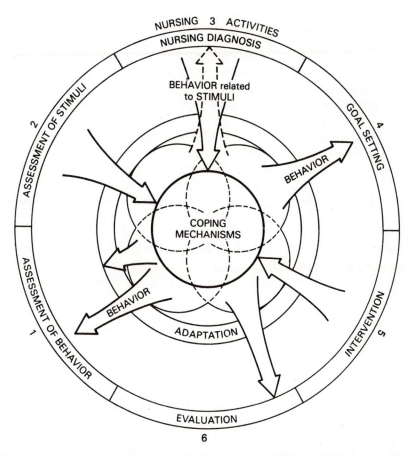

Figure 12-1. Diagrammatic conceptualization of the Roy Adaptation Model. (*Reproduced with permission from Andrews, H. A., & Roy, C. [1986]. Essentials of the Roy Adaptation Model. Norwalk, CT: Appleton & Lange.*)

Not only did the diagrammatic conceptualization prove invaluable at the time of the curriculum revision project in assisting faculty members to achieve familiarity with the concepts associated with the model, it facilitated implementation in other ways. It served to clarify for the beginning student and nurses unfamiliar with the model the interrelationships of the concepts described in the model and to assist in the identification of core concepts for the purposes of curriculum development; it became the tool through which focus on the nursing model was maintained throughout the curriculum planning process.

Since the inception of the Roy model at the school of nursing, the diagrammatic conceptualization has been used as an orientation tool for students in diploma, baccalaureate, and graduate level programs; new faculty members; and others not familiar with the model, including nursing practice personnel in clinical agencies.

Local Material Development

Another planning strategy identified during the change agent studies and closely associated with the affective perspective of teacher attitudes was local material development. As McLaughlin (1976) pointed out, such activity created a sense of involvement and the opportunity to learn by doing. It broke down the traditional isolation of the teacher and provided participants with a sense of professionalism and cooperation.

As has been mentioned earlier, faculty members were actively involved in the curricular implementation of the Roy model. During the development of courses, faculty members, in turn, served on course development teams related to their areas of interest and expertise. The details of subsequent application of the model—including the development of lectures, assignments, teaching aids, and examinations in the respective instructional areas—became the responsibility of each instructor.

Although project implementation strategies played an important role in both short- and long-term success of change initiatives, they did not complete the picture. Institutional leadership had a significant contribution to make.

Institutional Leadership

The change agent studies, as reported by McLaughlin and Marsh (1978), demonstrated that different administrative personnel affect the change process differently. Whereas an effective project director enhanced the implementation of the innovation, the support and interest of central office staff and the support and involvement of the principal enhanced continuation of the project. Supportive school climate was also an important influence on continuation.

Effectiveness of Project Director

The change agent studies identified the effectiveness of the project director, as perceived by the teachers, as having an important but short-term and circumscribed effect on project implementation.

In the curriculum revision project being described, the project director, as such, consisted of a team of four individuals—the director of the program, the assistant director, and two faculty members who had been released from their instructional responsibilities to serve in a full-time capacity as curriculum developers. The general objective of this steering committee was to "initiate and coordinate curriculum development activities and to direct and provide for continuity and integration in the design of the curriculum." Specific committee objectives were also derived.

The committee was very effective in its functioning; each member contributed a unique set of capabilities and strengths. It was viewed as a credible team by the faculty members and , as a result, performed an effective role in the direction and coordination of activities related to the curriculum revision.

An initial step taken by the committee members was the achievement of a working knowledge and competence in application of the Roy model. This enabled committee members to share their knowledge in assisting faculty members in their individual pursuit of competence in clinical application of the model; they were viewed by faculty members as an important resource in relation to interpretation and application of the model.

Although the effect of the project director was determined in the change agent studies to be an important influence on the implementation process, it was a factor that appeared to have only a short-term and circumscribed role. There was no demonstrated relationship with continuation or teacher change.

Central Office Staff

One institutional leadership factor that did enhance continuation of the change projects was the support and interest of central office staff. The support demonstrated by these individuals served to convey to the teachers the commitment of the "decision makers" to the change initiative.

The concept of "central office staff" as it relates to nursing education is somewhat different than that applying to public education; however, some similarities exist.

In the curriculum revision situation being described, the controlling institution (the body through which educational funding was channeled) was a large active treatment hospital in an urban setting. Approval for the revision project was obtained from this body. In addition, the accreditation body for the school of nursing was required to evaluate the proposed revision with the objective of granting approval for the project to be carried out. Both bodies were enthusiastic and supportive of the project. The controlling institution was required to demonstrate its support financially, because enrollment in the nursing program was cut back during the implementation phase and some revisions to staffing patterns were required as the curriculum was being developed and when the new program was implemented. It was possible, on occasion, for some of these "central office personnel" to be involved in curriculum development activities such as total faculty meetings and workshops. Further commitment to the project was evidenced by the participation of selected individuals from the clinical agency in many of the curriculum development activities. Not only was the commitment of the controlling agency evident, the participation of nursing service personnel provided a liaison between education and practice that would have otherwise been missing.

Principal Support

Principal support was another leadership factor identified in the change agent studies that was positively related to project continuation. In the case of the school of nursing, the director occupied this role. In this curriculum revision project, the vision of the new program can be attributed to the director; she was very involved in and supportive of the project from its inception. Evidence of this tangible support has been provided in the previous discussion.

School Climate

Another important influence on the continuation of the project was identified in the change agent studies (McLaughlin & Marsh, 1978) as being school climate. Good working relationships among teachers enhanced implementation and promoted continuation. Particular factors that comprised this supportive school climate were participation, a supportive organizational environment, and a strategy of teacher participation in the project development.

The impression should not be given that this curriculum revision project was without conflict and problems at some points in time. The demands placed on faculty members during a project such as this type of curriculum revision represents a significant investment of time, energy, patience, and cooperation. At times, all of these run in short supply. The important consideration is that differences of opinion be permitted—even encouraged—so that points of view can be considered, evaluated, and a decision as to the best way to proceed can be made.

A number of factors contributed to a positive school climate in this situation, some of which have been identified in previous discussion. Provision was made for participation of faculty members throughout the process, decisions were achieved through democratic procedures, efforts were made to compensate for additional time faculty members were investing in their particular developmental responsibilities, and consideration was given to particular areas of expertise and interest when developmental assignments were being made. Much of the credit for these arrangements rests with the administrative ingenuity of the director.

Another factor that boosted school climate was the opportunity on several occasions to have Sister Callista Roy visit the school for purposes of meeting with the faculty and providing input regarding the Roy Adaptation Model. The opportunity to become acquainted with the developer of the selected nursing model and to witness her enthusiasm about the project contributed to the faculty's sense of purpose relative to the project.

Teacher Characteristics

The fourth and final category of factors influencing the change process arising out of the change agent studies relates to characteristics of the teachers involved in the project.

McLaughlin and Marsh (1978) reported a number of interesting findings related to teacher characteristics and their effect on the process of change. Years of experience, verbal ability, and "sense of efficacy" were three important variables related to teacher characteristics that appeared to influence change project outcomes.

Years of Experience

An interesting relationship was observed in the change agent studies relative to teachers' years of experience: the number of years of experience was negatively related to all dependent variables except continuation of the change, where no relationship was observed; older teachers appeared to be less willing to change.

In the curriculum revision project being addressed, there were a number of teachers who demonstrated difficulty in integrating the Roy Adaptation Model into their instruction practice, but the relationship of variables such as age to this phenomenon is unclear and does not appear to be consistent. Without further research, it is not possible to make a statement regarding years of experience of nursing instructors and their tendencies to personally adopt and integrate a nursing model into their practice. The observation has been made, however, that it is much easier for a beginning student to become comfortable in the use of a nursing model, because the model is the student's initial contact with nursing-related concepts. For the experienced faculty member, this is a more difficult process. The new model represents a change in thinking; customary nursing practice must be aligned with a new vocabulary and possibly a new method of processing nursing information. This process has been equated with learning a new language—a task that is never easy.

Verbal Ability
A second factor related to teacher characteristics has been identified as the verbal ability of the teacher. This factor was significantly related to total improvement in student performance.

It is recognized that the ability to communicate the concepts inherent in the model is an important factor in student perception of the utility of the model as the framework for their nursing care. Students are very aware of the extent to which the instructor integrates the concepts in practice and instruction. In a research project recently completed (Andrews, 1987), it was noted that those instructors who are able to clearly articulate the concepts in the Roy model and how these influence the manner in which they teach students in the classroom and clinical setting are more likely to be implementing the nursing model in practice, as opposed to those instructors who are vague and nebulous in their description of the model. The latter group does not appear to be using the model in their interactions with students.

Sense of Efficacy
The factor that McLaughlin and Marsh (1978) labeled "sense of efficacy" demonstrated a strong positive relationship to all project outcomes. Teachers' attitudes of professional competence and the belief that the innovation would enhance student learning proved to be a major influence on teacher support of the project. This finding was observed by Leithwood and MacDonald (1981) as well. Their research on curriculum choices of teachers uncovered the importance of providing convincing evidence of student interest and learning. Teachers were attracted to the changes they perceived as likely to enhance student achievement.

As mentioned earlier in the chapter, there is increasing commitment on the part of nurse educators to base nursing education programs on one conceptual description of nursing. Nursing models have been regarded as a factor that can assist in the elimination of educational concerns related to curricular problems such as lack of direction, unnecessary repetition of content, diversity of approaches to the study of nursing, and seeming irrelevance of support courses. Through the framework provided by the nursing model, the presentation of nursing knowledge can be progressive; evaluation of students is facilitated. Continuity and consistency within the nursing program is achieved. The decision to adopt a nursing model is thus based on the perception on the part of faculty members and supported in the nursing literature that student learning will be enhanced.

The effect of the adoption of a nursing model as the conceptual basis for a nursing program on student achievement is yet to be determined. An internal, unpublished follow-up study involving graduates from both the "old" and the "new" Roy-based nursing program was done in 1986, but the results of the study were inconclusive due to the presence of a number of extraneous variables.

Staff and Administrative Turnover

One factor not yet mentioned but very important to all phases of the change process was identified by Fullan (1982)—staff and administrative turnover. The attrition of experienced personnel and the subsequent introduction of inexperienced and "unsocialized" faculty members represents a special challenge, particularly in relation to maintaining a change such as the implementation of a nursing model as the conceptual basis for a curriculum.

This factor was identified as an important concern relative to the integration of the Roy Adaptation Model in the new curriculum. A number of interventions were designed to assist in the maintenance of this curricular emphasis. Initially, commitment to the use of the Roy model is obtained from prospective faculty members before they are considered for a position at the school of nursing. Once hired, new faculty members undergo extensive orientation that focuses on the Roy Adaptation Model and the manner in which it has been integrated into the nursing program. Expectations regarding the use of the model in the instructional situation are explicated. In addition, "buddying" of new faculty members with experienced personnel assists with the integration of the new framework into personal practice. Finally, in an encompassing effort to emphasize the importance of application of the model throughout the curriculum, evaluations of each faculty member address the effectiveness with which the model is applied in instructional responsibilities.

The fact that personnel are continuously being introduced to an innovative program, even though the project may have been institutionalized for an extensive period of time, points to the continuity of the change process; it is nonlinear and never-ending. Factors that at one point in time enhanced the implementation of the innovation cannot be neglected once it is in place. They must become an integral part of the day-to-day functioning of the organization.

SUMMARY

This identification and illustration of factors influencing the implementation of change in education is not intended to be exhaustive; there are many other considerations that have not fallen within the scope of this categorization. This chapter has addressed some factors related to the categories of institutional leadership, teacher characteristics, and staff and administrative turnover. A very important consideration in the assessment of educational change not addressed in this chapter is the degree of implementation of the innovation and the effect of that factor on continuation and student performance.

It was not the intent of this chapter to suggest that the findings of the change agents studies are generalizable to nursing education; nor was it the intent to suggest that these are the only factors that influence the change process. Rather, this was an attempt to explore some research findings from a related discipline as a potential framework for investigation of a change initiative in nursing. The extent of generalizability will be evident only as replicative research is undertaken in nursing.

ENDNOTES

1. The Rand Corporation Change Agent studies of the mid-1970s were sponsored by the United States Office of Education to study federal programs supporting educational change. The conceptual model, methodology, and results of the first year of the study are reported in four volumes: *A Model of Education Change* (R-1589/I-HEW); *Factors Affecting Change Agent Projects* (R-1589/2-HEW); *The Process of Change* (R-1589/3-HEW); and *The Finding in Review* (R-1589/4-HEW).

REFERENCES

Andrews, H. A. (1987). The Roy Adaptation Model and its curricular application: An implementation study. Dissertation.

Andrews, H. A., & Roy, S. C. (1986). *Essentials of the Roy Adaptation Model.* East Norwalk, CT: Appleton-Century-Crofts.

Berman, F., & McLaughlin, M. W. (1976). Implementation of educational innovation. *Educational Forum, 40*(3), 345–370.

Bevis, E. M. (1982). Curriculum building in nursing: A process. St. Louis: Mosby.

Bloom, B. S. (Ed.). (1956). *Taxomony of educational objectives: The classification of educational goals. Handbook I—*Cognitive domain. New York: David McKay.

Chater, S. S. (1975). A conceptual framework for curriculum development. *Nursing Outlook, 32,* 428–433.

Fullan, M. (1982). *The meaning of educational change.* Toronto: Ontario Institute for Studies in Education.

Leithwood, K. A., & MacDonald, R. A. (1981). Reasons given by teachers for their curriculum choices. *Canadian Journal of Education, 6*(2), 103–116.

McLaughlin, M. W. (1976). Implementation as mutual adaptation: Change in classroom organization. In W. Williams & R. F. Elmore (Eds.), *Social program implementation.* New York: Academic Press, pp. 167–180.

McLaughlin, M. W., & Marsh, D. D. (1978). Staff development and school change. *Teachers College Record, 80,* 69–94.

Roy, C. (1976). *Introduction to nursing: An Adaptation Model.* (1st ed.). Englewood Cliffs, NJ: Prentice-Hall.

Roy, C. (1984). *Introduction to nursing: An Adaptation Model* (2nd ed.). Englewood Cliffs, NJ: Prentice-Hall.

King's General Systems Framework and Theory

Imogene M. King

Several individuals have published their own perceptions of my conceptual framework and my theory. The problem with each critique is that it is just that, one individual's perception. The critiques have tended to "lump" the conceptual framework and theory into something called a conceptual model. This tends to blur the differences between a framework and a theory. Some have implied that my theory is the process of interactions that lead to transactions, and this presents only one aspect of the theory. The critiques failed to identify differences between my conceptual framework, my theory, and a model of transactions.

Multiple telephone calls and letters from graduate students have indicated that some of the publications about theory generally and some of the critiques specifically have confused the scientific movement in nursing and my theory, and I agree with them. Each publication makes some contribution and at the same time adds to the confusion about the nature of theory and its primary purpose. The primary purpose of theory is to generate hypotheses or research questions, to design studies to test the hypotheses and answer the questions, and to produce knowledge that describes, explains, and predicts events in nursing.

This chapter was written to provide some clarification of the nature of my conceptual framework, my theory, and my model of transactions as the process component of the theory. An update is given on progress related to the use of my theory and conceptual framework in nursing education, nursing practice, and nursing research.

KING'S CONCEPTUAL FRAMEWORK

My conceptual framework is a general systems framework (King, 1971). General systems theory is defined as a "complex of elements standing in interaction (Von Bertalanffy, 1956, p. 33)." In the past, science reduced phenomena to small elementary units for the purpose of studying the parts of the phenomena. Recently, scientists have been concerned with the "wholeness" of phenomena. Wholeness deals "with problems of organization, phenomena not resolvable into local events, dynamic interactions manifest in the difference of behavior of parts when isolated, i.e., systems of various orders not understandable by investigation of their respective parts in isolation (Von Bertalanffy, 1968, p. 37)." Von Bertalanffy noted that "general system theory, therefore, is a general science of 'wholeness' which up till now was considered a vague, hazy, and semimetaphysical concept. In elaborate form it would be a logico-mathematical discipline, in itself purely formal but applicable to the various empirical sciences (p. 37)." General systems theory was created for sciences concerned with "organized wholes."

When I was studying systems research in the late 1960s, this movement in general systems theory provided information for me to think about the complexities and variability in the field of nursing. I know of no other discipline that deals with knowledge that is so vitally essential in the empirical world of application to practice as the knowledge we expect nurses to have for decision making for immediate action in many situations. If one analyzes the knowledge required for nurses to function in the complex world of practice, that knowledge is composed of concepts in every discipline in higher education. This is what motivated me to identify those concepts in other disciplines that give nurses specific knowledge that is applied in real world situations. This was done by using a technique called *content analysis*, whereby nursing literature and textbooks were analyzed for terms that were used consistently. From this analysis, a list of concepts was derived. A reconceptualization of the initial long list of words provided the concepts for my framework.

Because the focus of nursing is human beings interacting with their environment, nursing is conceived to be an open system. Open systems have several distinguishing characteristics. One characteristic is that the system has a goal. Systems exhibit other characteristics such as structure, functions, resources, and decision making. My conceptual framework has these characteristics. The goal for nursing is health. This means that nurses are concerned with the health of individuals and groups which make up a society. In designing my framework the following questions were formulated:

1. What kind of decisions are nurses required to make in the course of their roles and responsibilities?
2. What kind of information is essential for them to make decisions?
3. What are the alternatives in nursing situations?
4. What alternative courses of action do nurses have in making critical decisions about another individual's care, recovery, and health?
5. What skills do nurses now perform, and what knowledge is essential for nurses to make decisions about alternatives? (King, 1971, pp. 19–20)

My conclusion from responses to these questions was that nurses work with individuals who come from families and reside in a community. The result of the analysis of literature and thinking about the world of nursing practice was the design of my conceptual framework shown in Figure 13-1. Nursing phenomena are organized within three dynamic interacting systems: (1) personal systems (individuals); (2) interpersonal systems (dyads, triads, and small and large groups); and (3) social systems (family, school, industry, social organizations, and health care delivery systems).

My conceptual framework provided structure for nursing as a discipline and as a profession. It is so comprehensive that multiple theories may be generated from it. This framework helps one organize a multitude of facts into a system of wholes (King, 1986, pp. 75-76). The facts from the concrete world provide the ingredients for one's concepts. Concepts represent one's knowledge. Concepts are the organizing components of the framework. From my long initial list of concepts mentioned earlier, those shown in Table 13-1 were selected as essential to provide basic knowledge from many fields of study that is relevant for nurses.

The concepts are so interrelated in the interactions of human beings with their environment that the placement within each of the three systems is an arbitrary decision. It offers one approach to place primary emphasis on specific concepts essential for learning about the self as an individual and about other individuals. As you view the concepts, you can identify the multiple disciplines

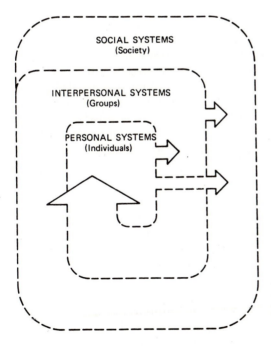

Figure 13-1. A general systems conceptual framework: dynamic interacting systems. (*Reproduced with permission from King, I.M. [1981]. A theory for nursing. New York: Wiley, p. 11.*)

TABLE 13–1. SELECTED CONCEPTS IN THE SYSTEMS FRAMEWORK

Focus	=	Person	Environment	
Goal	=	Health, a functional state		
Systems	=	Personal	Interpersonal	Social
Major concepts	=	Perception	Interaction	Organization
Subconcepts	=	Body image	Communication	Decision making
		Self	Stress	Power
		Learning	Role	Authority
		Time	Transaction	Control
		Space		Status
		Growth and development		
Nursing	=	Person	Environment	Health

Reproduced with permission from King, I.M. (1986). Curriculum and instruction in nursing. East Norwalk, CT: Appleton-Century-Crofts, p. 79.

from which they have been selected and studied. The knowledge we have used from other disciplines over the years is available for all to use. The question to be asked in nursing is "how do we put this all together from a nursing perspective?" Since nurses work in a world of "organized complexities" of great variability, how do we develop a curriculum to help students learn the essential knowledge and skills to use in the empirical world? The focus is on individuals whose interactions in groups within social systems influence behavior within the systems.

Because systems have goals, the goal of my conceptual system for nursing is health. Nurses help individuals attain and maintain their health, and if there is some disturbance such as illness or disability, nurses' actions are goal directed to help individuals regain health or live with a chronic illness or a disability. This idea implies that health is a dynamic state of an individual in which change is constant and an ongoing process. This explanation of health rejects a linear continuum of wellness-illness. Concepts have been identified as essential knowledge for nurses and the dynamic interacting systems with these concepts provide a way of organizing one's knowledge, skills, and values.

Concepts

The concepts have been identified that cut across all three systems and are interrelated. This demonstrates a characteristic of a general systems framework. The concepts identified here have been defined conceptually from analysis of studies related to the term (King, 1981). A few ideas are presented here as a demonstration of interrelationships.

Perception is a comprehensive concept in personal systems. Perception varies from one individual to another because each human being has different backgrounds of knowledge, skills, abilities, needs, values, and goals. Knowledge of perception is essential for nurses to understand self and to understand other individuals, such as a patient in a hospital and a family or group with a health problem. Perceptions of nurses and patients influence their interactions. Assessment of the perceptions of patients will help nurses understand a patient's point of view and will facilitate planning for care. Perception is a characteristic of a human process of interaction, and along with communication provides a channel for passage of information from one person to another. Concepts of self, growth and development, learning, body image, time, and space also relate to individuals as personal systems.

Interaction is a comprehensive concept in interpersonal systems. Knowledge of interaction is essential for nurses to understand a fundamental process for gathering information about human beings. Purposeful interactions lead to transactions. Related concepts are communication, transactions, role, and stress. However, knowledge of the concepts identified in personal systems is also used to understand interactions.

Organization is a comprehensive concept in social systems. Knowledge of organization is essential for nurses to understand the variety of social systems within which individuals grow and develop. Related concepts are power, authority, status, decision making, and control. All the concepts from personal and interpersonal systems provide knowledge for use within social systems. These concepts provide essential knowledge for nurses to understand human beings and their interactions with their environment.

Knowledge of the concepts of the general systems framework is applied in nursing through the interaction-transaction process model in King's theory. The process in this framework is defined as a "dynamic interpersonal process in which nurse and patient are viewed as a system with each affecting the behavior of the other and both being influenced by the factors within the situation (Daubenmire & King, 1973, p. 513)." This definition provides a theoretical basis for the nursing process as a method (Yura & Walsh, 1988) whereby nurses assess, plan, implement, and evaluate nursing care.

The conceptual framework is a system of processes which include processes of perception, communication, purposeful interactions, information, and decision-making. Specific skills are inherent in these processes. King defined nursing as a "process of action, reaction, and interaction whereby nurse and client share information about their perceptions in a nursing situation. Through purposeful communication they identify specific goals, problems or concerns. They explore means to achieve a goal and agree to means to the goal (1981, p. 2)." In viewing this process as a system, nurses collect data that include nurse variables, patient or client variables, and situational variables. Skills in observation and measurement are essential in using this process in nursing situations.

Purpose of a Conceptual Framework

The purpose of the general systems framework described here is to organize comprehensive concepts that cut across disciplines and give students substantive knowledge for use in nursing situations. My framework has served this overall purpose. This framework may be used to generate theories for nursing and for any discipline in higher education, and for any profession in which human beings are the focus of study or of practice. Knowledge is similar but the way each professional group uses knowledge is different.

USE OF KING'S CONCEPTUAL FRAMEWORK

The general systems framework explained in this chapter has been used in curriculum development, in organizing the delivery of nursing services in hospitals and health care agencies, and in developing a theory for nursing. Several faculty groups have used the dynamic, interacting systems framework to develop a curriculum leading to a baccalaureate degree, a master's degree, and an associate degree. One hospital program in Canada has used the framework to develop a curriculum.

The concepts identified in each of the three systems, shown in Table 13-1, provide substantive knowledge throughout the courses in the program. Some of the concepts help faculty members identify skills such as communication, perception, interaction, growth, and development. Some concepts help faculty members identify values. The development of a concept of self by students helps them begin to understand self as a human being, and then to translate knowledge of human beings to the concept of role as a professional nurse. The concepts in this framework provide a unique approach to curriculum development (King, 1986). One advances one's knowledge at each level of the educational program.

One of the ways this framework helps nurses in hospitals and community health agencies is that it gives a focus for the delivery of nursing services to individuals within families. Individual nurses have reported the use of the goal-oriented nursing record (GONR) to document nursing care related to goals for each client (King, 1984). The GONR is an information system that, if implemented, demonstrates a way to document nursing care and to measure the effectiveness of care.

The value of viewing nursing within this general systems framework is a special way of looking at phenomena—holistically, yet with a specific focus based on the situation. This general systems framework was developed prior to formulating my theory for nursing.

KING'S THEORY FOR NURSING

The nature of nursing can be described in many ways by many individuals. My theory for nursing was derived from my conceptual framework. The focus for the theory was on the interpersonal systems, because I believe that it is what we do with and for individuals in the role of nurse that makes the difference between nursing and any other health profession. This does not discount knowledge from other sciences as essential, but this does focus on holism—that is, the total human being's interactions with another total human being in a specific situation. The goal for nursing has been identified as helping individuals maintain a state of health. Although the primary point of interest in the theory relates to interpersonal systems of an individual in the role of caregiver and an individual in the role of recipient of care, the goals to be attained relate to the individual receiving the care. The care is provided in a health care system within society or in the home of an individual.

The theory of goal attainment is a general systems theory because it displays the characteristics of general systems, such as goal(s), structure, functions, resources, and decision making. The goal of the theory is health. Health, as a construct, is related to individuals and their health, to groups and their health, and to society and health.

The structure of the theory indicates some semipermeable boundaries of two or more individuals interacting in a health care system for a purpose that leads to goal attainment. This shows elements in interaction connected by communication links and this describes a general systems theory.

Functions of the theory relate to its usefulness. The theory has been used to generate hypotheses that have been and are being tested in research. It has been used as a guide to help individuals organize the delivery of nursing services in health care systems. The theory has been used in curriculum development, for teaching in higher education, and with undergraduate and graduate students to plan, implement, and evaluate nursing care, and it has been used by individuals in their practice. These are a few of the functions of this specific theory which, generally speaking, assists individuals to organize a multitude of facts into meaningful wholes.

Material and human resources are essential in open systems. The human resources in this theory relate to individuals and groups. The material resources are the things, objects, and technology that assist individuals to function in their world. This may include money, goods, and services.

Decision making is an essential characteristic in an open system. In this theory of goal attainment, decision making is a shared collaborative process in which client and nurse give information to each other, identify goals, and explore means to attain goals; each moves forward to attain goals. This is identified in the theory as a critical independent variable called *mutual goal setting*. This is a process variable.

The process of interaction that leads to transaction has been formulated in a descriptive study (King, 1981, p. 150). Transaction cannot be defined in and of itself but is defined when the six elements in the interaction are present as described in a model of transactions (King, 1981, p. 156). The transaction model operationalizes one major concept in the theory. This involves other concepts in the theory as well, such as perception, communication, self and role, stress, growth and development, and time and space. These concepts are interrelated in every nursing situation. The next time the reader is functioning in the role of nurse and interacting with a patient in the hospital or a person in the home, he or she is challenged to test these out informally.

All of the concepts of the theory have been conceptually defined (King, 1981). Only the concept of transaction has been operationally defined thus far (King, 1981, pp. 150–151). The operational definition of transaction with its classification system and model may be used in designing studies, in teaching students, and in nursing practice. The concept of transaction defines a process whereas the theory defines outcomes in the form of goals to be attained. One applies the knowledge of the concepts in practice, one does not apply the theory because the theory is abstract and one cannot apply an abstraction. When the relationships among the concepts have been identified and tested in research, the knowledge from the research may be applied in practice. Austin and Champion (1983) have identified some relationships among the concepts of my theory, as shown in Figure 13-2. When one uses knowledge of the concepts of this theory with the primary focus on interpersonal systems, one must recognize and use knowledge of the concepts of personal and interpersonal systems.

SUMMARY

My approach to the organization of a general systems framework for nursing was to review the empirical world of nursing. This resulted in the identification of the conceptual model shown in Figure 13-1, which shows three levels of abstraction called personal systems, interpersonal systems, and social systems, in dynamic interaction. Concepts that cut across disciplines in higher education were selected following analysis of nursing research literature and books.

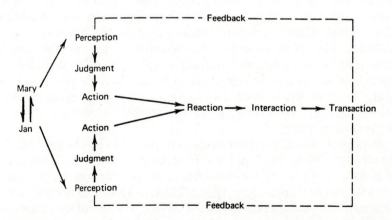

Figure 13-2. Relationships of concepts specified in the propositions. (*Reproduced with permission from Chinn, P.L.,* Advances in nursing theory development. *Rockville, MD:* Aspen, [*1983*]. *p. 54-55, 58.*)

These concepts were placed within each of the three levels of abstraction primarily for a focus yet recognizing that the concepts cut across the levels of abstraction.

Subsequent to identifying a general systems framework (King, 1971), a theory of goal attainment was derived with a focus on interpersonal systems. A look at the empirical world of nursing, the basic unit of behavior, the nursing act (King, 1964), was identified within the interpersonal systems. The basic unit of behavior was identified as interactions between nurse and recipient of care. These phenomena are represented in the major concepts and subconcepts that comprise the theory of goal attainment. These concepts are perception, interaction, communication, transaction, self, role, growth and development, stress, time and space (King, 1981, p. 145). These concepts cut across many disciplines, and when put together in this theory form a wholeness for my personal perception of nursing as a discipline and a profession. Wholeness is one of the aims of general systems theory.

A transaction model was developed as a result of a descriptive study of nurse-patient interactions in a hospital situation (King, 1981, p. 145). This model describes the elements in the interactions fo two individuals (nurse and patient) and indicates how mutual goal setting (decision making) is the process that leads to goal attainment. Process describes ongoing functions of systems. My theory demonstrates a general system that is a set of elements joined together by communication links with goal-directed purposeful behavior. The need for theory development and testing is important for description, explanation, and prediction in nursing. Research that tests theoretical ideas will result in identification of relevant concepts and basic principles that are valid throughout the body of knowledge essential for professional nursing.

Postscript I

The economic situation in society, in health care systems, and in the health professions makes it imperative to document the effectiveness of care. My theory helped me define an information system for nursing called a goal-oriented nursing record system (GONR). The problem-oriented medical record (POMR) provided a systematic way for physicians to document their care. The GONR has provided a systematic way for nurses to document their care and also to measure the effectiveness of the care provided for each person. When the outcomes are stated in terms that represent behavior expected in the recipient of care, these become the criteria for measuring the effectiveness of care.

This record system was described briefly by me in 1981 (King, p. 163). I have operationalized this system for use in renal dialysis units in hospitals (King, 1984). This system can be adapted for use in any hospital unit and in home health care.

Postscript II

The few ideas about measurement of goal attainment in the management literature and in community mental health literature were inadequate for me to use
in designing a study of goal attainment in nursing. An opportunity was provided
in a continuing education program sponsored by the University of Maryland,
from 1983 to 1985, for me to develop an instrument with the guidance of the experts in measurement. I wanted to cover the whole universe of nursing but
found out rather quickly in the project that I had to define the domain
specifically. My interest for years had been to devleop an instrument to assess
functional abilities in human beings (other than the physiological dimensions).
So my domain objectives were stated to identify categories within which I
would write items to represent the categories adequately. An instrument was
developed that is called a criterion-referenced measure of goal attainment
(King's goal attainment scale). The measure is valid and the initial reliability is
0.99. As individuals use the instrument, they are sending me their reliability
data. Three studies have been designed using this instrument to test hypotheses
related to goal attainment in nursing situations with different samples of
patients.

  If you are interested in networking in research to test the theory, wel-
come aboard.

REFERENCES

Austin, J. K., & Champion, V. L. (1983). King's theory for nursing: Explication and
    evaluation. In P. L. Chinn, (Ed.), *Advances in nursing theory development.* Rockville,
    MD: Aspens.
Daubenmire, M. J., & King, I. M. (1973, August). Nursing process models: A systems ap-
    proach. *Nursing Outlook, 21*(8), 512–517.
King, I. M. (1964, Oct.). Nursing theory: Problems and prospects. *Nursing Science 2,* 394.
King, I. M. (1971). *Toward a theory for nursing.* New York: Wiley.
King, I. M. (1981). *A theory for nursing.* New York: Wiley.
King, I. M. (1984, April). Effectiveness of nursing care: Use of a goal-oriented nursing
    record system in end stage renal disease. *American Association of Nephrology Nurses
    and Technicians* (AANNT), 11–17.
King, I. M. (1986). *Curriculum and instruction in nursing.* East Norwalk, CT: Appleton-
    Century-Crofts.
Von Bertalanffy, L. (1968). *General systems theory.* New York: Braziller.
Yura, H., & Walsh, M. (1988). *The nursing process* (5th ed.). New York: Appleton &
    Lange.

Evaluation of the Nursing Theory of Imogene M. King

Patricia B. DiNardo

Many nursing theories are now being developed and refined by nursing theorists. Where do these theorists get their basis for theory building? "Imogene King began her theory building for nursing by developing a conceptual framework (Chinn, 1983, p. 50)." She uses a framework based on three open, interacting systems. Systems theory is often used in the behavioral sciences to enable us to look at things more easily and gain a better understanding of them (Ruben & Kim, 1975). King, it seems, used her knowledge and research of systems theory as a foundation for her own theory of nursing.

The three systems described in King's conceptual framework are the personal system (individual), the interpersonal system (groups), and the social system (society). Her *Theory for Nursing* is based on these three interacting systems and the relationships between them.

In an attempt to understand what King describes as an individual, group, or society, we can refer back to other theorists used by King herself in the formation of "a conceptual frame of reference for nursing (King, 1971, p. ix)." Undoubtedly, numerous theorists have contributed to King's understanding and conceptualization, and are even quoted or mentioned in her descriptions of her three basic concepts; but Ralph Linton, a noted anthropologist, appears to have contributed substantially to King's idea of what an individual, group, and society are.

The Individual

"An individual at any point in time is a product of a very complex interaction between his genetically determined physical and psychological potentialities and his environment (Linton, 1962, p. 37)." An individual comes to know himself or herself through perceptions of self over time and by acknowledgement of the perception of others. Individuals possess the capacity for independent thought, feelings, and actions. They are molded in their personalities and behaviors by past experiences (Linton, 1962). Concepts relevant to King's personal system are: perception, self, body image, growth and development, and time and space.

Groups or Interpersonal Systems

Groups are comprised of individuals—as few as two or as many as infinity allows. Cultural elements lend control to the social interactions of individuals in a group. There are those that are "conscious statements as to the way in which individuals in different social positions should behave (Linton, 1962, p. 37)." These are the various roles assigned to the individuals of a group. There are also those generalized patterns of response that may be termed "value-attitude systems," often unconscious and unverbalized but exerting tremendous emotional effect and influencing overt behavior (Linton, 1962).

Groups are usually assembled in order to achieve a group goal, which in turn requires group problem solving. Within the group there must be acceptance of the group goal. "By acceptance of a goal is meant that the group member believes that his outcome will be improved when the task is in the state designated by the goal (Thibaut & Kelly, 1959, p. 271)."

Interpersonal systems are the main focus of King's theory, in particular the dyad formed by the nurse and the patient or client. The concepts of role, interaction, communication, transaction, and stress are the very basis of her theory of goal attainment.

Social Systems

According to Linton, a society is an organized group of individuals. Although an individual has a limited life span, "societies and cultures, on the other hand, are continual with no predetermined duration (Linton, 1962, p. 29)." Society exists to meet the needs of the individuals comprising it.

There are two fundamental processes involved in the formation of a society. These are the adaptation and organization of the behavior of the component individuals, and the development of a group consciousness or feeling of unity (Linton, 1936, p. 92). The members of a social system are held together by economic interdependence, strong emotional ties based on affection and habitual association, and a shared culture.

Social systems make up the last of King's interrelating systems. "Concepts of organization, power, authority, status, and decision making are characteristics of social systems that have relevance for nursing (King, 1981, p. 115)."

The following is an internal and external evaluation of King's *Theory for Nursing*. The format used is the one presented by Barbara J. Stevens (1984) in her book *Nursing Theory: Analysis, Application, Evaluation.*

INTERNAL EVALUATION

I. Commonplaces
Stevens (1984) states that most all nursing theories address common topics, or commonplaces. Six commonplaces have been defined by Stevens. These are the patient, nurse or nursing acts, health, nurse-patient relationship, patient to health, and nursing acts to health.

King describes at length all six of these commonplaces throughout her book *Theory for Nursing*. The following lists the commonplaces and the various definitions and meanings assigned to them by King.

A. Patient
1. One with a decreased control over environment and space.
2. One with decreased personal space.
3. Participant in active communication, interaction, and transaction.
4. Participant in mutual goal setting.
5. One who expressed concerns, problems, and disturbances in health.
6. One with a perception of a problem.
7. One who supplied information about self.

B. Nurse or nursing acts
1. Nurse.
   a. Increase knowledge of self.
   b. Understand self in relation to personal space.
   c. Initiator and facilitator of communication.
   d. Communicator of attitudes and information.
   e. Individually demonstrate power when interacting with patient.
2. Nursing acts.
   a. Action, reaction, and transaction.
   b. Goal setting.
   c. Teach, guide, counsel, and give care.
   d. Data gathering and analysis.
   e. Assess verbal and nonverbal communication.
   f. Maintain open communication with patient, other health care members, and family.
   g. Assist patient in coping with health problems, health concerns, and stressors.
   h. Help patients make decisions to choose between alternatives in their care.
   i. Assess patient's perception of space, time, self or body image, role and the health problem or concern.

C. Health
1. The way one deals with stresses of growth and development.
2. A harmony and balance with the environment.
3. A dynamic life experience; continuous adjustment to internal and external stressors through optimum use of one's resources to achieve maximum potential for the activities of daily living.

        4. An ability to function in social roles; a state that permits functioning in roles.

   D. Nurse-patient relationships
      1. Verification of perceptions.
      2. Mutual goal setting and decision making.
      3. Collaborative exploration of means to meet goal.
      4. Help each other grow in self-awareness and understanding of human behavior.
      5. Interaction, transaction to meet goal.
      6. Reciprocal communication; sharing of information.

   E. Patient to health
      1. Perception of health problem, concern, or disturbance.
      2. Inability to continuously adjust to internal and external stressors in a positive manner.
      3. Acceptance—internalizes change in role and self-image.
      4. Disruption of harmony and balance with the environment.

   F. Nursing acts to health
      1. Attain, maintain, or restore health.
      2. Assistance in coping with perceived health problems or concerns (nurse and patient perceptions).
      3. Exploration of resources to achieve maximum potential for activities of daily living.
      4. Concern for health of individuals and health care of groups.

II. Consistency
   A. Terms. Other concepts and terms are presented in King's theory, although the following appear to be the dominant ones. The terms listed below have been operationally defined and their meaning remains the same throughout the theory development.

      PERCEPTION: Each being's representation of reality; major concept in theory of goal attainment.

      INTERACTION/INTERPERSONAL RELATIONSHIP: A concept involving perception, communication, role, and stress. In nursing, most concentrated upon interaction is one between nurse and patient or client. Usually formed to identify goals and ways to achieve goals.

      TRANSACTION: A concrete activity humans actively participate in to obtain movement to achieve goals bringing about change in an individual.

      SYSTEMS: Systems theory used to explain interrelationships between three open systems: personal, interpersonal, and social. Major scope of nursing theory is interpersonal systems; dyads.

      COMMUNICATION: Described as verbal and nonverbal; occurring between persons or from persons to environment.

      GOALS/GOAL ATTAINMENT: The theory itself. Product of actions, interactions, and transactions. Participation of both nurse and pa-

tient in mutual goal setting and the use of a dyad to attain mutually satisfying goals.
  B. Interpretation
      "An essential interpretation is one in which the nursing phenomenon is explained by reference to the circumstances in which it occurs (Stevens, 1984, p. 33). "King's theory of goal attainment meets the criteria of an essential interpretation because it is based on interaction and transaction, the conceptual framework of interpersonal systems.
  C. Principles
      1. The primary principle in King's theory is action, interaction, and transaction.
      2. The overall assumption is that the "focus of nursing is human beings interacting with their environment leading to a state of health for individuals, which is an ability to function in social roles (King, 1981, p. 143)."
          This overall assumption is based on specific assumptions about human beings and nurse-client interactions. Although King (1981) admits that a personal philosophy of human beings influenced development of her conceptual framework and her theory, the specific assumptions do form a deductive framework for the overall assumption.
          Examples:
      1. Individuals are social beings. Therefore, interaction between nurse and patient appears logical.
      2. Perceptions of nurse and of client influence the interaction process. Therefore, perceptions of both nurse and patient must be verified through interaction to lead to mutual goal setting and attainment.
  D. Method
      The logistic method was used in this theory development. In this method, parts are used to organize the whole. The parts are the systems. The whole is the interrelationships.
  E. Approach
      There is a consistent approach in the organization of structures throughout the theory. Refer to the reasons stated in II-C, II-D, and IV.
III. Adequacy
      The theory appears adequate in any nursing situation where a nurse-patient interaction can occur and mutual goal setting can be accomplished through *reciprocal* communication. The theory is limited, however, where communication, and therefore transaction, is not possible by the patient (for example, comatose patients, irrational patients, and infants).
IV. Logical development
      A deductive argument is used in King's nursing theory. Assumptions are based on concepts; propositions are based on assumptions. There is a predictive nature generated from the concepts of the theory.

Example: "If perceptual accuracy is present in nurse-client interactions, transaction will occur (King, 1981, p. 149)."

V. Level of theory development

The level of theory development is explanatory and predictive. The theory predicts what future interactions of the same phenomenon will produce.

Example: "If nurse and client make transactions, goals will be attained (King, 1981, p. 149)."

VI. Clarity

The terms are consistent and have a denotative meaning in the theory. The logistic method of thinking is clear and easy to follow. Deductive reasoning is built in the same manner as the logistic method of thinking and is also clear and easy to follow.

EXTERNAL EVALUATION

I. Reality convergence

  A. Principle. The basic premise of theory is the interrelationship of nurse and patient or client through action, interaction, and transaction to achieve mutual goal attainment. Knowledge of the personal systems (the nurse self and the patient self), interpersonal systems (the dyad comprised of the two), and social systems (the system the dyad operates in) is essential to understanding the interactions between them. An overall assumption for the theory of goal attainment is "that the focus of nursing is human beings interacting with their environment leading to a state of health for individuals, which is the ability to function in social roles (King, 1981, p. 143)." This author agrees with the principles identified by King as an adequate representation of reality.

  B. Interpretation. Refers to action, interaction, and transaction. King interprets the nursing world as a world of interactions and reactions between personal, interpersonal, and social systems. The nursing process and its components involves actions on the part of one or more systems, interactions between systems, and transactions among systems.

   ASSESSMENT: Must involve verification of perceptions of both nurse and patient or client (action, reaction, interaction).

   DIAGNOSIS: Nursing action in "organizing diagnostic categories that deal with personal and interpersonal systems (King, 1981, p. 176)."

   PLANNING: Interactions between the nurse and the patient for setting mutual goals and exploring means of goal attainment.

   IMPLEMENTATION: Transaction between the nurse-patient dyad and often involving other social systems to obtain movement to achieve goals in bringing about change in an individual.

EVALUATION: Must again involve verification of perceptions of both nurse and patient interaction.

C. Method. Refers to the theory, which is based on the logistic method. It appears relatively easy to implement experimental studies to test the general hypotheses generated from this theory.

Example: Interactions—Person to person and/or person to environment, which are directly observable, provide the raw data to be analyzed to identify transactions made and, hopefully, goals attained.

II. Utility

The main principle of action, interaction, and transaction can be used in most nursing situations where the patient or client can communicate. There are some situations where this may not be the case, however. Examples of these are newborns, very young children, entubated patients, comatose or neurologically impaired patients, trauma patients, and irrational patients.

III. Significance

A. As stated by Stevens (1984), most all nursing theories address common topics, or commonplaces. King's theory is based on the interactions of the nurse or nursing acts commonplace with the patient or client commonplace in attaining the goal of health. Therefore, the theory is based in the heart of nursing and is basic and essential to issues in the profession.

B. This theory contributes to nursing knowledge in that research is easily generated. The research stemming from this theory should "predict and ultimately control those factors that comprise the essential aspects of nursing (Stevens, 1984, p. 69)."

Example: If nurse-client interactions lead to transactions (which are concrete, active movements by humans to achieve a predetermined goal), research can be generated to find out which interactions produce the greatest amount of transaction and, in turn, goal attainment. Effectiveness of nursing care and nurse-client interactions could be measured.

IV. Discrimination

Action, interaction, and transaction can occur in any social exchange, and in any of the behavioral sciences. This in itself does not bind the theory to nursing. However "interactions are limited to a licensed professional nurse and to a client in the need of nursing care (King, 1981, p. 150), "the theory discriminates itself from other social and behavioral sciences and from other health care professionals.

V. Scope

King's theory is limited in scope—that is, it is limited to situations where reciprocal communication can take place between nurse and client. Refer also to point II.

VI. Complexity

King's *A Theory for Nursing* (1981) achieves an appropriate balance between complexity and parsimony. The main essence of the theory can be grasped by the terms and concepts listed in the internal evaluation. Additional concepts relating to each of the three open systems allow for greater variability and therefore greater complexity in the interactional nursing process.

SUMMARY

Because nursing theories are now being developed and refined by nursing theorists, we must familiarize ourselves with them and evaluate them as to their relevance, practicality, and worth to the nursing profession. An internal and external evaluation of King's *A Theory for Nursing* (1981) was presented here.

King's theory is a systems theory that uses three interacting open systems. These are the personal system, the interpersonal system, and the social system. The basic premise of the theory is the interrelationship of the nurse and the patient or client through action, interaction, and transaction to achieve mutual goal attainment.

The definitions of King's three systems seem to correspond with the definitions Linton assigns to an individual, group, and society. It is possible that King used Linton's theory as one reference in developing her own.

REFERENCES

Chinn, P. L. (Ed.). (1983). *Advances in nursing theory development.* Rockville, MD: Aspen.

King, I. M. (1981). *A theory for nursing.* New York: Wiley.

King, I. M. (1971). *Toward a theory for nursing.* New York: Wiley.

Linton, R. (1936). *The study of man.* New York: Appleton-Century Company.

Linton, R. (1962). *The tree of culture.* New York: Knopf.

Ruben, B. D., & Kim, J. Y. (Eds.) (1975). *General systems theory and human communication.* Rochelle Park, NJ: Hayden.

Stevens, B. J. (1984). *Nursing theory analysis, application, evaluation* (2nd ed.). Boston: Little, Brown.

Thibaut, J. W., & Kelley, H. H. (1959). *The social psychology of groups.* New York: Wiley.

A Baccalaureate Nursing Curriculum Based on King's Conceptual Framework[1]

M. Jean Daubenmire

The aim of baccalaureate education for nursing is to provide a curriculum, a climate for life-long learning, and resources whereby students acquire values, knowledge, and skills used in practicing theory-based nursing. In the rapidly changing world of health care, it becomes increasingly important to educate students who will be able to create and assume new and emerging roles of nursing in the twenty-first century. The challenge for nurse educators is clearly one of creating and implementing curricula that will facilitate the development of our future nurse leaders in theory, research development, and practice.

This chapter describes the use of King's (1971) theory in the development and implementation of a baccalaureate curriculum in nursing at Ohio State University, College of Nursing. The curriculum was implemented in 1970 and for the past 15 years the curriculum model and conceptual framework based on King's theory have remained essentially the same.

Curriculum evaluation is viewed as an ongoing process with continual evaluation and updating of knowledge and skills as well as expansion of models and refinement of teaching strategies. Additionally, there have been two National League for Nursing accreditation reviews and a university internal review program, all of which were very positive. Based on both internal and external evaluation, it is clear that King's framework continues to provide a viable curricular strategy for the education of baccalaureate nurses. Extensive curriculum revision is extremely costly in terms of faculty time and energy, which can be better used in conducting research, service, and other scholarly endeavors. A curriculum model which is conceptually based allows for updating content and skills without the necessity for major curriculum change.

The faculty elaborated upon King's work to develop a framework for nursing (Table 15–1). The framework provides the structure and delineates the con-

TABLE 15-1. THE OHIO STATE UNIVERSITY COLLEGE OF NURSING BACCALAUREATE PROGRAM CONCEPTUAL FRAMEWORK

Health is the goal of nursing.

Individual is the focus of nursing.

  Three systems of function—Personal, Interpersonal, and Socio-cultural—include the concepts of—Perception and Health, Interpersonal Relations, Social Systems and Health.

Nursing process is Action-reaction-interaction-transaction, whereby the nurse utilizes the elements of the methodology to systematically study the nurse-client interaction within the nursing situation.

Nursing situation is an interaction of nurse and individual, with the goals of health.

Systems approach is a way of viewing the interconnections of the conceptual framework.

tent for the undergraduate program in nursing. The nursing process provides the basis for integration of the content. In this framework health is the goal of nursing. The individual is the focus of nursing. The individual functions in three systems: personal, interpersonal, and sociocultural. These three systems are identified as the levels of analysis used for learning the concepts of the curriculum. Four concepts that cross all systems are perception, interpersonal relations, social systems, and health.

The student views the nursing process as a dynamic, interpersonal process in which nurse and client are each affected by the behavior of the other and by factors in the system in which they operate (Daubenmire & King, 1973).

The systems approach is used as a way of viewing the interconnections of the conceptual framework. This approach provides a method for studying the individual as an open, complex, living system. The systems approach is also used to logically organize the content in the curriculum. How this was accomplished can be seen in the following discussion of the curriculum model.

Students are admitted to nursing as sophomores, having completed required courses in the natural and behavioral sciences as well as liberal arts courses.

The curriculum model is the foundation for the undergraduate curriculum at the Ohio State University College of Nursing (Fig. 15-1). This model is presented in a time frame delineating the focus for each year of the program. Both the individual student and client are viewed as bio-psycho-social beings who function in personal, interpersonal, and sociocultural systems. This unique way of studying nursing focuses on nursing students and their behavior and actions, as well as on the client in the nursing situation. This focus is continued throughout the 3 years and is equally distributed between the system of the nursing student and the system of the individual client.

The nurse and client are brought together in the nursing situation. Thus, the dynamic interaction of the nurse-client dyad is the major focus for applying the content of the curriculum. It is the nursing situation, comprised of the dyad, that becomes the essential experience (E = experience: E_1 through E_n) for applying the nursing process. The nursing situations are defined as core experiences in which all students participate throughout the nursing program.

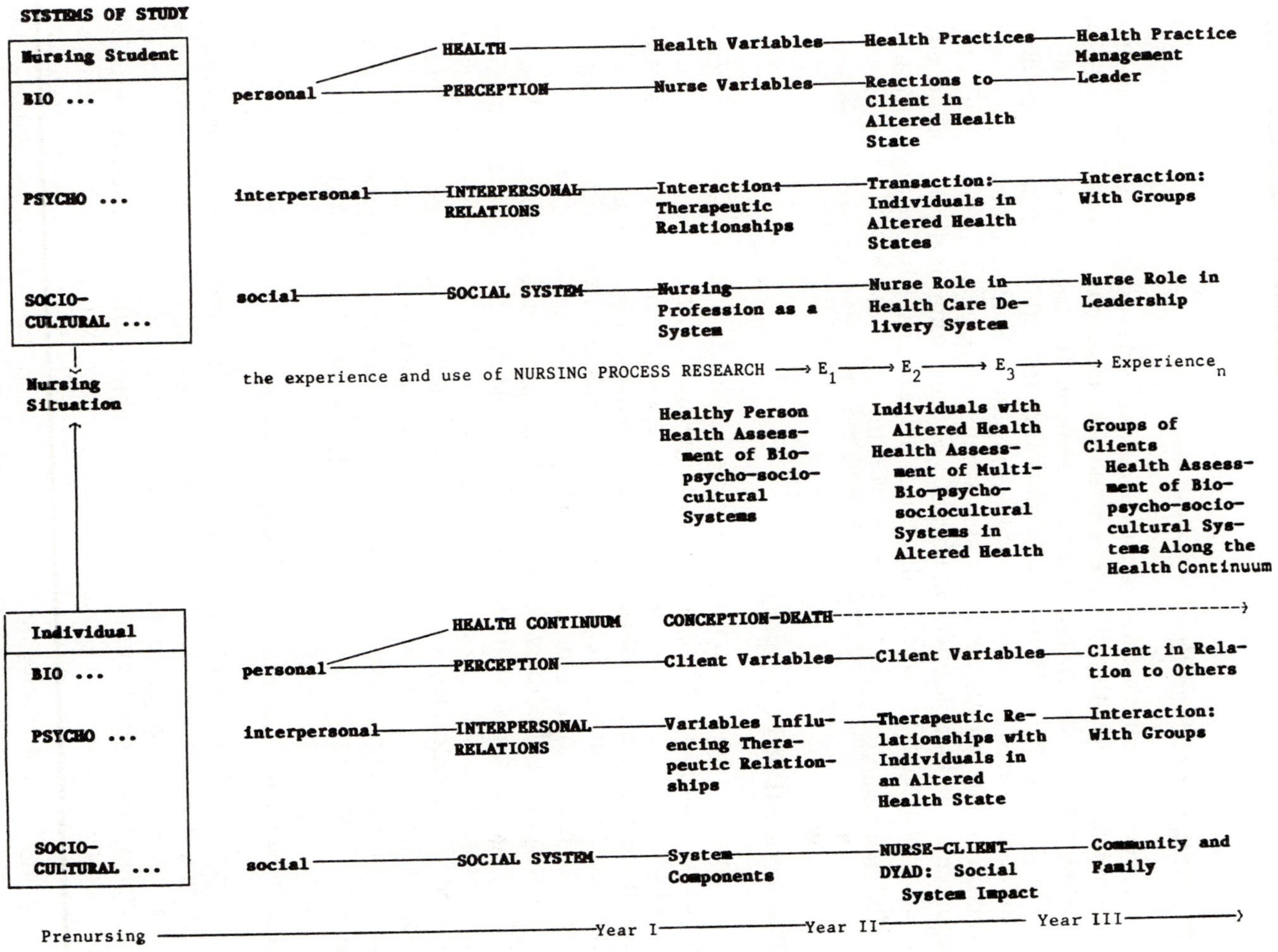

SYSTEMS OF STUDY

Nursing Student
- BIO ...
- PSYCHO ...
- SOCIO-CULTURAL ...

→ Nursing Situation ←

Individual
- BIO ...
- PSYCHO ...
- SOCIO-CULTURAL ...

personal —— HEALTH —— Health Variables —— Health Practices —— Health Practice Management

PERCEPTION —— Nurse Variables —— Reactions to Client in Altered Health State —— Leader

interpersonal —— INTERPERSONAL RELATIONS —— Interaction: Therapeutic Relationships —— Transaction: Individuals in Altered Health States —— Interaction: With Groups

social —— SOCIAL SYSTEM —— Nursing Profession as a System —— Nurse Role in Health Care Delivery System —— Nurse Role in Leadership

the experience and use of NURSING PROCESS RESEARCH $\longrightarrow E_1 \longrightarrow E_2 \longrightarrow E_3 \longrightarrow$ Experience$_n$

Healthy Person Health Assessment of Bio-psycho-socio-cultural Systems —— Individuals with Altered Health Health Assessment of Multi-Bio-psycho-sociocultural Systems in Altered Health —— Groups of Clients Health Assessment of Bio-psycho-socio-cultural Systems Along the Health Continuum

HEALTH CONTINUUM —— CONCEPTION-DEATH

personal —— PERCEPTION —— Client Variables —— Client Variables —— Client in Relation to Others

interpersonal —— INTERPERSONAL RELATIONS —— Variables Influencing Therapeutic Relationships —— Therapeutic Relationships with Individuals in an Altered Health State —— Interaction: With Groups

social —— SOCIAL SYSTEM —— System Components —— NURSE-CLIENT DYAD: Social System Impact —— Community and Family

Prenursing —— Year I —— Year II —— Year III

Figure 15-1. The curriculum model of the Ohio State University College of Nursing.

169

Based on the curriculum model, the student is introduced to the framework, nursing theory and nursing process, and the four concepts early in the sophomore year. The concepts then become substantive content for study throughout the 3 years.

The Concept of Health

The concept of health at the student's personal level is designed to assist the student in knowing health parameters, identifying his or her own health practices, and planning for health practice management. The focus for the concept of health at the client level during the sophomore and junior years addresses both health and altered health states of the individual. Students reexamine health behavior again during the senior year when it is expected that they can better appreciate the complexity of the health concept. Additionally, the model emphasizes that students broaden their knowledge of health by expanding from an understanding of the individual to working with the health of groups of clients.

The Concept of Perception

The concept of perception is considered essential to the framework because it influences the nurse's ability to assess, diagnose, plan, implement, and evaluate client care. "Perception is a process of organizing, interpreting, and transforming information from sense data and memory. It is a process of human transactions with environment. It gives meaning to one's experience, represents one's image of reality, and influences one's behavior (King, 1981, p. 24)."

The concept of perception at the student's personal level continues to emphasize that students will understand variables influencing their own perceptions and will be able to examine their perceptions of clients experiencing altered health states. Perception of self as a leader is emphasized in the senior year. At the client level, the concept of perception focuses on client variables during the sophomore and junior years and is expanded during the senior year to imply that students consider group influences on client perceptions.

The Concept of Interpersonal Relations

The concept of interpersonal relations at the nursing student level is developed such that students are first introduced to the nursing process as an interpersonal process and begin to develop therapeutic communication skills. By the end of the junior year, they are expected to be able to effect transaction with individual clients, and during the senior year, they are expected to be able to effectively interact with groups of individuals. The emphasis during the senior year is on caring for and managing nursing care for groups of clients. Long-term health problems that influence individuals, families, and society are also a focus of study during the senior year. At the client level, the concept of interpersonal relations is developed to show the expectation that students will develop increasingly complex interpersonal skills. They are first expected to work with individuals in simple nursing situations and then with individuals experiencing more complex health alterations at the various levels of health along the health continuum. Finally, students interact with groups of clients to assist in the recovery from illness and to promote practices that will improve health states.

The Concept of Social Systems

A major concept of study in all 3 years is social systems, progressing from the level of individual, to family, to community, and to other large social systems. In the sophomore year the student studies the components of a system and examines nursing as a profession. Students are introduced to the qualities needed to become contributing and accountable members of the nursing profession. During the junior year and part of the senior year, the nurse-client dyad is the major focus, with the emphasis on how the health care delivery system and the client's family influence the relationship of the nurse and the client. A secondary focus is to understand the nurse's role within the health care delivery system. The community system is a primary focus during the senior year. The client's family and the health care delivery system are considered significant subsystems in studying the community. In addition, the nurse in leadership roles is studied in the senior year.

The conceptual framework is based on the philosophy of nursing and the philosophy of learning. It is then reflected in all terminal objectives and course objectives. Tables 15-2 through 15-4 illustrate how theory, concepts, nursing process, technical skills and development through the life cycle are studied throughout the curriculum. Required nursing and support courses can also be viewed.

In the sophomore year (Table 15-2) the major system of study is the personal system. Students are introduced to the science and discipline of nursing and to nursing theory and research (Nursing 340). Historical development of the nursing profession and nursing education provides a basis for later discussions of the roles of the professional nurse. Students also learn to understand general systems theory and the purpose and function of nursing models for nursing practice with emphasis on King's (1986) conceptual framework.

In the second course (Nursing 341) the primary emphasis is on the study of health and its relationship to life style application of teaching, learning, and nursing process in health promotion through the life span.

In Nursing 342, students study perception in personal, interpersonal, and social systems. Perception is considered a key concept in establishing professional and all interpersonal relationships. Communication and culture are studied as mediators of perception.

Nursing process, health assessment, and technical skills are included in all courses. In Nursing 400, students are introduced to a study of nursing in acute

TABLE 15–2. OVERVIEW OF SOPHOMORE LEVEL CURRICULUM

Autumn Quarter		*Winter Quarter*		*Spring Quarter*	
Anatomy 200	6 credits	Physiology 311	5 credits	Physiology 312	5 credits
Nursing 340	5 credits	Nursing 341	5 credits	Nursing 342	5 credits
Nursing 335	3 credits	Nursing 336	3 credits	Nursing 400	3 credits

Nursing 340, 341, 342—Introduction to Theory and Nursing Process

System of study	*Personal*			*Personal*		*Personal*	
	Nursing theory	Nursing process	Health	Nursing process	Interpersonal relations	Perception
			Nursing process			
	Health assessment				Technical nursing skills	

Nursing 335, 336—Process of Human Adaptation

Developmental stage	Conception → Preschool age	School age → Youth	Young adult → Elderly
	Bio-psycho-social development		

health care delivery systems, with a focus on the practice of psychomotor skills. Nursing 335 and 336 emphasize the bio-psycho-social development of the individual through the life cycle.

In the junior year (Table 15–3) the concept of health alterations become the primary focus in all of the courses. The concepts of interpersonal relations, perception, and social systems are secondary foci of study. Again, nursing process, health assessment, and technical skills are developed across courses. Students practice with clients at all stages of the life cycle.

The senior year (Table 15–4) is considered to be an integrative year with the system of study changing with each course. For example, in Nursing 520 the personal system is again studied as the student learns about role and skills related to leadership with groups of clients. He or she also studies organizational theory and learns to analyze contemporary issues in nursing.

In Nursing 521, the system of study is the interpersonal system as the student studies nursing process with a focus on mental health throughout the life cycle at personal, interpersonal, family, and community levels.

In Nursing 522, the primary focus is on social systems as the student studies the concepts of health in community systems and nursing process with individuals, groups, and families in the community. Students also have courses in statistics and the research process and its relevance to the advancement of nursing theory and practice.

The curriculum was designed to encourage students to pursue specific areas of interest and to promote a liberal education. Nursing students take a

TABLE 15-3. OVERVIEW OF JUNIOR LEVEL CURRICULUM

Autumn Quarter		*Winter Quarter*		*Spring Quarter*	
Nursing 432	8 credits	Nursing 431	8 credits	Nursing 430	8 credits
Pharmacy 470	4 credits	Microbiology 509	5 credits	Nutrition 310	5 credits

Nursing 430, 431, 432—Health Alterations and Nursing Process

System of study	*Personal*	*Personal*	*Personal*
Major concept focus	Health alterations in selected body systems	Health alterations in selected body systems	Health alterations in selected body systems
Minor concept focus	Interpersonal relations	Interpersonal relations	Interpersonal relations
	Perception	Perception	Perception
	Social systems	Social systems	Social systems
		Nursing process	
	Health assessment and technical nursing skills		
Developmental stage	Adult → Elderly	Childhood	Fetus → Middle adult

minimum of 34–35 credit hours of electives. For those interested in specific topics related to nursing, a series of nursing electives and independent study courses are available to enrich their studies in nursing. For those students interested in areas other than nursing, an arrangement with the Colleges of Arts and Sciences allows them to pursue a minor in liberal arts in more than 50 subjects. Nursing students may structure their elective courses to receive a minor in liberal arts that will be posted on their transcript at graduation.

It is important to emphasize that although specific concepts are delineated as the focus of study in nursing courses, students are always encouraged to use all concepts in expanding or enhancing their knowledge and understanding of themselves and their clients. This is facilitated through the use of the nursing process methodology. While King's conceptual framework delineates the structure and content of the curriculum, the components of the framework also provide the foundation of the conceptual model of nursing process as shown in Figure 15-2. As illustrated in the model, nursing process is a method of integrating systems concepts and framework concepts.

The nursing process methodology (Table 15-5) is utilized to systematically direct student interactions with clients. It is based on the proposition that the interaction process of nurse and client is a basic practice phenomenon that

TABLE 15-4. OVERVIEW OF SENIOR LEVEL CURRICULUM

	Autumn Quarter		*Winter Quarter*		*Spring Quarter*	
	Nursing 520	10 credits	Nursing 521	8 credits	Nursing 522	8 credits
	Statistics	3-5 credits	Nursing 540	3 credits		

Nursing 520, 521, 522—Health Alterations and Nursing Process

System of study	*Personal*	*Interpersonal*	*Social*
Major concept focus	Health Perception Interpersonal relations	Health Perception Interpersonal relations	Health Perception Social systems
Minor concept	Social systems	Social systems Nursing process Technical nursing skills Leadership skills	Interpersonal relations
Developmental	Childhood → Elderly	Adolescent → Elderly	Infant → Elderly

Nursing 540

Nursing research

provides the vehicle for giving nursing care. Through this methodology students are assisted to understand themselves as well as the clients. They have the opportunity to synthesize their learning in increasingly complex situations. Students use the same nursing process evaluation tool throughout their own strengths, weaknesses, and progression, as well as expansion of the knowledge base with each new experience. The nursing process, then, is a process of inquiry and self-learning, a conceptual and perceptual process. The faculty member operates at the interface of the process, helping the student to identify skills that have been mastered; potential data collection and interpretation errors; and diagnosis, planning and evaluation skills. As a part of the process, students are expected to become intelligent consumers of research and to utilize relevant research findings in their care of clients. The nursing process provides a methodology that permits the student to update knowledge and to evaluate the effectiveness of interventions, and thus a foundation for life-long learning process.

In summary, as a faculty chooses or develops conceptual frameworks as a basis for a curriculum, it is important to remember that student learning and concept development is a personal process. Students should not be limited by frameworks or faculty, but be encouraged to go beyond or transcend present

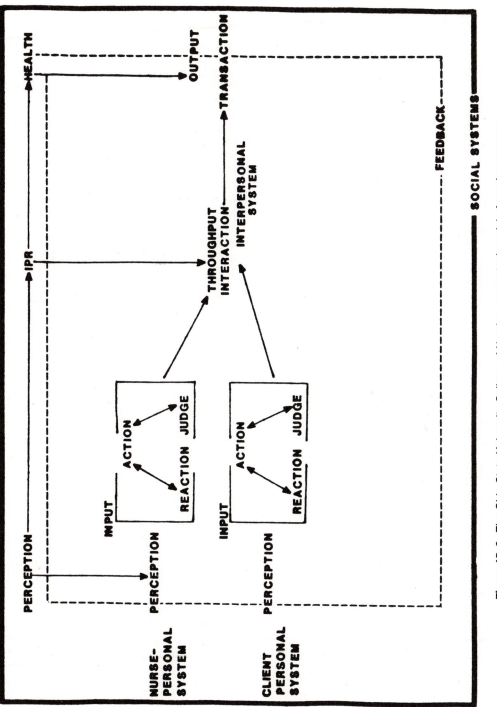

Figure 15–2. The Ohio State University College of Nursing conceptual model of nursing process.

TABLE 15–5. NURSING PROCESS METHODOLOGY: A GUIDE TO NURSING PROCESS

Step	Purpose
I. ASSESS	
1. Collects data	1. Data are collected continuously and systematically throughout the nursing process to identify client* and nurse strengths and limitations and environmental influences in the nursing situation
2. Accumulates knowledge	2. Knowledge is accumulated and applied throughout the process and provides a foundation for the collection and interpretation of data about the client's health state, perceptions, interpersonal relations, and social systems
3. Makes inferences	3. Inferences are made to provide preliminary assumptions based on collected data and knowledge
4. Verifies data and inferences	4. Verification is accomplished through the process of questioning and confirming to insure the accuracy of data and inferences
II. DIAGNOSE	
1. Organizes data	1. Data are organized to cluster behaviors representing client strengths and limitations
2. Formulates nursing diagnostic statements	2. Nursing diagnostic statements are formulated to name the clusters of client behaviors in the nursing situation
3. Verifies nursing diagnostic statements	3. Nursing diagnostic statements are verified to insure that the proper diagnoses have been formulated and is accomplished through the process of questioning and confirming
4. Establishes priorities	4. Priorities are established for diagnoses to plan care according to the clients most immediate needs in the nursing situation
III. PLAN	
1. Identifies goals and expected outcomes	1. Behavioral goals and expected outcomes are mutually defined between the nurse and client to maximize strengths and alter limitations
2. Identifies strategies and nursing orders	2. Strategies are actions identified to achieve goals and expected outcomes in the nursing situation
3. Identifies rationale	3. Rationale is identified to support or explain goals, expected outcomes, and strategies
IV. IMPLEMENT	
1. Implements plan	1. The plan is implemented to carry out the strategies

(cont.)

TABLE 15–5. (CONTINUED)

Step	Purpose
V. EVALUATE	
1. Evaluates achievement of goals and expected outcomes	1. Evaluation determines the extent of goal achievement in the nursing situation
2. Evaluates steps of the process	2. Each step is examined to determine its completeness and effectiveness
3. Evaluates variables	3. Variables are identified to examine their influence upon the process and include the client, nurse, and environment
4. Revises	4. Steps of the nursing process are revised as necessary to insure that the process is effective

*Client refers to an individual, family, or community.

nursing theory. King's framework provides a mechanism for students to continue this life-long learning process.

Integration of the content studied under the previously identified concepts occurs in the nursing situations, or core experiences, which are provided for all students. Students begin their experiences with a focus on health before being exposed to health alterations. They examine the variables that influence perception, develop increasing skill in interpersonal relationships, and utilize the concept of social systems to study the nurse-client dyad, the family, the health care delivery system, the community, and the nursing profession. Students have experiences with individuals at all stages of the life cycle.

Students are exposed to a variety of health care agencies in the central Ohio area and have multiple opportunities to collaborate with other health care providers. They develop leadership skills through working with other health team members and through the formal study of group process. They are provided with opportunities to examine the past, present, and emerging roles of the nurse and are assisted in becoming accountable beginning practitioners.

Nursing, taught in this environment of higher education, supports the study of nursing as a professional discipline, grounded in both science and caring and tested in the real world of practice.

END NOTES

[1] The author wishes to acknowledge the contributions of the Ohio State University College of Nursing faculty in the development of materials presented in this chapter.

REFERENCES

Daubenmire, M. J., & King, I. M. (1973, August). Nursing process models: A systems approach. *Nursing Outlook, 21*(8), 512–517.

King, I. M. (1971). *Toward a theory for nursing.* New York: Wiley.

King, I. M. (1981). *A Theory for nursing: Systems, concepts, process.* New York: Wiley.

King, I. M. (1986). *Curriculum and instruction in nursing concepts and processes.* East Norwalk, CT: Appleton-Century-Crofts.

Part 3

Developmental Models for Nursing Practice

Four models are placed in this section: the theories constructed by Rogers, Watson, Parse, and Chrisman and Riehl. The Rogers model is described in Chapter 16 and is critiqued by Burd and Cerilli in Chapter 17. In Chapter 18, Ference provides an application of the Rogerian framework with the theory of dying. And in Chapter 19, Barrett examines the Rogers model with a focus on the theory of power for nursing practice.

Watson's model (Chapter 20) is a new addition to this text and is a fairly new arrival on the nursing model scene. Watson writes as an existentialist. Because this philosophy is grounded in an individual's experience of existence having being in time and space, Watson's model was a better fit in this unit than in the others. Watson's model is critiqued by Ryan in Chapter 21, and Clayton reports on research that addresses the phenomena of caring with the elderly in Chapter 22.

Parse's model (Chapter 23) provides another perspective that employs the existentialist philosophy. Her model is also a new addition to this book. It is critiqued in Chapter 24 by Pugliese, who is an acquaintance of Dr. Parse. As a result, Parse had the opportunity to read and make suggestions to Pugliese regarding the content of the chapter. This was not the case with any of the other model critiques. All the evaluators selected the model they wished to write about. The only limitation was that they use Stevens' criteria. This was important for consistency in the book's format. In the last chapter on Parse's model (Chapter 25), Smith addresses research and the application of practice related to man-living-health.

There are two final chapters in this unit. Chapter 26, a reprint from the first edition, is called the systems-developmental-stress model and was written by Chrisman and Riehl. It is included because the first edition is out of print, yet professional nurses are implementing the model today. Only one example of the model's use is included here, however. Although the model was not developed per se, elements of it are evident in the Riehl interaction model reported in the second as well as the present edition of this text. No separate critique is included of the earlier model, but the fact that it is in current use indicates that for some the model is evaluated positively. Chapter 27 illustrates the model's application in Canada where John English utilizes the framework in a psychiatric setting.

Nursing: A Science of Unitary Human Beings

Martha E. Rogers

Nursing's evolution from prescience to science is emerging out of accelerating change on all fronts. Scientific and technological wonders abound. New world views multiply. Diversification marks the fields of business and industry. A cashless society is on the horizon. Low-tech robots for home and hospital are in the making. Space towns and moon villages may be only a few decades away with galactic grocery stores, educational centers, health services, recreational opportunities, and the like as inevitable inclusions in a space-bound world society. The liberal arts and sciences including extraterrestrial matters are essential bases for learned professional education in any field.

THE EMERGENGE OF NURSING

Evidence of the space age surrounds us. In a *Time* magazine article written in the mid-1980s, Chairman Paine of the National Commission of Space was quoted as saying that someone would be mining on the moon by the year 2005. His question was what language will the people there be speaking. On the political scene, bills have been presented before congress to establish space colleges with scholarships in a system similar to earlier agricultural colleges. The first national conference on nursing in space was presented in April, 1988 under the aegis of the University of Alabama at Huntsville School of Nursing. It was so well attended that a second conference is scheduled for 1989.

Fritz Capra writes in his book *The Turning Point:* (1982, pp. 15–16) "We are trying to apply concepts of an out-dated world view to a reality that can no longer be understood in terms of these concepts."

Sheldrake stirred the biological world with *A New Science of Life* (1981). David Bohm (1980) has proposed *Wholeness and the Implicate Order* (1980). Thomas Kuhn's (1957, 1962, 1970, 1977) paradigm shift is undergoing many opinions.

Larry Laudan (1977), discussing a theory of scientific growth, proposes three guiding priniciples:

1. In the case of competing scientific research traditions, if one of the traditions is compatible with the most progressive world view available, and the other is not, then there are strong grounds for preferring the former.
2. If both traditions can be legitimized with reference to the same world view, then the rational decision between them may be made on entirely "scientific" grounds.
3. If neither tradition is compatible with a progressive world view, their proponents should either articulate a new progressive world view which does justify them, or develop a new research tradition which can be made compatible with the most progressive extant world view. (pp. 132–133)

A new world view compatible with the most progressive knowledge available is a necessary prelude to studying human health and the determining modalities for its promotion. Such a view focuses on people and their environments. Space exploration has opened new avenues. Communication technology provides new means.

An abstract system identifying a new reality evolves out of a synthesis of fact and ideas. Definitions of specificity contribute clarity and precision. The future of nursing will be within the context of rapid change, diversity, new knowledge, and new horizons.

For nurses to fulfill their social and professional responsibilities demands an organized body of abstract knowledge specific to nursing—a substantive theoretical base.

Nursing is considered a learned profession and as a learned profession is both a science and an art. A science is defined as an organized body of abstract knowledge arrived at by scientific research and logical analysis. The art of nursing is the imaginative and creative use of this knowledge in human service. Historically the term "nursing" has been used as a verb to signify "to do." When nursing is perceived as a science, the term nursing becomes a noun signifying a "body of knowledge." The education of nurses has identity in transmission of nursing's body of theoretical knowledge. The practice of nursing is the use of this knowledge in service to people. Research in nursing is the study of unitary human beings and their environments.

The uniqueness of nursing, like that of any other science, lies in the phenomenon central to its purposes. Nursing's long-established concern with human beings and the world they live in is a natural forerunner of an organized abstract system encompassing people and their environments. The irreducible nature of individuals, as different from the sum of the parts and the integralness of human and environmental fields, coordinates a universe of open systems to identify the focus of a new paradigm and initiate nursing's identity as a science.

An abstract system constitutes the substantial base of a science of nursing. Such a system is arrived at by the creative synthesis of facts and ideas and is an emergent—a new product. Theories derive from this system and are tested in the real world. A science has many theories. However, theories deriving from one abstract system cannot be mixed with theories deriving from a different world view.

The purpose of nursing is to help all people wherever they are to achieve maximum well-being within the potential of each individual, family, and group.

The abstract system basic to nursing's science of unitary human beings is rooted in a progressive world view coordinate with current and emerging knowledge theories. A science has many theories. A science's open-ended definitions of specificity identify the phenomena of concern to nurses. Unitary human beings and their environments are identified as irreducible energy fields (*see* the glossary on page 183). The study of nursing, then, is the study of unitary human beings and their environments.

The study of nursing is not the study of nurses or what nurses do. Neither is it the study of biology, physics, psychology, sociology, engineering, medicine, nor is it any combination of these. This does not negate the need for all educated persons to have a foundation in the liberal arts and sciences, but these are not the science of nursing. The study of nurses and what nurses do can provide useful knowledge; but just as the study of what biologists do is not the study of biology, neither is the study of what nurses do the study of nursing. A science is a synthesis of facts and ideas—a new product—an emergent.

NURSING'S SCIENTIFIC LANGUAGE

Definitions play an important part in the development of a science and are necessary for precision, clarity, communication, and for replication of research. A language of specificity—nursing's scientific language—derives from the general language. Definitions specific to one field of study are not valid for a different field of study. Consequently it is important to note that terms not defined with specificity in the science of nursing are used in their general language definition. See glossary below.)

Glossary

LEARNED PROFESSION: A science and an art.
SCIENCE: An organized body of abstract knowledge arrived at by scientific research and logical analysis.

ART: The imaginative and creative use of knowledge.

ENERGY FIELD: The fundamental unit of the living. Field is a unifying concept. Energy signifies the dynamic nature of the field. Energy fields are infinite.

PATTERN: The distinguishing characteristic of an energy field perceived as a single wave.

FOUR DIMENSIONAL: A nonlinear domain without spatial or temporal attributes.

CONCEPTUAL SYSTEM: An abstraction. A representation of the universe or some portion thereof.

UNITARY HUMAN BEING (human field): An irreducible, four-dimensional energy field identified by pattern and manifesting characteristics that are specific to the whole and that cannot be predicted from knowledge of the parts.

ENVIRONMENT (environmental field): An irreducible, four-dimensional energy field identified by pattern and integral with the human field.

Nursing's abstract system is a synthesis of facts and ideas organized into a meaningful pattern specific to nursing's focus. Some building blocks included in developing nursing's abstract system are postulated to encompass energy fields, a universe of open systems, pattern, and four dimensionality. Although some definitions of specificity for these appear in the glossary, some additional comments should be made. Definitions taken from other fields are incorrect for nursing's abstract system.

People and their environments are perceived as irreducible energy fields integral with one another and continuously creative in their evolution. The proposed paradigm is humanistic and not mechanistic. Moreover, this is an optimistic model, though not a utopian one. Further, it is postulated that people have the capacity to participate knowingly and probabilistically in the process of change.

Unitary human beings are specified to be irreducible wholes. Moreover, a whole cannot be understood when it is reduced to its particulars. Unitary human beings are not to be confused with current popular usage of the term *holistic*, generally signifying a summation of parts, whether few or many. A science of unitary human beings is unique to nursing as well as having relevance for other fields. The explication of a body of abstract knowledge concerning unitary persons requires an organized conceptual system from which to derive unifying principles and hypothetical generalizations basic to description, explanation, and prediction.

Energy fields are postulated to constitute the fundamental unit of both the living and the inanimate. Field is a unifying concept. Energy signifies the dynamic nature of the field. Energy fields are infinite. Two energy fields are identified: the human field and the environmental field. Specifically, according to this view, human beings and the environment do not *have* energy fields, they *are* energy fields. The human and environmental fields are not biological, physical, social, or psychological fields. Human and environmental fields are irreducible.

The universe of open systems indicates that energy fields are infinite. They are open—not a little bit or sometimes—but continuously open. The human and environmental fields are integral with one another. A closed-system model of the universe is contradicted. Such concepts as equilibrium, adaptation, homeostasis, and steady-state are outdated. Causality is invalid. The universe is not running down. Rather, open systems are characterized by growing complexity and diversity.

Pattern identifies energy fields. It is the distinguishing characteristic of a field and is perceived as a single wave. The nature of the pattern changes continuously and innovatively. Each human field pattern is unique and is integral with its own unique environmental field.

The evolution of unitary human beings is a dynamic, irreducible, nonlinear process characterized by increasing diversity of energy field patterning. Manifestations of patterning emerge out of the human-environmental field mutual process and are continuously innovative. Pattern is an abstraction that reveals itself through its manifestations.

The nature of unitary field patterning is probabilistic and creative. Change is relative and increasingly diverse. Some manifestations of relative diversity in field patterning are noted below on a continuum.

Lesser Diversity	. . . .	Greater Diversity
longer rhythms	shorter rhythms	seem continuous
slower motion	faster motion	seem continuous
time experienced as slower	time experienced as faster	timelessness
pragmatic	imaginative	visionary
longer sleeping	longer waking	wakefulness

Four dimensionality is defined as a nonlinear domain without spatial or temporal attributes. All reality is postulated to be four dimensional. The relative nature of change becomes explicit. Human and environmental fields are *not* becoming four dimensional; they *are* four dimensional. This implies a new way of perceiving reality that differs from the traditional view of a three-dimensional reality.

Nursing's abstract system encompassing people and their world postulates a new reality commensurate with today's knowledge. Principles and theories derive from the totality of the abstract system. Characteristics and manifestations of unitary human beings are specific to the whole. They are manifestations of the whole.

The unitary human being (human field) is defined as an irreducible, four-dimensional energy field identified by pattern and manifesting characteristics different from those of the parts and which cannot be predicted from knowledge of the parts. The *environmental field* is defined asan irreducible, four-dimensional energy field identified by pattern and manifesting characteristics different from those of the parts. Each environmental field is specific to its given human field. Both change continuously and creatively.

Principles and theories derive from the conceptual system.The principles of homeodynamics postulate the nature and direction of change.

PRINCIPLES OF HOMEODYNAMICS

- Principle of resonancy—The continuous change from lower to higher frequency wave patterns in human and environmental fields.
- Principle of helicy—The continuous, innovative, probabilistic, increasing diversity of human and environmental field patterns characterized by nonrepeating rhythmicities.
- Principle of integrality*—The continuous, mutual human field and environmental field process.

The testing of the principles of homeodynamics is ongoing. Violet Malinski's book titled *Explorations on Martha Rogers' Science of Unitary Human Beings* (1986) reports a range of studies completed in this area.

A theory of accelerating evolution deriving from this conceptual system puts in different perspective today's rapidly changing norms in blood pressure levels, children's behavior, longer waking periods, and other events. Higher frequency wave patterns of growing diversity portend new norms coordinate with accelerating change. Labels of pathology based on old norms generate hypochondriasis and iatrogenesis. *Normal* means "average." Normal (average) blood pressure readings in all age groups are notably higher today than they were a few decades ago. Evidence that these norms are jeopardizing the public health are insubstantial. It is interesting to note that astronauts and olympic champions are reported to have higher than average blood pressure readings. Norms are changing rapidly and suggest evolutionary emergence rather than pathology according to outdated world views.

Not only has the average waking period lengthened but sleep-wake continuities are increasingly diverse. Developmental norms have changed significantly in recent years. Gifted children and the so-called hyperactive not uncommonly manifest similar behaviors. It would seem more reasonable to hypothesize hyperactivity as accelerating evolution than to denigrate rhythmicities that diverge from outdated norms and erroneous expectations.

---

*Formerly called the principle of complementarity.

Manifestations of a speeding up of human field rhythms are coordinate with higher-frequency environmental field patterns. Radiation increments of widely diverse frequencies are common household accompaniments of everyday life. Atmospheric and cosmological complexity grows. Environmental motion has quickened.

Human and environmental fields evolve together. The doom-sayers who would have it that people are destroying themselves are in error. On the contrary, there is a population explosion, increased longevity, escalating levels of science and technology, and multiple other evidences fo human's developmental potentials in the process of actualization.

With increased longevity growing numbers of older persons move into the picture. Contrary to a static view engendered by a closed system model of the universe, which postulates aging to be a running down, the science of unitary human beings postulates aging to be a developmental process. Aging is continuous from conception through death. Field patterns become increasingly diverse and creative. The aged need less sleep and sleep-wake frequencies become more varied. Higher frequency patterns give meaning to multiple reports of time perceived as racing. Aging is not a disease nor is it analogous to the "one-hoss shay" of literary lore.

Facts have meaning within the context of theory. The observations noted above need new examination within the context of a new world view. New questions must be asked, new theories derived, and new investigations pursued.

A nonlinear domain points up the invalidity of chronological age as a basis for differentiating development. In fact, as developmental diversity continues to accelerate, the range and variety of differences between individuals also increase. The more diverse field patterns evolve more rapidly than the less diverse. Populations defy so-called normal curves as individual differences multiply.

Paranormal phenomena are recognized increasingly as valid areas of serious scientific research. Nonetheless, there has been a paucity of viable theories to explain these events. The abstract system presented here does provide a means for deriving testable hypothesis in this area. The potential for creative health services using noninvasive modalities is great. Alternative forms of healing are increasingly popular and some are surprisingly effective. Meditative modalities bespeak beyond-waking manifestations. Therapeutic touch, developed by Dolores Krieger (1981), is documentally efficacious. Further implications for research in paranormal phenomena may well include criteria for selection of astronauts. Several years ago there was a report that persons who made the best aquanauts had histories of multiple health problems as they were growing up. Is it possible that travelers to outer space may evidence higher-frequency diversity? Will space dwellers of the future need support systems in reverse to visit planet Earth?

Research findings support the nature of change postulated in the principles of homeodynamics. Investigations into the nature of human and environmental field patterning with its continuously changing manifestations are under way. Unitary human field attributes are necessary adjuncts to studying questions arising out of a world view that is different from the traditional view. A number of tools already exist and others are in the process of development.

Nursing is concerned with the dying as well as with the living. Unitary human rhythms find expression in the rhythmicity of the living-dying process. And just as aging is deemed developmental, so is dying hypothesized to be developmental. Interest in the dying process and after-death phenomena has gained considerable public and professional interest in recent years. Yet rejection of the dying person continues to be all too common. Questionable practices in securing organs for transplantation have led to legislative action. The right to die with dignity is being written into final testaments. Concomitantly, reports of near-death and after-death experiences are listed among the bestsellers. The dying process should be studied. The continuity of field patterning after death will be a difficult area to investigate, although it should be by no means impossible.

The practice of nursing is rooted in the science of nursing—the Science of Unitary Human Beings. There is a critical need for greater individualization of services as diversity continues to accelerate. Noninvasive modalities, positive thinking, innovative delivery of health services, emphasis on promotion of health, and a good sense of humor are necessary adjuncts.

The potentialities of this paradigm are several. It is logically and scientifically tenable. It is flexible and open ended. It is researchable. The practical implications for human health and welfare are already demonstrable.

Seeing the world from this viewpoint requires a new synthesis, a creative leap, and the inculcation of new attitudes and values. Guiding principles are broad generalizations that require imaginative and innovative modalities for their implementation. A science of unitary beings identifies nursing's uniqueness and signifies the potential of nurses to fulfill their social responsibilities in human service.

REFERENCES

Bohm, D. (1980). *Wholeness and the implicate order.* Boston: Routledge & Kegan Paul.

Capra, F. (1982). *The turning point.* New York: Simon & Schuster.

Krieger, D. (1981). *Foundations for holistic nursing practices: The renaissance nurse.* Philadelphia: Lippincott.

Kuhn, T. S. (1957). *The Copernican revolution.* New York: Vintage.

Kuhn, T. S. (1962, 1970). *The structure of scientific revolutions.* Chicago: University of Chicago Press.

Kuhn, T. S. (1977). *The essential tension.* Chicago: University of Chicago Press.

Laudan, L. (1977). *Progress and its problems: Toward a theory of scientific growth.* Berkeley, CA: University of California Press.

Malinski, V. (Ed.). (1986). *Explorations on Martha Rogers' science of unitary human beings.* East Norwalk, CT: Appleton-Century-Crofts.

Sheldrake, R. (1981). *A new science of life.* Los Angeles: Tarcher.

An Analysis of Martha Rogers' Nursing as a Science of Unitary Human Beings

Karen Cerilli
Susan Burd

This chapter is a critique of Martha E. Rogers' conceptual framework of nursing as a Science of Unitary Human Beings. The criteria used to analyze Rogers' conceptual framework were found in Stevens' *Nursing Theory: Analysis, Application, and Evaluation* (1984).

Commonplaces and Nursing Domain

The commonplaces in Rogers' conceptual framework appear to be person-other and the environment, with person here defined as a unitary being only to be examined as a whole. The environment is seen as a four-dimensional energy field in constant contact with the energy fields of unitary human beings. This is evidenced in the principles of homeodynamics upon which her framework is based. The constant flow of waves between people and the environment is the basis for nursing intervention in relation to Rogers' framework.

A goal of the nursing domain in Rogers' conceptual framework is for the nurse to aid the patient in the redirection of life events to patterns that lead to optimal health (Whelton, 1979). This exemplifies the enhancement theory of nursing, which sees nursing as a means of improving the quality of the patient's existence in regards to health, totality, or some aspect of his or her being (Stevens, 1984). Rogers' (1970) belief that nursing's task is to promote symphonic interaction between people and their environment, and that unitary human beings always progress towards increasing diversity and uniqueness, further supports this classification.

INTERNAL EVALUATION

Clarity

Rogers' conceptual framework seems to possess a high degree of clarity in the authors' opinions. Her basic building blocks are simply stated, and the five assumptions of her conceptual framework appear strongly supported on those building blocks. Rogers' use of connotative meanings, which indicate what it is that the denoted objects have in common (Stevens, 1984), is evident in her principle of resonancy. It is here that she states that the human field and environmental field are propagated by wave patterns (Rogers, 1970). Her conceptual framework attempts to explain the life process by means of the constant interaction of these wave patterns. Although the terms Rogers uses are abstract and often foreign to the reader, if Rogers' work is read slowly from beginning to end, one forms a clear picture of her conceptual framework.

Consistency

Rogers defines the terms of her conceptual framework in a logical manner, and then consistently refers to those terms in the same manner throughout her writing. She maintains the same meanings in regards to the four building blocks and her principles of homeodynamics. If one is familiar with her early writings, when a later work is read, one is completely tuned in to the terms she is referring to.

In regard to principle, Martha Rogers appears to be comprehensive. Her consistent view of unitary human beings as greater than the sum of their parts has not been altered with the updating of other areas of her conceptual framework.

In interpretation, Rogers' conceptual framework is transcendental, beyond human experience, with an ontic type of interpretation. Rogers' views of person as being a four-dimensional energy field, and her belief in the unidirectional movement of unitary human beings interacting with a four-dimensional environmental field seems to further support the classification of her paradigm as ontic. This position is also evident in the principles of homeodynamics. By understanding these principles, one sees how the nature and direction of unitary human development is probabilistic and creative (Rogers, 1963). Because person and environment are evolving and changing together, the experience is larger than life.

Rogers utilized a dialectic method to present her conceptual framework. Rogers exhibits this in an understanding of the first of her five basic assumptions of persons, as well as in an understanding of her definition of unitary human beings. As Rogers (1986) states, "Unitary human beings are specified to be irreducible wholes. A whole cannot be understood when it is reduced to its particulars (p. 4)." Rogers' conceptual framework certainly describes not only the individual person but can be applied to all of society and remains consistent with her views of person as a whole greater than the sum of the parts.

Adequacy

Rogers' conceptual framework appears to possess a great deal of adequacy. She approaches nursing with an understanding of the patient in the immediate present. Her focus is on people, their environment and development in regard to changes in their lives. Rogers' conceptual framework accounts well for the subject matter of unitary human beings, explaining all aspects of human existence. The principles of homeodynamics are extensive enough to cover the broad scope of her conceptual framework.

Logical Development

The science of unitary human beings is logically developed and is done using the deductive method, meaning that the conclusions—the principles of homeo-dynamics—necessarily follow from Rogers' basic assumptions and building blocks. She steadily and systematically builds on her terms to lead to an understanding of the major components of the conceptual framework.

Level of Theory Development

Rogers' conceptual framework appears to move through levels I and II of theory development. Her framework begins at a simple descriptive ad hoc level in which she states basic assumptions concerning human beings. She then moves into the categorical level in which she begins to provide an interrelationship between person and environment. This is evidenced in the four building blocks of her framework, where she identifies energy fields, open systems, patterns, and four-dimensionality. All are components of both human and environmental fields.

Rogers' conceptual framework then moves into level II. In this explanatory level, a theory should explain how its given constituents relate to and with each other (Stevens, 1984). The explanatory level is evidenced in her principles of homeodynamics. It is here that Rogers explains the relationship of human beings and their environment to each other.

The conceptual framework can be viewed as predictive in that it attempts to show how, by means of the understanding of wave patterns of person and environment, one can predict changes in person and environment. The principle of resonancy provides us with an understanding of this predictive component.

It can also be situation-producing in that the framework lends itself to the hope that redirectioning of wave patterns can produce a desired situation. This final level of theory development has already undergone various research studies that attempt to produce a desired outcome through altered wave patterns.

EXTERNAL EVALUATION

Reality Convergence

In relation to terms, Rogers' conceptual framework lacks reality convergence. Her terminology does not lend itself well to the real world of nursing, persons, and health. Words such as helicy, resonancy, and homeodynamics are not present in the average professional nurse's vocabulary. Rogers' terms serve as a limitation to her conceptual framework as they are difficult to operationalize and understand (Falco & Lobo, 1985). The fact that Rogers has had to change her terms ("complementarity" to "integrality") or expand on her definition (four-dimensionality) shows the confusion that developed in regards to her conceptual framework. An important point to note is that Rogers has attempted through articles and books to update and increase the accuracy and clarity of her terms.

Because Rogers' conceptual framework is presented in such a way that the conceptual ideas of unitary human beings are related to process (Kim, 1983), one would agree that reality convergence in relation to principle is present. The conceptual framework is built upon basic assumptions that are accepted and further reflected in the four building blocks and principles of homeodynamics. Although her work is sometimes quickly discarded as being too abstract, the principles of homeodynamics and her transcendental ontological interpretation of person as a unitary whole provide a refreshing concept with which to view the world.

The intrepretative level of reality convergence appears to lack adequacy. Rogers' world of fluctuating waves, changing human and environmental boundaries, and bioelectrical phenomena (Stevens, 1984), lacks appropriate interpretation for nurses. It is important to note, however, that her world stresses the importance of human-environmental interaction, which is the focus of nursing.

Rogers' method of dialectic thought certainly does not fall in synchrony with the current popular scientific method of today. This is not viewed as a detriment to her conceptual framework, but is seen as a probable path for nursing to follow. The limitations of the scientific method have been stated more and more, and Rogers' dialectic method of looking at the whole as greater than the sum of the parts provides a unique and useful way in which the nursing community can view human beings (Rogers, 1963). Although the methodology utilized by Rogers does not lend itself to research using the scientific method per se, dialectic reasoning can be utilized in research by means of the problematic or the logistic modes (Stevens, 1984).

Utility

The usefulness to the practitioner in work is apparent. The nurse views the human being in regards to self and environment. The nurse's interventions are geared toward changes in the environment leading to changes in the human being. Unfortunately, although the potential is there, the lack of operationalized definitions and measurable outcomes makes it difficult to utilize her conceptual framework in practice (Meleis, 1985). This is not seen as a deficit to Rogers' conceptual framework, but simply as a lack of sophistication in our development of tools with which to measure her proposals. Operational definitions are needed for development of hypotheses that test theoretical concepts and for selection of tools to adequately measure concepts. Without tools, the ability to utilize or test the conceptual framework's success is impossible (Falco & Lobo, 1985). As Meleis (1985) states "researchers who have been inspired by Rogers' theory and theoretical propositions have found innovative ways to test and support some theory propositions (p. 227)."

Significance

In reference to addressing the essential issues in nursing, the science of unitary human beings is significant. It performs the most important task necessary in nursing today in that it gives nursing a unique way of viewing human beings. The growing use of therapeutic touch is an example of how Rogers' framework has been utilized by other researchers. The knowledge that changes in the patient occur simultaneously with changes in the environment directs the nurse to focus interventions toward the environment. This leads to predicting a change in the patient as he or she interacts with the changed environment (Whelton, 1979). The essential issue in nursing is changing patient behavior to lead to optimal health. Rogers' framework addresses this issue.

Capacity for Discrimination

Although Rogers' conceptual framework is applicable to all aspects of society, she does exhibit a capacity for discrimination of nursing from nonnursing acts. From the examination of Rogers' conceptual framework, one can see the central interest is unitary human beings, and nursing is seen as the only discipline in which one focuses on the whole being (Fawcett, 1984). It is nondiscriminatory in that her conceptual framework can be applicable to all situations. It does not limit human beings to being viewed strictly as a nurse would view them, but rather humans can be viewed by all sciences. Rogers' human being is an ever-changing person whose characteristics are not predetermined by genetics, destiny, or preset patterns of growth. Rather, people are influenced in dynamic ways by the changing nature of their environment, the changing nature of self, and the continuous interaction between them (Kim, 1983).

Scope

Rogers' conceptual framework is wide in scope as it attempts to describe life processes that result from human and environmental energy field interaction

(Meleis, 1985). Her conceptual framework, as stated earlier, can be applied to a variety of phenomena. The explanation of human and environmental wave patterns being in constant interaction allows for application to various situations. This can be demonstrated in the wide variety of research generated from her conceptual framework, from examining the relationship between mystical experience and creativity (Cowling, 1986) to researching the relationship between visible light waves and the experience of pain (McDonald, 1986).

Complexity Versus Parsimony

Rogers seems to achieve a good balance between simple and complex, although she tends to utilize complex terms and abstract concepts. Her attempts to explain interactions by the use of wave patterns allows for interrelationship of the variables, but the abstract nature of the conceptual framework produces complexity in the framework. As stated by Fitzpatrick (1986) when giving a critique of Rogers' conceptual framework, "Rogers' conceptualization, even in its complexity in terminology and essence, has simplicity in form and structure (p. xxv)."

SUMMARY

The Science of Unitary Beings is a refreshing way to view nursing. It is hoped that instead of dismissing it as too abstract, more students of nursing will be encouraged to explore this conceptual framework, and that more research will be done to lend support to Rogers' views. This unique framework has strong significance for both the nursing community and for society in general. The theories generated from Rogers' conceptual framework have great potential to alter the way unitary human beings examine themselves and the world around them.

REFERENCES

Cowling, W. R., III. (1986). The relationship of mystical experience, differentiation and creativity in college students. In V. Malinski (Ed.), *Explorations on Martha Rogers' science of unitary human beings* (pp. 131–142). East Norwalk, CT: Appleton-Century-Crofts.

Falco, S., & Lobo, M. (1985). Martha Rogers. In J. George (Ed.), *Nursing theories: The base for professional nursing practice* (2nd ed., pp. 214–232). Englewood Cliffs, NJ: Prentice-Hall.

Fawcett, J. (1983). Rogers' life process model. In J. Fawcett (Ed.), *Analysis and evaluation of conceptual models of nursing* (pp. 211–214). Philadelphia: Davis.

Fitzpatrick, J. (1986). Introduction. In V. Malinski (Ed.), *Explorations on Martha Rogers' science of unitary human beings* (pp. xxiii–xxvii). East Norwalk, CT: Appleton-Century-Crofts.

Kim, S. (1983). *The nature of theoretical thinking in nursing.* East Norwalk, CT: Appleton-Century-Crofts.

McDonald, S. (1986). The relationship between visible lightwaves and the experience of pain. In V. Malinski (Ed.), *Explorations on Martha Rogers' Science of unitary human beings* (pp. 119–129). East Norwalk, CT: Appleton-Century-Crofts.

Meleis, A. (1985). *Theoretical nursing: Development and progress.* Philadelphia: Lippincott.

Rogers, M. E. (1963). Building a strong educational foundation. *American Journal of Nursing, 6,* 94–95.

Rogers, M. E. (1970). *An introduction to the theoretical basis of nursing.* Philadelphia: Davis.

Rogers, M. E. (1986). Science of unitary human beings. In V. Malinski (Ed.), *Explorations on Martha Rogers' science of unitary human beings* (pp. 3–8). East Norwalk, CT: Appleton-Century-Crofts.

Stevens, B. (1984). *Nursing theory: Analysis, application, evaluation* (2nd ed.). Boston: Little, Brown.

Whelton, B. (1979). An operationalization of Martha Rogers' theory throughout the nursing process. *International Journal of Nursing Studies, 16,* 7–20.

Comforting the Dying
Nursing Practice According to the Rogerian Model

Helen M. Ference

Nurse A leaves the patient's room and confer's with her colleague, saying, "The patient is seeing ghosts! He is hallucinating! He thinks that I'm his daughter. It's spooky. He scares me!"

Nurse B tries to explain her fears by responding, "Oh, he's just dying. Give him some morphine, or maybe a sedative, and those behaviors will go away."

Nurses are very powerful. We control behaviors and make patients comfortable. Yet, are we making our clients comfortable or is it our own comfort to which we are attending?

HUMAN ENERGY FIELD TRANSFORMATION

Dying, according to the Rogerian Science of Unitary Human Beings (Rogers, 1970, 1986), is an energy transition. It is a transformation of the pattern of the human energy field. In a broad sense, it can be said that we begin dying immediately after birth.

We have concentrated so much of our attention on three-dimensional living and a three-dimensional life, that we have neglected comparable attention to three-dimensional dying.

By definition, three-dimensional dying is the absence of life. It is what happens when we no longer live. As in all nature, there usually are opposites, or frequency variations, that provide a natural dynamism or motion for a comfortable balance that we operationally define as health. Dying is the opposite of living three-dimensionally. In fact, if we attend to dying four-dimensionally in a different relative space-time, it is a function of living through the life process.

According to the Science of Unitary Human Beings, the human energy field

197

is the fundamental unit (Rogers, 1970, 1986). The pattern is the mosaic of waves (Ference, 1979) observable in the visible light wave spectrum. When we are sharply "in focus" we are "in tune" with living or very much "alive." When we appear to "slow down" or "speed up" excessively, our relative space-time changes and we appear or manifest ourselves to the very 'alive' as less alive. We have called these "less alive" patterns diseases, syndromes, and negatively value-laden patterns. These patterns are only tolerated in society when they are short-term.

There is a romantic fear of death and dying that is evident in our literature, our many cultures, and our religions. It has only been recently that it has been appropriate to study dying scientifically, because the sciences of living have altered our so-called "natural processes" of three-dimensional dying. By extending living, we have have extended dying. The challenge is before us to understand the meaning of the living and dying process as evolutionary processes. It is the intent of this chapter to offer explanations of this phenomenon, so important to humankind, through the Science of Unitary Human Beings as proposed by Martha E. Rogers (1970, 1986).

Nurses tend to underestimate their important role in understanding human experiences such as dying. No other profession sees so much death and dying from common work experiences, such as those shared by this author, in acute care settings, especially emergency rooms, critical care units, and other settings of hospitals in which the elderly "had pathology."

With the assertive efforts of medicine to treat natural transition processes as pathology and to perform elective procedures to extend life, nurses are faced with opportunities and situations to view people in more crises than ever before. Technology has extended our lives and made dying a longer process. People today are accompanied by artificial hearts, artificial kidneys, and other artificial organ systems and transplanted body parts.

The notion of out-of-body experiences has become a three-dimensional technical reality, in that our bodies are separate and distinct from the artificial parts appended to us. If you lose a body part, it can usually be substituted. If you have cancer, the affected body part can usually be removed or eradicated. The person affected must spend time informing family and friends that the cancer they had is not related to dying.

Losses of body parts, or aberrations and abnormalities such as tumors, form our systemic association of dying. We are beginning to define ourselves as something different from our physical image or reality. This may be likened to discarding the high-frequency parts that are "out of synch" with the rest of our self. This differentiation is helping us to understand the meaning of living and of dying. Death of parts is now accepted.

Systemic death, or major energy field transformation, today remains outside our general comprehension. So to focus on the dying process, we must neutralize the values we have associated with dying or passing on.

Reflecting on a working experience, much is to be gained towards a major professional endeavor, comforting the dying. This comprehension of the experience of the dying is achieved through the Rogerian nursing science according to the principles of homeodynamics.

APPLICATIONS OF ROGERIAN NURSING SCIENCE

The theory of dying is a multidimensional transformation of the human energy field in which patterning falls outside of the visible light wave spectrum. It can be systematically described from a four-dimensional, negentropic perspective.

The human being is an energy field, not comprised of parts as we have learned in a three-dimensional reality, but rather complete and whole in its image. We know this by the descriptions that people give during crises or near-death experiences. Out-of-body experiences are whole. They are a microcosm of the image of that unified energy field. Multiple manifestations, such as a person appearing in two different relative space-times, reveal the person in their wholeness rather than a leg, an arm, or a part. The image is whole. This might be described as 2 three-dimensional places in the same clock-time. Yet it connotes, more rationally, a defined field that is comprehended by its wholeness. The field cannot be reduced to its parts.

According to Rogers (1986), there are four concepts, logically linked, that serve as a framework in this nursing science. First, there are energy fields, both the human energy field and the environmental energy field. We identify the field through the second concept, its pattern. The third concept is openess, referring to the relationship between the person and environmental energy fields. Four-dimensionality is the fourth concept, referring to the relative space-time in which the fields exist.

Three principles guide the direction of human and environmental development (Fig. 18–1). Resonancy describes the direction of change; helicy describes the nature of change, and integrality provides for the continuous mutual process between the energy fields.

That which we can see is the pattern of wave frequency that is within our visible light wave spectrum. When we refer to those "living," the reference is usually for those within that same light wave spectrum. Wave frequencies outside of that spectrum exist, but are not as easily detected (Fig. 18–2).

The field is much greater than that which we can perceive. To illustrate, observe the dotted pinwheels in Figure 18–3. The pinwheels represent a mosaic of

Resonancy: The energy field evolves in the direction of higher frequency, shorter wave length from lower frequency, longer wave length.

Helicy: The pattern of the field evolves multidirectionally toward greater complexity and diversity.

Integrality: The human and environmental fields are in continuous mutual process.

Figure 18–1. Principles of homeodynamics. (*Adapted from Rogers, 1986, p. 6.*)

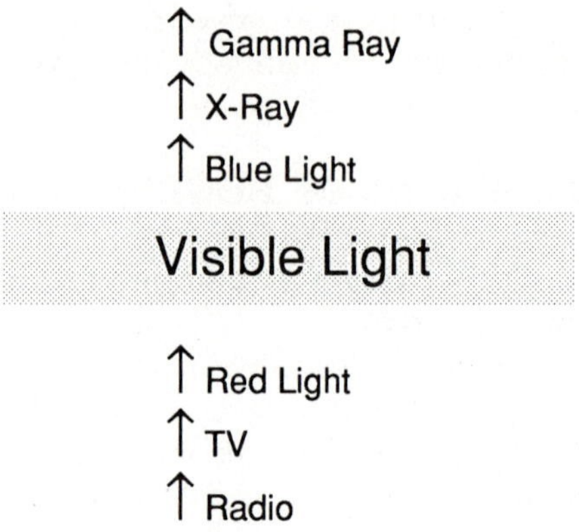

↑ Gamma Ray

↑ X-Ray

↑ Blue Light

Visible Light

↑ Red Light

↑ TV

Figure 18–2. Electromagnetic wave spectrum.   ↑ Radio

waves on the field pattern. Just as in observing an impressionistic painting, the close-up discloses small dots, whereas a more distant view exhibits a pattern that has shape and form. One energy field depicted in Figure 18–3 might be the human field. A second might be the environmental energy field.

The energy field is open, not relatively open with the environment. More is known about the human energy field than the environmental energy field. Nurses are the environmental energy field in the Science of Unitary Human Beings. When care is being planned in the science with the client, it is interpreted as patterning the environmental energy field.

This demands that we have an understanding of the four-dimensional relative space-time. Schematic representations of energy fields as in Figure 18–3 serve to illustrate clinical situations in which patients may be seeing loved ones who are not presently there, because their relative space-time, or their energy field, is not within a spectrum that the nurse may be able to perceive. Nevertheless, in delivering care, it is important to be cognizant of the patient's environment and relative space-time.

Figure 18–4 illustrates further facets of a person's relative space-time. Four-dimensionality is more than just the three dimensions of space and time.

● Energy Fields

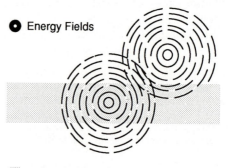

Figure 18–3. Energy fields and visible light.   Visible Light

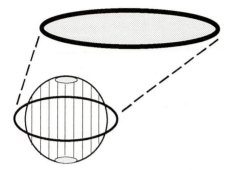

Figure 18-4. Schematic of two different relative space-times.

Schematically Figure 18–4 contrasts two different relative space-times: (1) an astronaut orbiting earth, where the time in orbit during each revolution to cross the globe is relatively short; and (2) where the time to encircle the same vast segments of earth on the ground, or even in a low-flying, slow plane like the Voyager, takes days rather than minutes.

The electromagnetic train, in proposed development, conceptualizes energy fields in different relative space-times. The train would travel coast-to-coast in a draft-free tunnel within 30 minutes. Outside, near the tunnel, the train and the passengers could not be perceived as it passed by at extraordinary speed. In the passenger compartments, people would converse and enjoy the exciting trip. Space-time would be distinctly different within and outside of the train, illustrating that the clock time is simply an artifact in a three-dimensional orientation of ourselves.

To illustrate that the relative space-time or the environment of an individual might be at a higher frequency, it can be surmised that persons sometimes are able to see ghosts, and perhaps unidentified flying objects, when their frequency slows sufficiently that they can be perceived within the visible light wave spectrum. Appreciably, this illustration can be likened to persons experiencing a different relative wave frequency who are dying, or in crisis, who are considered beyond our normal or average wave frequency.

When nurses provide care in the Rogerian framework it is important to comprehend that the nurse may not be patterning the environment of the patient or client, so much as the nurse's own physical environment. To insure that more is being accomplished than merely thinking the nurse is making a difference for the patient, strategies are adopted to assess the patient's environment. Such strategies include human field touch, and, with particular reference to this discourse, imaging. The Rogerian nurse continually appreciates that positions with reference to the patient are multidimensional.

In the Science of Unitary Human Beings *reality is the image*, or fantasy. In a three-dimensional sense such imaging is descriptive of thinking, whereas the *performance* is reality. Contrast the downhill skier anticipating success in the difficult gates before the performance; the golfer's perception of the arcing, long drive before the swing; and the diver's intricate midair positions conceived before the first springboard step. In a four-dimensional sense imaging is the reality. The performance that we see is the *manifestation* of that reality, much as the first light of a new galaxy first reaching the radiotelescopes of earth from the distant past of the universe. Similarly, in dying and then in death, the pattern transformation is a reality; physiological death is simply a manifestation of that reality.

Helicy, the third principle of the Rogerian Science of Unitary Human Beings, focuses on the nature of the human and environmental change. In part it is probabilistic and mulitdirectional. The pattern and organization of the field changes so that in pattern A, for example, the intent through imaging is not to return to a prior pattern, but to be innovative and influence a creative, probabilistic pattern such as B, which will never be the same. By way of differentiating between functioning in a three or four-dimensional sense in actual practice settings, the "Oh, he's just dying. Give him some morphine, or maybe a sedative, and those behaviors will go away." depicts three-dimensional practice. Making those behaviors go away with sedatives is an attempt to revert apparent abnormality or aberrations to a state that is considered more "healthy." In a four-dimensional sense the behaviors described in the introduction represent a transition in field pattern and organization from what is considered normality into a distinctly different zone, or a second pattern, B, in an effort to make a probabilistic change.

The standard methodology of nursing process can be used to develop care plans in the Rogerian framework. The terminology is slightly modified to match the framework. The goal is the manifestation of the four-dimensional reality, which is the new and innovative image. The indicants of whole human beings are assessed, not the body parts. The environmental field is patterned, which is the implementation strategy. The indicants of the whole person are evaluated, such as the person's manifestations of the field, as well as comfort levels, to determine successful repatterning. The goal of the person is quite important, because the goal is the image of living in relative space-time. The manifestation of the image is what is termed four-dimensional reality. Without determining the image, the nurse's care plan would be useless, while appearing to be a satisfactory bit of work.

CLINICAL VIGNETTES

Actual work experiences are helpful in portraying situations in which patterning nursing care can effect a pattern change in the human field. Moving through different relative space-times requires a pattern change, serving to aid and comfort the dying.

Case One. A 55-year-old woman entered a midwestern medical center, complaining of intermittent pain in both legs, for an elective aortofemoral bypass graft. Despite claudication in her legs, she was active, walking, and alert. Following surgery she experienced acute renal failure and adult respiratory distress syndrome. Her breathing was maintained by a mechanical ventilator. She became comatose during a seven-day effort by the medical team to wean her from the ventilator and reverse the renal failure. After five more days in the intensive care unit, she was transferred to an intermediate care unit, because the medical team could not do more assist her.

The registered nurses caring for the patient were operating from the medical model. They informed the patient's husband that there was nothing more the physicians could do, and that the husband should begin to accept this loss. They offered him help in his grief.

This author, together with nursing students capable of assisting in a critical care setting, took a fresh look at this situation. A goal of assisting the patient with a comfortable death was not established, even when, to many, it seemed there was little else to do.

We tried to envision the environment of this patient. What was her four-dimensional relative space-time? We knew it was not the unfamiliar critical care unit her body was in. We also knew she entered the center for elective surgery with the full intent of returning home. Her husband detailed what a usual day was like in her home as we tried to ascertain the nature of that environmental field. She read the newspaper each morning; tended her many flowers; and cared for the cat, among her many activities. With the information about her fundamental relative space-time, a care plan was developed to pattern the environmental field.

Through the principle of integrality, there is a continuous mutual process with the environment and the human energy field. As the patient was comatose, we could only focus on what we thought was her relative space-time and endeavor to keep that same pattern within the visible light wave spectrum. In contrast, repatterning to help move the patient outside that spectrum would assist her in dying.

With the assistance of the students and other nurses we proceeded to repattern the field in concert with what was thought to be her goal. The same local newspapers were read to her daily. Her flowers were discussed, as though they were in our visible light wave spectrum. At the same times as she was being turned and range of motion exercises were being applied to her body parts, we talked of her usual events in an average day. After two weeks she began moving her eyelids on command, and gradually appeared to be functional in our relative space-time.

Eventually she walked out of the hospital. The medical team could not ascribe a reason for her recovery. It has left a lasting impression that the energy field was repatterned to manifest an energy field transformation of life, which was her intended goal.

Nurses have a very powerful set of strategies. This clinical experience demonstrates how nurses can enhance the nature of living and dying processes. It is imperative that nurses practice within a framework in which probabilistic outcomes can be predicted. Otherwise, the learned profession is a practice without responsibility.

Case Two. This clinical experience exemplifies a person who was ready to make a transformation of the energy field in a situation that many would not consider timely.

A man in his 80s had patchy gangrene in his lower leg from small vessel occlusions. Physicians spent days trying to convince him of the need for an amputation. He perceived that a loss of a body part was a loss of life. He could not imagine what it would be like to live or function without his leg. He also reflected on the many achievements he had accomplished in a lifetime; everything he had wanted to do.

He wanted to see his family as often as possible. Often he seemingly aggravated nurses by insisting his daughter be called in to talk with him very late at night. The patient began having multiple manifestations of the daughter being present when she actually was not in the hospital.

We discussed his manifestations with the daughter. Using the Rogerian framework, he was helped to imagine a reality of comfort. He was then able to reminisce with the daughter and prepare himself for what he termed "passing on."

A week passed by; he was thoroughly prepared. Restating his aversion to an amputation, he confided in the author that not only did he not want to live without a body part, but he also did not want to involve his loved ones in such a loss. Without a distinct physiological reason, he died that night.

Case Three. A young couple, engaged to be married, were in an automobile accident. Comatose from severe head injuries, they were both in the critical care unit, yet some distance apart, separated by more than a partition. The young man was very unstable; the woman, not as seriously injured, had generally stable vital signs.

For several days, each time the man's vital signs shifted, her signs changed in a like manner. Nurses could sense something curious, yet the parallel changes in vital signs remained inexplicable. When he died, her vital signs were normal. She died three hours later.

Excepting that this couple had the same relative space-time, these concurrent events do not have a satisfactory explanation. Both cases two and three exhibit characteristics outside of, or apart from, the physical manifestations of what we know as our reality.

CARE PLAN DESIGN CONSIDERATIONS IN THE ROGERIAN FRAMEWORK

The care plan design is a conceptual method for organizing a powerful set of strategies to direct and repattern the environmental field, facilitating a comfortable transition for the dying patient.

To comprehend a patient's relative space-time and the nature of the patient's environment, together with the goal or image intended by the patient, an array of implements are useful to assess field pattern. These consist of human field motion; pain-comfort levels; the number and characteristics of multiple manifestations; a diagnosis, which may be a pattern transformation; breathing patterns and activity display, such as rapid-shallow breathing and fidgety, continuous movements; and the presence and character of out-of-body experiences. The latter two areas tend to be associated with crisis-related situations when dying is not imminent.

Dying persons often experience multiple manifestations, such as seeing and talking to loved ones who are not physically present or who may have even died. The loved ones are there in four-dimensional reality, the relative space-time having expanded for that person. The direction for the energy field is toward greater complexity and diversity, and an expanded field. These manifestations are an important experience in helping a person die, or remain alive.

In interventions, the nurse never directly interacts with the patient. Based upon the principle of integrality, there is continuous mutual process, so the nurse is the environment energy field and modifies the environmental energy field. Certain intervention strategies may be of considerable use.

Multiple manifestations should be encouraged by conversationally exploring their meaning to the patient. Patients will articulate who they are talking to, and what they are talking about, together with how this is important to them. It is comforting for the patient to have the opportunity to go through these experiences. Blue light in the environmental energy field does make a difference in pain and comfort (Ludomirski, 1984; McDonald, 1981). Imagery is quite helpful in visualizing a new environment as well as assisting a patient with repatterning. The image is the new pattern that one is trying to manifest, so the person actually has that perception of his or her energy field.

Evaluation may include the human field motion test, a semantic differential tool that measures high and low frequency. Levels of comfort are measured from experiential interactions with the patient. The evaluation should include the extent to which fear has been alleviated for the patient with multiple manifestations, and whether these have become meaningful and comfortable ones. This enables the patient to comprehend that the field is changing, that there is changing pattern and organization, and that there is changing pattern and organization, and that the transition is comforting to the dying.

Nurses have available these extraordinary, powerful strategies that remain virtually unexploited. With continued movement beyond the rendering of nursing care in a medical model into a true nursing model, nurses will be able to thoroughly enjoy the gratification to be obtained in directing and repatterning the environmental field.

REFERENCES

Ference, H. M. (1979). *The relationship of time experience, creativity traits, differentiation, and human field motion: An empirical investigation of Roger's correlates of synergistic human development.* New York University doctoral dissertation, University microfilms publication no. 80–10, 281.

Ludomirski-Kalmanson, B. (1984). *Relationship between the environmental energy wave frequency pattern manifest in red and blue light and human field motion in adults with visual sensory perception and total blindness.* New York University doctoral dissertation.

McDonald, S. F. (1981). *A study of the relationship between visible lightwaves and the experience of pain.* Detroit: Wayne State University doctoral dissertation. University microfilms publication no. 81–17, 084.

Rogers, M. E. (1970). *An introduction to the theoretical basis of nursing.* Philadelphia: Davis.

Rogers, M. E. (1986). Science of Unitary Human Beings. In V. M. Malinski (Ed.), *Explorations on Martha E. Rogers' Science of Unitary Human Beings.* East Norwalk, CT: Appleton-Century-Crofts.

19

A Nursing Theory of Power for Nursing Practice
Derivation from Rogers' Paradigm

Elizabeth Ann Manhart Barrett

Power is the capacity to participate knowingly in the nature of change characterizing the continuous patterning of the human and environmental fields as manifest by awareness, choices, freedom to act intentionally, and involvement in creating changes. Power, a continuous theme in the flow of life experiences, dynamically describes the way human beings interact with their environment to actualize some development potentials rather than others and thereby share in the creation of their human and environmental reality. Power is being aware of what one is choosing to do, feeling free to do it, and doing it intentionally. Depending on the nature of the awareness, the choices one makes, and the freedom to act intentionally, the range of situations in which one is involved in creating changes as well as the manner in which one knowingly participates vary. It is the interrelationship of the concepts of awareness, choices, freedom to act intentionally, and involvement in creating changes that constitutes power.

Background

Since the days of Nightingale, nursing has been concerned with the human-environment interaction. During the past decade nurse theorists seem to be evolving toward concensus that the human being viewed from a wholistic perspective is the phenomenon on which nursing focuses (Gordon et al., 1978). Rogers' (1976) Science of Unitary Human Beings distinguishes the phenomenon of concern to nursing as the unitary human being who as a whole cannot be understood as a summation of knowledge of the parts. If one accepts Rogers' thought, then other frameworks and their measurement tools have limited usefulness for answering questions about the unitary human being in continuous, mutual process with the environment.

207

In previous basic research, a new theory of power was derived from Rogers' paradigm, and an instrument designed to measure theoretically proposed field behavior was developed and tested (Barrett, 1984). Current efforts to translate this power theory to a model that can be applied and tested in nursing practice continues the search for answers to Rogers' question concerning the human being's capacity to participate in changing the pattern of the human and environmental fields (Rogers, 1970). Both the power theory and the "power as knowing participation in change test" (PKPCT) are useful in nursing practice and represent avenues for operationalizing nursing science.

The pervasiveness of power emphasizes the importance of a nursing theory of power that enhances the understanding of people and their world. By providing another parameter for understanding wholeness, power instruments can serve as assessment, planning, intervention, and evaluation tools. Clients, by participating in nurse-initiated teaching and counseling that encourages field exploration, can identify their power patterns and, in a knowing manner, change.

Derivation of the Power Model for Practice

Consistent with the Rogerian building blocks of energy fields, openness, pattern, and four-dimensionality, power was defined as the capacity to participate knowingly in the nature of change characterizing the continuous, innovative patterning of the human and environmental fields (Fig. 19–1). Like energy, power can be neither directly observed nor measured. However, the field behaviors that characterize power can be operationalized. These field manifestations of power are awareness, choices, freedom to act intentionally, and involvement in creating changes. The hypothesis that human field motion, and index of unitary human development (Ference, 1979), would be related to power, the capacity whereby humans knowingly participate in the nature of that development, was supported (Barrett, 1984). As a four-dimensional experience of position, human field motion is an indicator of the continuously moving position and flow of the human field pattern. Human field motion is an experience of process, change, and wave frequency that is postulated to transcend time and space as well as movement and stillness.

Hypothesis testing resulted in statistically significant canonical correlations which accounted for 40 percent of shared variance. Construct validity and reliability studies indicated adequate psychometric properties of the Barrett power tool (PKPCT) and the Ference human field motion test. As theoretically predicted, age, sex, and education were not important predictors of power or human field motion.

The Power Theory

Interest in power dates back 25 centuries (Dahl, 1968). According to Webster, *power* derives from a Latin word meaning "to be able" and means capacity, ability, being able to do something (Webster's Third New International Dic-

209

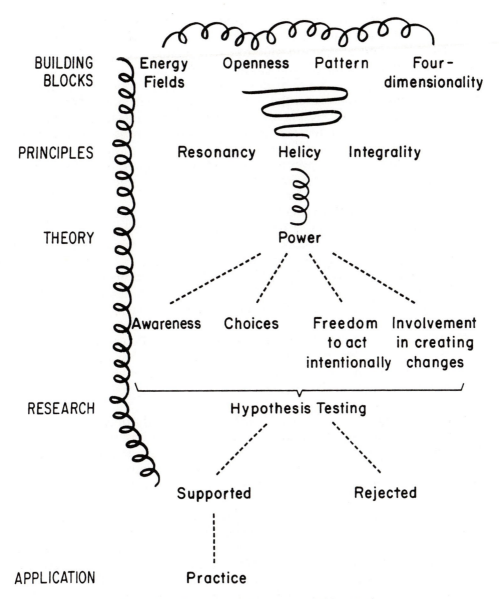

Figure 19-1. Derivation of the power model for practice.

tionary, 1976). To substantiate the proposition that this is a new power theory unique to nursing science required both differentiation from the perspective of other disciplines and connection with the existing literature to validate that the theory is descriptive of power and not another phenomenon.

Despite varying theoretical and operational definitions, the themes of change and causality permeate the power literature. This power theory connects with the literature in relation to change; it departs in relation to causality. Instead, the principle of helicy postulates that change is probabilistic, innovative, and creative (Rogers, 1970). The literature offers limited support for a noncausal conceptualization of power (McClusky, 1975; Olsen, 1970). Acausality allows for the idea of knowing participation. Power is an emergent manifestation of wholeness and reflects the mutually participatory process of the human and environmental fields. In accordance with the Science of Unitary Human Beings, power can be examined from the perspective of the human field, the environmental field, or the two fields in interaction. It is postulated that power is the same phenomenon regardless of the perspective from which one views it. Although there is a growing body of literature that is similar to this theoretical-empirical view of power, the perspective from Rogers' paradigm is different.

Life is a flow of experiences. To be alive is to experience this flow, and thus to move and to change. To change is to become irreversibly more complex, diverse, and differentiated in pattern (Rogers, 1976). Power, a continuous theme in the flow of life experiences, dynamically describes the way human beings interact with their environment to actualize some development potentials rather than others and thereby share in the creation of their human and environmental reality.

Rogers' notion of knowing participation is the central axiom in this theory. Power is being aware of what one is choosing to do, feeling free to do it, and doing it intentionally. Depending on the nature of the awareness, the choices one makes, and the freedom to act intentionally, the range of situations in which one is involved in creating changes as well as the manner in which one knowingly participates vary.

The intensity, frequency, and form in which power manifests itself differ. Outcomes are innovative, creative, and probablistic. Power as a natural potential of development is neither intrinsically good nor evil. However, the form in which power manifests can be labeled destructive or constructive, depending on the interpretation of the specific power form according to various value systems. The theory does not value the various power forms; it recognizes differences. Particular power forms that characterize how one knowingly participates are yet to be theoretically specified.

IMPLEMENTING THE POWER MODEL IN NURSING PRACTICE

This theory has potential for widespread use in nursing practice, because power is everywhere we find people in the world. If the professional nurse is knowledgeable in the Science of Unitary Human Beings and understands the power theory, then creative imagination and consistency with the assumptions of Rogers' system are all that are required to implement the model in practice. Use is not limited to a particular setting or client population.

The theory, like the Rogerian paradigm from which it derives, has meaning wherever and whenever nurses are caring for people, sick and well. The focus is on optimizing wellness rather than treatment of illness. Although the power theory itself does not vary, the way the professional nurse applies the theory does vary depending on the nature of the treatment setting, frequency and duration of nurse-client encounters, and the unique pattern manifestations of individual clients and families.

Application of the theory with critically ill clients will be different than with clients who are in crisis. Use of the theory in an outpatient or long-term facility will differ from use in a short-term acute care hospital setting. Likewise, within settings there will also be differences. Furthermore, the nurse will use the theory differently for the same client at different times.

Research has not yet described the fluctuation of the human field power pattern during illness, although the theory postulates that there is change within a more consistent range of variability. One might anticipate lower-frequency power manifestations during illness, although during developmental transition periods there may be pattern shifts to higher-frequency power. Such transition may or may not be associated with crisis or illness.

Every person and environment are not only unique, they are ever-changing. Whatever situation is presenting is continuously new and different. Hence the baccalaureate and higher-degree nurse draws on nursing science in innovative and novel ways. There are no rules of thumb.

Rogers' paradigm can also provide the theoretical basis for a nursing private practice in health patterning. In working with clients who experience difficulties in living, the power theory has been useful for clients whose presenting issues have included hopelessness with suicidal ideation, hypertension and obesity, drug and alcohol dependence, grief and loss, self-esteem issues, adolescent turmoil and other phase-of-life manifestations, cultural relocation trauma, career conflicts, marital discord, desire for major life style change, and a variety of other health problems (Barrett, 1985).

Lower-frequency power, although often initially not recognized or verbalized, is a common theme as it is in many conditions for which clients seek nursing services. Clients are often "stuck" and need help in accelerating field pattern diversity.

Although the mutual process interventions used in health patterning are not primarily didactic, clients learn to exercise options and maximize participation in their desired, probabilistic health outcomes. In the early phase of their care, most clients do not feel free to act intentionally and may resist acknowledging their involvement in creating changes. Power in some clients manifests in forms such as dependency and manipulation. The objective is not to set goals for clients, but rather to facilitate pattern evolution based on clients' awareness that they have the capacity to participate knowingly in change. When clients acknowledge that their involvement in the world is a mutual process and that they participate in a manner in which they choose, they often no longer need nursing counseling services.

It is crucially important to avoid orienting people to think themselves sick or helpless. Compliance is not encouraged and may represent lower-frequency power. For many people, noncompliance represents a more favorable prognosis, especially on a long-term basis. This phenomenon is indicative of the shift from illness care to the promotion of health and wellness movements that focus on the role that the individual plays in health and healing (Bezold, Carlson, & Peck, 1986). Many clients are shocked and sometimes dismayed when they discover that "Aha!" experience in relation to their own power. This framework presents clients with a different perspective for viewing their momentary, day-to-day and ongoing year-to-year existence in the world and facilitates identification and exploration of their human and environmental field patterns.

Now, shift gears and consider a different example of implementing the power model in nursing practice. This illustration is more structured, with particular emphasis on client teaching. The model is not, however, a recipe. There is no cookbook for the Science of Unitary Human Beings. Nevertheless, the ingredients are practical and can be creatively applied. Use of the power model represents one dimension of the nursing services. The power model, as it is envisioned, could be applied in various settings with different client populations.

To assist the nurse and the client in identifying the client's power pattern, clients are invited to complete the PKPCT. Informed consent includes a contract that findings from this confidential assessment will be discussed and that the information will be used by the nurse and client in planning and implementing nursing care. To prevent biased responses the nurse, prior to testing, does not use the word "power," nor does the word power appear on the instrument. Following instruction in semantic differential scaling technique, the client indicates the field behaviors that characterize his or her power as manifest by awareness, choices, freedom to act intentionally, and involvement in creating changes. One scale is repeated on each concept. This retest item allows the nurse to appraise consistency (reliability) of the client's response. Completion of the assessment requires about 15 minutes.

Initial assessment of the power pattern is determined by scores for each of the four power concepts, and the total of the concept scores is the overall power score. For each concept, each bipolar scale is scored from 1 to 7 depending on whether the rating is in the direction of lower or higher frequency. Using a scoring guide (Fig. 19–2A) where blue represents higher frequency and red represents lower frequency enables the nurse to accurately score the tool in less than ten minutes. The score range (Fig. 19–2B) is from 12 to 84 on each concept, with a total power score range from 48 to 336. These scores are recorded on the nursing history form and are used for mutual planning with clients.

Next, the nurse informally introduces the power theory to the client. About 30 minutes should be allowed for this dialogue. Teaching begins with the defini-

My involvement in creating change is:

	1	2	3	4	5	6	7	
constrained	1	2	3	4	5	6	7	FREE
ORDERLY	7	6	5	4	3	2	1	chaotic
unpleasant	1	2	3	4	5	6	7	PLEASANT
worthless	1	2	3	4	5	6	7	VALUABLE
IMPORTANT	7	6	5	4	3	2	1	unimportant
INTENTIONAL	7	6	5	4	3	2	1	unintentional
superficial	1	2	3	4	5	6	7	PROFOUND
following	1	2	3	4	5	6	7	LEADING
shrinking	1	2	3	4	5	6	7	EXPANDING
INFORMED	7	6	5	4	3	2	1	uninformed
SEEKING	7	6	5	4	3	2	1	avoiding
ASSERTIVE	7	6	5	4	3	2	1	timid
VALUABLE	7	6	5	4	3	2	1	worthless

Figure 19-2A. Scoring guide. Words typed in capitals represent higher-frequency end of scales. On a color chart, higher frequency is represented by blue and lower frequency is represented by red.

My involvement in creating change is:

	position		score
constrained	X	FREE	2
ORDERLY	X	chaotic	3
unpleasant	X	PLEASANT	3
worthless	X	VALUABLE	2
IMPORTANT	X	unimportant	5
INTENTIONAL	X	unintentional	4
superficial	X	profound	3
following	X	leading	5
shrinking	X	expanding	2
INFORMED	X	uninformed	5
SEEKING	X	avoiding	7
ASSERTIVE	X	timid	5
+ VALUABLE	X	worthless	
			46

Figure 19-2B. Example of scoring. Note that the retest item indicates the same response on the scale as when the item appeared earlier in the rating of this concept. The retest item is not included in the score. The correlation of retest items constitute a separate analysis design as an estimate of reliability.

tion of power and continues until the client understands the four major manifestations of power as representing dimensions of participating knowingly in change. The nurse emphasizes that involvement in creating changes seems to require the feeling of freedom to act intentionally, which in turn is related to the kinds of choices one makes. The nurse tells the client that awareness is important. Yet, more than awareness is necessary, because power also means involvement in creating change. The nurse views the client as a knowing, feeling, willing, and doing human being and shares this perception.

It is essential for the nurse to validate that the client's understanding of the power theory is accurate. Misinterpretations need to be clarified. The nurse can then begin to facilitate the client's application of the theory to his or her existence in the world. For example, a client's recent surgery and involvement in the recovery process provides meaningful opportunity for exploring the extent to which the client experienced freedom to act intentionally and whether the choices that were made were viewed as powerful or powerless. As the client begins to understand his or her power pattern, ideas for knowing participation in actualizing particular developmental potentials will emerge.

Scores on the power test are reviewed with the client as an integral aspect of the teaching. Scores are considered as a relative, tentative assessment of the dynamic nature of the client's field pattern in relation to power. It is important that the nurse suspend value judgments in relation to the client's scores. Clients are provided with information so that they are in an optimal position to participate knowingly in changing their power pattern, if they choose to do so.

The nurse's role in health education is that of advocate. Unquestioned compliance is antithetical to the Rogerian perspective. Optimal use of the power model involves the nurse as facilitator and the client as knowing participant. The client is assisted in exercising options in a manner that is consistent with his or her individually defined health practices. If the client so chooses, the nurse participates in optimizing movement toward the higher-frequency direction of the scales representing increased pattern diversity.

From this world view, there is no causality. Power is a noncausal phenomenon. It is helpful for clients to recognize that neither they nor the environment control anything. This awareness attenuates resentment and remorse while clarifying responsibility. Clients are comforted as they explore ideas of a mutual process where both fields continuously participate in change. The notion of *knowing* participation in that change constitutes the rationale for teaching clients the power theory.

During the nurse-client interchange, the nurse asks both "yes and no" and "open-ended" type questions. Questions that the client answers with a "yes" or "no" create an opportunity for the nurse to provide general knowledge from the Rogerian world view. Conversely, open-ended questions allow for clients to use this knowledge in exploring themselves and their world: "What kinds of choices are open to you now?" "How do you exercise your freedom to act intentionally in making decisions?" "In what ways are you involved in creating changes in your life?" Questions such as these lead to exploration of the pattern context of people's existence. Although choices may be quite limited, there is often a wider range of choices available than one recognizes. Awareness and freedom to act intentionally may be the knowing and willing that guide participation in choices and involvement in creating changes. Awareness, choices, freedom to act intentionally, and involvement in creating changes are manifestations of pattern that characterize the phenomenon of power.

The focus is not on giving information provided by a nursing expert but rather on eliciting client description, incorporating information concerned with the client's current dilemma, and helping people work through the complexities of their current situation. The nurse is aware that change is an ongoing process. It does not proceed on steady, linear increments; it flows in relativistic spurts (Ferguson, 1980). The nurse considers that it may be possible that the universe is "brought into being" in some strange sense by the participation of those who participate. "The vital act is the act of participation (Wheeler, Thorne, & Misner, 1973, p. 1273)."

Another modality that can assist in implementing the power model is creative imagery. A guided imagery exercise, recorded on audiotape, can provide continuity between visits. Of course, audiovisual materials are not a substitute for human caring and contact and for other nursing modalities such as therapeutic touch or exploring dreams as beyond-waking experiences. The purpose of the taped imagery exercise is to provide an imaginative experience of higher-frequency power within the context of continuous change. Words from the bipolar adjective scales provide direction. Clients are asked to imagine making choices that evolve from timid, unintentional, and constrained to assertive, intentional, and free. Awareness of themselves and their world can be profound, orderly, and expanding as opposed to superficial, chaotic, and shrinking. Clients are given the message that they are free to act intentionally and that they can consider this important and valuable rather than unimportant and worthless. Finally, clients are invited to explore their involvement in creating changes and to imagine their actions as evolving from avoiding, unpleasant, following, and uninformed, to involvement in creating changes that are seeking, pleasant, leading, and informed.

This exercise allows clients to envision optimal wellness and perhaps to experience the synergistic felt cognizant activity of power. Such a power encounter is an affective feeling of strength, a volitional and cognitive recognition of choices, and behavioral activity expressing freedom to act with intent in creating changes.

Nursing research needs to be a planned integral aspect of nursing practice. An experimental design could be used to study changes in health status in relation to intervention based on the power model. Changes in clients' power scores over time also need to be investigated.

SUMMARY

If we accept that nursing is a science, then nursing practice concerns use of the body of knowledge that constitutes nursing science. A basic foundation in general education with emphasis on the biological, physical, psychological, social, economic, and political sciences provides preparation for the study of nursing science. However, knowledge from other particulate sciences is insufficient for understanding the phenomenon of concern to nursing, people, and their world (Rogers, 1970). Knowledge of the open-ended science of unitary human beings allows for creative interventions that reflect the discipline of nursing. In situations where professionals are prepared with baccalaureate and higher degrees in nursing, nursing knowledge is required to provide nursing services.

The Science of Unitary Human Beings is complex and cannot be simplified by attempting to simplify unitary human beings. Nursing practice based on nursing science allows for application of principles, theories, and facts from that science allows for application of principles, theories, and facts from that science. This knowledge is different from the tools of practice used to implement knowledge.

Theory is practical and guides creative practice. What nurses do flows from what nurses know and reflects their commitments and personhood. Excellence in nursing practice integrates nursing's scientific knowledge with compassionate human caring for the benefit of people.

Rogers has challenged the thinking of the nursing community and provided a paradigm for nursing scholars to derive theories that can be tested through research and applied in practice. Theories derived from the science of unitary human beings are bridges from the science to practice. Research tests these bridges in the real world. During the next decades nursing scholars will continue to build and test bridges. Professional knowledge claims that allow for predictable, probabilistic outcomes in nursing practice have their roots in the science of the nursing discipline.

REFERENCES

Barrett, E. A. (1984). *An empirical investigation of Martha E. Rogers' principle of helicy: The relationship of human field motion and power.* Ann Arbor: Dissertation Abstracts International, *45*(2), no. 8406278.

Barrett, E. A. (1985, August 24). *A Rogerian power theory for nursing practice.* Paper presented at the Nursing Theory in Action International Congress. Boyle, Letourneau and Associates, Edmunton, Alberta.

Bezold, C., Carlson, R. J., & Peck, J. C. (1986). *The future of work and health.* Dover, MA: Auburn.

Dahl, R. A. (1968). In D. L. Sills (Ed.), *International encyclopedia of the social sciences* (Vol. 12). New York: MacMillan & The Free Press.

Ference, H. M. (1979). *The relationship field of time experience, creativity traits, differentiation, and human field motion: An empirical investigation of Rogers' correlates of synergistic human development.* Ann Arbor: Dissertation Abstracts International.

Ferguson, M. (1980). *The aquarian conspiracy.* Los Angeles: Tarcher.

Gordon, M., Johnson, D. E., King, I., et al. (1978). *Future directions in nursing theory* [Audiotape]. Chicago: Teach 'em.

McClusky, J. E. (1975, September). *Power without control: Exemplary power.* Paper presented at the annual meeting of the American Political Science Association, St. Louis.

Olsen, M. E. (1970). Power as a social process. In M. E. Olsen (Ed.), *Power in societies.* New York: Macmillan.

Rogers, M. E. (1970). *An introduction to the theoretical basis of nursing.* Philadelphia: Davis.

Rogers, M. E. (1976, Fall). *Lecture given during the course "Science of Man."* New York University, Division of Nursing.

Webster's Third New International Dictionary (4th ed.). (1976). Springfield, MA: Merriam.

Wheeler, J. A., Thorne, K. S., & Misner, C. (1973). *Gravitation.* San Francisco: Freeman.

Watson's Philosophy and Theory of Human Caring in Nursing[1,2]

Jean Watson

> Within man is the soul of the whole,
> which the wise silence, the universal
> beauty, to which every part and particle is
> equally related; the eternal ONE. And this
> deep power in which we exist and whose
> beatitude is all accessible to us, is not
> only self-sufficing and perfect in every
> hour, but the act of seeing and the thing
> seen, the seer and the spectacle, the
> subject and object are one.
>
> *Ralph Waldo Emerson, "The Oversoul."*

Ironically, Ralph Waldo Emerson's view of humanity and nature are timeless and consistent with new revelations in nursing and science. For example, if we are seeking greater depths and power in the nurse caring transactions, and trying to connect nursing care to health or healing and wholism, then concepts such as the presence of a higher spiritual element in humanity and the inseparable connections among persons and between person and nature are essential to the quest for a nobler view of person—beyond the person as patient or object and beyond the person as separate from nature.

The ideas and ideals associated with my philosophy and theory of human caring are concerned with spirit rather than matter, flux rather than form, inner knowledge and power, rather than circumstance; these are not final thoughts but my own reflective, evolving process of thinking. Such a reflective process, however, testifies to the existence of permanent values and moral imperatives that undergird nursing philosophy, theory, science, education, research, and practice. Embedded within these perspectives is a particular stance and starting point, along with a certain dynamic of human transactions that flow between

219

and connect the one-caring-for with the one-cared-for. Often this human caring transaction is not made articulate, nurtured, or acknowledged as foundational and basic to the professional nursing caring relational process and health and healing. Rather, much of nursing has focused on matter and form.

Thus, the essence, moral imperatives, and core of nursing have largely remained unarticulated, have been taken for granted, and have appeared seemingly invisible, resulting in their being largely disregarded and unattended in nursing education, research, and practice. However, the recent phenomena of nursing theory development, along with changing views of science and the universe, provide new opportunities to attend to human caring as a serious epistemic, ethical, and practical endeavor. Transforming perspectives on caring-person-nature-health-healing allows us to pursue notions of spirituality, holographic energy fields, and new ethics of caring. These activities are all part of a new dynamic and consciousness within nursing science and society at large.

The process of human-to-human caring illuminates the mystery of humanity and the possibility of a higher power, order, or energy in the universe that can be activated through the nurse caring process, that can in turn potentiate healing and health and facilitate self-knowledge, self-reverence, self-control, self-care, and possibly even self-healing. Such an orientation requires a certain assumption—that fundamental clinical, technological competencies and knowledge underpin nursing practice. The human caring process goes beyond the basic educational competency level toward higher-level, professional care processes that potentiate health and healing in persons and society.

Universal spirit and a central cosmic unity are identified as essential to human caring. A theory of caring must admit that parts are related to the whole. "A leaf, a drop, a crystal, a moment of time is related to the whole and partakes of the perfection of the whole (Emerson, 1982)." Each caring transaction is a microcosm that faithfully renders the likeness of the whole; yet each human caring moment creates a field of its own that is more complex than any one component. Thus, I am proposing ideas about how nursing connects with the whole and serves people, which in turn advances nursing's contributions to the welfare of humanity.

In this theory, human caring is viewed as the moral ideal of nursing. Human caring consists of transpersonal, intersubjective attempts (1) to protect, enhance, and preserve humanity by helping a person find meaning in illness, suffering, pain, and existence; and (2) to help another gain self-knowledge, self-control, and self-healing. As a result, a sense of inner harmony may be restored regardless of the external circumstances. The nurse is a coparticipant in a process in which the ideal of caring is the human-to-human, subject-to-subject transaction. Because of the human nature of nursing, its moral, spiritual, and metaphysical components cannot be ignored. These components are inherent in the nursing process, operating directly or indirectly, and therefore, need to be acknowledged as part of a theorist's world view, belief system, or philosophy. In a sense, the metaphysical beliefs of a nursing theory provide the passion for nursing and keep it alive, changing, and open to new possibilities.

This particular theory of nursing is therefore metaphysical, in that it goes beyond the rapidly emerging existential-phenomenological approaches in nursing, to perhaps a higher level of abstraction and sense of personhood, incorporating the concept of the soul and transcendence. The notion of a human soul is nothing new. It is, however, unusual to include it in a theory. In psychology and nursing, the concepts that are closest to soul and transcendence are self, inner self, I, me, and self-actualization. The bold attempt to acknowledge and try to incorporate a concept of the soul in a nursing theory is a reflection of an alternative position that nursing is now free to take. This position breaks from the traditional medical science model and also reflects a scientific paradigm shift. The evolution of the history and philosophy of science now allows some attention to metaphysical views that would have perhaps been unacceptable at an earlier point in nursing science.

SCIENCE AND DISCIPLINE OF NURSING

Nursing in this context may be defined as a human science of health-illness-healing experiences that are mediated by professional, personal, scientific, aesthetic, and ethical human care transactions. Such a view not only requires the nurse to be a scientist, scholar, and clinician but also a humanitarian and moral agent who is engaged as a coparticipant in the human care transactions. This science leans toward employing qualitative theories and research methods, such as existential-phenomenology, literary introspection, case studies, philosophical-historical work, and other approaches that allow a close and systematic observation of one's own experience, and that seek to disclose and elucidate the lived world of health-illness-healing experience and the phenomena of human caring.

Because nursing involves intersubjective caring, the nursing process becomes transpersonal and metaphysical. When these aspects of nursing are acknowledged and incorporated into our science, then nursing can cultivate a fuller access to the intuitive, aesthetic, quasirational modes of thought, feeling, and action. Thus, there can be greater use of our geist or spirit (higher sense of self) in relating to others in a way that rational, Western scientific culture often inhibits.

This position does not discount scientific method or Western thought; rather it seeks to elucidate and acknowledge other dimensions—dimensions that are important to the understanding of the idea of the person, nursing, human care, and healing processes in health and illness.

ASSUMPTIONS RELATED TO HUMAN CARING
VALUES IN NURSING (Watson, 1985, pp. 32–33):

1. Care and love are the most universal, the most tremendous, and the most mysterious of cosmic forces: They comprise the primal and universal psychic energy (De Chardin, 1967, pp. 7–8).

2. Often these needs are overlooked; or we know people need each other in loving and caring ways, but often we do not behave well toward each other. If our humanness is to survive, however, we need to become more caring and loving to nourish our humanity and evolve as a civilization and live together (De Chardin, 1967, pp. 7–8).

3. Because nursing is a caring profession, its ability to sustain its caring ideal and ideology in practice will affect the human development of civilization and determine nursing's contribution to society.

4. As a beginning we have to impose our own will to care and love upon our own behavior and not on others. It is necessary to treat oneself with gentleness and dignity before being able to respect and care for others with gentleness and dignity (De Chardin, 1967, pp. 7–8).

5. Nursing has always held a human-care and caring stance in regard to people with health-illness concerns.

6. Caring is the essence of nursing and the most central and unifying focus for nursing practice (Leininger, 1981).

7. Human care, at the individual and group level, has received less and less emphasis in the health care delivery system.

8. Caring values of nurses and nursing have been submerged. Nursing and society are therefore in a critical situation today in sustaining human care ideals and a caring ideology in practice. The human care role is threatened by increased medical technology and bureaucratic-managerial institutional constraints in a nuclear-age society. At the same time there has been a proliferation of curing and radical treatment cure techniques often without regard to costs.

9. Preservation and advancement of human care as both an epistemic and clinical endeavor is a significant issue for nursing today and in the future.

10. Human care can be effectively demonstrated and practiced only interpersonally. The intersubjective human process keeps alive a common sense of humanity; it teaches us how to be human by identifying ourselves with others, whereby the humanity of one is reflected in the other.

11. Nursing's social, moral, and scientific contributions to humankind and society lie in its commitment to human care ideals in theory, practice, and research.

WATSON'S VALUE SYSTEM

The value system set forth within the philosophy and theory of human caring consists of values associated with deep respect for the wonders and mysteries of life and an acknowledgment of a spiritual dimension to life and of the internal power of the human caring and healing process. Human care requires high regard and reverence for a person and human life, nonpaternalistic values that are related to human autonomy, and freedom of choice. There is a high value on the subjective life-world of the person experiencing health-illness-healing conditions. An emphasis is placed upon helping a person gain more self-knowledge, self-control, and readiness for self-healing, regardless of the external health condition. The nurse is viewed as a coparticipant in the human care process. Therefore, a high value is placed on the relational processes between the nurse and the person.

This value system is blended with Watson's ten carative factors, (Watson, 1979), such as humanistic altruism, sensitivity to oneself and others, and love for and trust of life and other humans and our own inner power. Underlying this value system is a call for a revaluing of the inner healing power of humans and the human caring process in theory, practice, and science.

THE BASIC PHILOSOPHY AND THEORY OF CARING

To provide a condensed version of my ideas for this theory book, I have drawn from key sections of my two earlier works (Watson, 1979, 1985). My theory of human caring begins with by philosophical and metaphysical view of personhood and human existence. What is essential in human existence is that the human has transcended nature-yet remains a part of it. The human can progress to higher levels of consciousness by finding meaning and harmony in existence through the use of the mind.

My conception of life and personhood is based on the notion that one's soul possesses a body that is not confined by objective space and time. The world as experienced is not distinguished by external and internal notions of time and space, but is shaped by its own sense of time and space, which is unconstrained by linearity. Notions of personhood, then, transcend the here and now, and acknowledge the capacity to coexist with past, present, and future all at once. This view has a great deal of respect and awe for the concept of a human soul (spirit, geist, or higher sense of self) that is greater than the physical, mental, and emotional existence of a person at any given time. The individual spirit of a person or of collective humanity may continue to exist throughout time, keeping alive a higher sense of humankind. Although a body may be diseased, infirm, or die, the soul or spirit lives on. However, the soul can be underdeveloped or dormant and in need of reawakening.

According to Jung (1968):

People will do anything, no matter how absurd, in order to avoid facing their own souls. They will practice yoga and all its exercises, observe a strict regime of diet, learn theosophy by heart, or mechanically repeat mystic texts from the literature of the whole world—all because they cannot get on with themselves and have not the slightest faith that anything useful could ever come out of their own souls. (pp. 99–101)

The belief that a person possesses a soul is to be regarded with the deepest respect, dignity, mystery, and awe because of the continuing, yet unknown, journey throughout time and space—infinite and eternal. The soul, then, exists for something larger, greater, and more powerful than physical life as we know it and could know it for time past, time present, and time future. This concept of the soul refers to the essence of the person, which possesses a greater sense of self-awareness, a higher degree of consciousness, an inner strength, and a power that can expand human capacities and allow a person to transcend his or her usual self. From a higher sense of consciousness one can more fully access the intuitive. Such access sometimes allows uncanny, mystical, or miraculous experiences, modes of thought, feelings, and actions—experiences that our rational, scientific cultures inhibit. One's ability to transcend space and time occurs in a similar manner through one's mind, imagination, and emotions. Our bodies may be physically present in a given location or situation, but our minds and related feelings may be located elsewhere.

The assumptions underlying this view of human life is that each of us is a magnificent spiritual being who has often been undernourished and reduced to a physical, materialistic being. We know both rationally and intuitively, however, that our human predicament may not be related to the external, physical world as much as to our inner world-as-lived. Awareness of oneself as a spiritual being opens up infinite possibilities.

Throughout time, poets, sages, and philosophers have advocated the self-knowledge, self-reverence, and self-control that comes through attention to the inner, spiritual life. The notion of a spiritual self and inner power requires a rethinking of our views of people, existence, and the world. The idea of transcendence is fairly alien to the Western world with its belief in a mind-body schism. Yet since ancient time, philosophers, and poets have written about self-transcendence, higher consciousness, over-soul, spiritual experience, mystical experiences, and so on.

Transcendence provides opportunities to grow and become more fully human. Inherent in these ideas is the notion of turning inward and regarding oneself and others with reverence and dignity, as spiritual beings capable of contributing to their own health and healing as well as the spiritual evolution of self and civilization.

Life

Human life is defined as being-in-the-world, which is continuous in time and space. This approach incorporates scientific views along with metaphysics, aesthetics, and a belief in the goodness of humankind. From these values and beliefs about life and personhood, it follows that access to the higher sense of self comes more readily through the human emotions, the mind, and the subjective world.

The locus of human existence is experience. The person exists as a living, growing gestalt, possessing three spheres of being—mind, body, and soul—that are influenced by the concept of self. The mind and the emotions are the starting point, the focal point, and the point of access to the subjective world. The self is the subjective center that lives within the whole of body, thoughts, sensations, desires, memories, life history, and so forth. The person is neither simply an organism, nor simply spiritual. Although a person is embodied in experience, in nature, and in the physical world, a person can also transcend the physical world by controlling it, subduing it, changing it, or living in harmony with it.

In developing a theory of nursing, it is helpful to clarify one's philosophical values and views of human life because they give direction and meaning to nursing, the human caring process, and other components of the nursing theory.

Human Caring Process

The human caring process in nursing is a special, delicate gift to be cherished. The shared moment of a caring transaction has the potential to transcend conventional notions of the physical world.

Each participant brings to the present moment a unique causal past.[3] Each experiential moment of "now" becomes incorporated into the causal past and helps to direct the future. All three phases of time (past, present, and future) can be, and usually are, operating in the subjective world. The inner world can transcend time through introspection, creative imagination, meditation, visualization, self-projection, dreaming, fantasizing, and perhaps other unconscious and possibly supraconscious processes not yet fully explored. Watson's ten carative factors (described later in the chapter) provide the epistemic dimensions for nursing science and the human caring process.

Illness

Illness is not necessarily disease. Illness is disharmony within a person's inner self. Illness may be a disease, for example, of the mind, body, or soul, either consciously or unconsciously. In a situation where one's "I" is separated from one's "me," the self is separated from the self. Illness connotes a felt incongruence between the self as perceived and the self as experienced.

A troubled inner self can lead to dis-ease, and dis-ease can result in pathology. Specific experiences (such as developmental conflicts, inner suffering, guilt, self-blame, despair, loss and grief, lack of self-love, and general or specific stress) can lead to dis-ease and result in pathology and disease. Disease itself in turn creates more disharmony.

Health

Health refers to unity and harmony within the mind, body, and soul—harmony between self and others and between self and nature. Health is also associated with the degree of congruence between the self as perceived and the self as experienced. Such a view of health focuses on the whole individual including physical, social, aesthetic, and moral realms instead of just certain aspects of human behavior and physiology. Such a view is referred to as an *eudaimonistic* model of health (Smith, 1983). In summary:

- I = Me - Health (harmony with world and open to increased diversity)[4]
- I ≠ Me - Dis-ease (in varying degrees and making the person less open to increased diversity). When I ≠ me for continuous periods of time, disease may be present.

Goal

The proposed goal of nursing is to help persons gain a higher degree of harmony within the mind, body, and soul, which generates self-knowledge, self-reverence, self-healing, and self-care processes while allowing increasing diversity. The nurse pursues this goal through the human caring process and transactions by responding to the person's subjective world in such a way that individuals can find meaning in their existence through exploring the meaning of their disharmony, suffering, and turmoil. This exploration promotes self-knowledge, self-control, self-love, choice, and self-determination in relation to health, illness, treatment, and healing decisions. The general goal is mental-spiritual growth for self and others as well as discovering inner power and self-control through caring. Achieving this goal can potentiate health, healing, and transcendence.

Agent of Change

In the theory of caring, the agent of change is not the physician, nurse, medication, treatment, or technology per se, but the person's internal, mental-spiritual mechanisms that allow the self to be healed. This self-healing can occur through various internal or external means. Such a view holds a commitment to a particular end beyond disease or pathology, to a moral ideal toward inner power of the self, choice, inner healing potential, and preservation of harmony with mind-body-soul. These actions, in turn, seek to maintain human dignity and integrity.

WATSON'S TEN CARATIVE FACTORS[5]

The carative factors are the factors the nurse uses for the delivery of health care. The carative factors provide a tentative epistemological foundation for the study and practice of human caring that nursing encompasses. The cognitive factors and the human process of caring need to be further delineated, expanded, and researched. Nevertheless, they provide the structure that forms the whole of nursing.

The carative factors in this theory involve the human caring process with full participation of the nurse and the person. Human care requires: (1) knowledge of human behavior and human responses to actual or potential health problems (ANA, 1980); (2) knowledge and understanding of individual needs; (3) knowledge of how to respond to others' needs; (4) knowledge of our strengths and limitations; (5) knowledge of the meaning of the situation for the person; and (6) knowledge of how to comfort, offer compassion and empathy. Human care also requires enabling actions—that is, actions that allow another to solve problems, grow, and transcend the here and now, actions that are related to general and specific knowledge of caring and human responses.

Efforts to establish or contribute to the knowledge of human care may be futile unless they contribute to a philosophy of actions. Gaut (1983) reported that caring action must be judged solely on the welfare of the person being cared for. She further indicated that the necessary and sufficient conditions for caring include:

1. Awareness and knowledge about one's need for care.
2. An invitation to act, and actions based on knowledge.
3. A positive change as a result of caring, judged solely on the basis of the welfare of others. There must be also be an underlying value and moral commitment to care, along with a will to care.

Thus, the identified carative factors related to the human care process require an intention, caring values, knowledge, a will, a relationship, and actions. This process entails a commitment to caring as a moral ideal directed toward the preservation of individual dignity and humanity. The process affirms the subjectivity of persons and leads to positive change for the welfare of others, while allowing the nurse to benefit and grow.

The ten primary carative factors (Watson, 1979) that form a structure for studying and understanding the caring process in nursing are

1. Formation of a humanistic-altruistic system of values.
2. Nurturing of faith and hope.
3. Cultivation of sensitivity to one's self and others.
4. Development of a helping-trusting, human caring relationship.
5. Promotion and acceptance of the expression of positive and negative feelings.

6. Use of creative problem-solving processes.
7. Promotion of transpersonal teaching-learning.
8. Provision for a supportive, protective, or corrective mental, physical, sociocultural, and spiritual environment.
9. Assistance with gratification of human needs.
10. Allowance for existential-phenomenological-spiritual forces.

The following sections provide a brief description of each carative factor.

The Formation of a Humanistic-Altruistic System of Values

Caring must be grounded on a set of universal humanistic and altruistic values. Humanistic values include kindness, empathy, concern, and love for others. They derive from childhood experiences and are enhanced by beliefs, cultures, and art. Altruistic values arise from commitment to and satisfaction from receiving through giving. They bring meaning to one's life through relationships with other people. (This does not mean sacrificial and self-denying attitudes and behaviors; rather, this refers to the extension of self resulting from maturity.) A humanistic-altruistic value system can also be developed through consciousness raising—a close examination of one's views, beliefs, and values. Humanistic-altruistic feelings and acts provide the basis of human caring and promote the best professional care, and as such, constitute the first and most basic factor for the science of caring.

Nurturing of Faith and Hope

The history of medicine is filled with documentation of the importance of a person's belief in faith and hope. For example, Hippocrates thought that an ill person's mind and soul should be inspired before one's illness was treated. In many other examples, medicine itself was secondary to magic, incantations, spells, and prayers. In this carative factor, patients' beliefs are encouraged and respected as significant influences in promoting and maintaining health. Regardless of what scientific regimen is required for the medical care of a person, the nurse should nurture faith and hope in one's self and one's potential, and the one cared for. Even when there is nothing left to do medically, the nurse can nurture a patient's faith and hope in something or someone beyond his or her self.

Cultivation of Sensitivity to One's Self and Others

To be human is to feel. All too often people allow themselves to think their thoughts but not to feel their feelings. The only way to develop sensitivity to one's self and to others is to recognize and feel one's feelings.

The development of self and the nurturing of judgment, taste, values, and sensitivity in human relationships evolve from emotional states. The development of feelings is encouraged by the humanities and compassionate life experiences.

Sensitivity to self is the recognition and acknowledgment of feelings—painful as well as happy ones. It is cultivated by looking into oneself and a willingness to explore one's own feelings. People who are not sensitive to and repress their own feelings may be unable to allow others to express and explore their feelings. Sensitivity to self not only leads to self-acceptance and psychological growth, but to sensitivity and acceptance of others.

Nurses who are sensitive to others are better able to learn about another's view of the world which, subsequently, increases concern for others' comfort, recovery, and wellness. Nurses who recognize and use their sensitivity promote self-development and self-actualization, and are able to encourage the same growth in others. Without this factor, nursing care would fail.

Development of a Helping-Trusting, Human Caring Relationship

The human caring relationship is a transpersonal one, in that it connotes a special kind of relationship: a reunion with another person, and a high regard for the whole person and their being-in-the-world. In the transpersonal human caring relationship, the nurse enters into the experience of another person, and another can enter into the nurse's experiences. It is an *ideal* of intersubjectivity in which both persons are involved. It is an *art* in which the nurse forms a union with another on a level that transcends the physical, freeing both from their separation and isolation. (This union of feelings can potentiate self-healing, discovery, and finding the meaning of existence.) It is a *moral-ideal* in which the nurse has the utmost concern for human dignity and preservation of humanity.

A helping-trusting human caring relationship evolves from a certain quality of communication. A person who feels that a nurse really cares about and really sees his or her individual needs and concerns is likely to establish trust in the nurse and see the nurse as helping. In addition to the previous carative factors, congruence, empathy, nonpossessive warmth, and attention to the principles of good communication are necessary nurse qualities and skills. The potential for facilitating health-seeking behaviors reside in this factor; this factor is foundational to transpersonal caring, which is discussed in a later section.

Promotion and Acceptance of the Expression of Positive and Negative Feelings

Because feelings alter thoughts, behavior, and experience, they need to be acknowledged and considered in the human caring process. A focus on feelings and the "nonrational" emotional aspects of an event is necessary for nurses engaged in the human caring process. (The caring relationship can move to a deeper, more honest level if the nurse acts on this carative factor.) Therefore, the acceptance and promotion of the expression of positive and negative feelings has been identified as a major carative factor, and part of nursing's core and the science of caring.

Use of Creative Problem-Solving Processes

Professional nursing employs the nursing process, which is a creative problem-solving method to help with decision making in all nursing situations. A creative problem-solving approach is the nurse's valuable tool for "pulling it all together." It is the focus of the nurse's orientation for practicing the art and science of caring.

Within the nursing processes of assessing, planning, intervening, and evaluating are the full use of self and all domains of knowledge, including empirical, aesthetic, intuitive, affective, and ethical knowledge. All knowledge is valuable and accessed within the caring process. The process is not strictly scientific or empirically based but calls on the creative imagination as well as a systematic problem-solving approach.

Promotion of Transpersonal Teaching-Learning

Nurses have long been clearer about their teaching role than the transpersonal learning that is critical in a caring relationship. Health teaching has always been one of nursing's main functions. Although the imparting of information is important in reducing stress and anxiety, the dialectic, transpersonal learning aspects of relationships are often overlooked. Learning is more than the receiving of information. It also depends on the nurse's ability to accurately assess another's perceptions, feelings, concerns, and understandings. The caring process requires openness to others' knowledge and creative problem-solving abilities and ideas.

In this carative factor, six phases are outlined that facilitate data gathering, decision making, and feedback. These phases include scanning, formulating, appraising, planning, implementing, and evaluating—all of which focus on the nurse as coparticipant and on *learning* (because without learning, there has been no teaching). The caring process draws on the transaction between the nurse and the one cared for. Both can be active coparticipants in the teaching-learning process.

Provision for a Supportive, Protective, or Corrective Mental, Physical, Sociocultural, and Spiritual Environment

The purpose of providing a supportive, protective, or corrective environment is quality health care. The factors relevant to providing such care are:

1. Comfort—such as removing noxious stimuli and maximizing choices and self-control.
2. Privacy—such as ensuring that one has time alone, and respecting the need for quiet times.
3. Safety—such as eliminating existing or potential hazards and explaining safety precautions.
4. Clean aesthetic surroundings—such as a clean, attractive environment incorporating art, music, and poetry according to one's needs and meaning.

The goal of this carative factor is to strengthen self-concept and self-worth through holistic attention to physical, mental, sociocultural, and spiritual aspects of the health-healing environment.

Assistance with Gratification of Human Needs

Assistance with the gratification of human needs is important to nursing's role of helping persons in their daily activities as well as facilitating their growth and development. A need is generally defined as a requirement of a person which, if supplied, relieves or diminishes distress or improves well-being. The ordering of needs believed to be most relevant to nursing as part of the human caring process are: survival (food and fluid, elimination, ventilation); functional (activity-inactivity, sexuality); integrative (achievement, affiliation); and growth-seeking (inter- and intrapersonal, spiritual development, and self-actualization). All of these needs operate interdependently, and demand that the nurse respond to the other as a unique individual, allowing the one cared for to assist in the identification of the most important needs. Although self-actualization is considered to be the highest-order need, all needs are equally important in nursing care and must be equally valued if knowledgeable caring is to promote health, growth, and harmony.

Allowance for Existential-Phenomenological-Spiritual Forces

Existential, phenomenological, and spiritual forces are closely related in that they all support a subjective appreciation of the inner world of the experiencing person and the meaning he or she finds in life. The incorporation of these forces into the science of caring is more of a philosophical approach to viewing the human predicament than any sort of technique. The clinical application of existential concepts is based on the assumption that each person must find his or her own meaning and solution to the problems of existence—separateness, aloneness, and death. A phenomenological orientation to nursing emphasizes understanding people from their frame of reference, from their own phenomenal world. The spiritual dimension refers to the inner self or essence, which allows for the development of a higher degree of consciousness and inner strength and transcendence of the usual self. The combination of the existential phenomenological and spiritual forces often help the nurse to understand another's internal human predicament. Attention to them as a carative factor not only helps the one cared for to transcend personal struggles and achieve meaning, but this factor brings focus and meaning to the nurse's personal and professional life as well. Awareness of oneself and others as existential-phenomenological and spiritual beings opens up infinite possibilities for growth, both intrapersonal and transpersonal.

All of these carative factors become actualized in the moment-to-moment human caring process in which the nurse is "being-with" the other person (whether administering an emergency intravenous treatment to a critical care patient or changing the linen of an unconscious patient). Although these views are ideals, different nurses and different moments allow higher levels of caring. The more one strives toward an intersubjective transaction, the more the caring process contributes directly to the preservation of the humanity of both self and other. The degree of caring is influenced by multiple, complex forces. The more human caring is actualized as an intersubjective moral ideal in each moment-to-moment caring occasion, the more potential the caring holds for human health goals to be met through finding meaning in one's own existence, discovering one's own inner power and control, and potentiating instances of transcendence and self-healing.

Finally, my theory of human caring proposes that nursing, individually and collectively, contributing to the preservation of humanity in an individual and society: The moral ideals and intersubjective human caring processes proposed here for nursing foster the spiritual evolution of humankind.

TRANSPERSONAL CARING[6]

Transpersonal human care and caring transactions incorporate all the carative factors—those scientific, professional, ethical, yet aesthetic, creative, and personalized care giving-receiving behaviors and responses that occur between two people (the nurse and the one cared for). Such transactions allow for contact between the subjective world of persons through physical, mental, or spiritual routes, or some combination. Transpersonal caring is the full actualization of the carative factors in a human-to-human transaction. The human care transactions include the nurse's unique use of self through movements, senses, touching, sounds, words, colors, and forms in which the nurse transmits and reflects the person's condition back to him or her. The nurse does this in such a way that allows for the release and flow of intersubjective feelings and thoughts, and pent-up energy. Such a transaction, in turn, helps to restore inner harmony, self-knowledge, and control, while also contributing to the nurse and the one cared for finding meaning in the experience. However, the origin of the meaning for both resides *within* rather than existing *without*. In this process the nurse is also attending to the dignity of the person as an important end in and of itself. A person has dignity when enabled to find one's own meaning and to create one's own integrity (Gadow, 1984).

Contact with the subjective world has the potential to go beyond bodily or mental-emotional contact or interaction, and to reach out and touch the higher, spiritual sense of self, or the soul. As such, transpersonal human care occurs in an I-Thou relationship. It can release inner power and strength and help the person gain a sense of harmony within, with others, and with nature; this contact and process in turn generates and potentiates the self-healing processes.

The two individuals (the nurse and the one cared for) in a caring transaction are both in a process of being and becoming. Both individuals bring to the relationship a unique life history and phenomenal field; both are influenced and affected by the nature of the transaction, which in turn becomes part of the life history of each person. In this sense of a caring transaction, caring is both a moral ideal and a caring process, rather than an interpersonal technique. It entails a commitment to a particular goal of protection, enhancement, and preservation of the person's humanity. This in turn helps to restore dignity, inner harmony, and potential healing.

An Event or Actual Caring Occasion

Two persons (the nurse and another) together with their unique life histories and phenomenal fields in a human care transaction comprise an event.[7] An event, such as an actual occasion of human caring, is a focal point in space and time from which experience and perception are taking place, but the actual occasion of caring has a field of its own that is greater than the occasion itself. As such, the process can go beyond itself, yet arise from aspects of itself that become part of the life history of each person, as well as part of some larger, deeper, complex pattern of life.

An actual caring occasion involves action and choice both by the nurse and the individual. The moment of coming together in a caring occasion presents the two persons with the opportunity to decide how to be in the relationship and what to do with the moment. Whatever is decided involves one manner and not another. If the caring occasion is indeed transpersonal and allows for the presence of the geist or spirit of both, then the event expands the limits of openness and has the ability to expand the human capacities. It thereby increases the range of certain events that could occur in space and time at the moment as well as in the future. The moment of the caring occasion becomes part of the past life history of both persons and presents both with new opportunities. Such an ideal of intersubjectivity between the nurse and patient is based upon a belief that we learn from one another how to be human by identifying ourselves with others or recognizing their dilemmas in our own. What we all gain from it is self-knowledge. The self we learn about or discover is every self: it is universal—the human self. We learn to recognize ourselves in others. The comparison shows us what we are, what humanness is, in general, and in particular.

The intersubjectivity keeps alive our common humanity and avoids reducing the human being to an object.

In transpersonal human caring, the nurse can enter into the experience of another person, and another can enter into the nurse's experience. The ideal of transpersonal caring is an ideal of intersubjectivity in which both persons are involved. This means that the value and views of the nurse, though not decisive, are potentially as relevant as those of the one cared for. A refusal to allow the nurse's subjectivity to be engaged by a another is, in effect, a refusal to recognize the validity of the other's subjectivity. The alternative to caring as intersubjectivity is not simply the reduction of the one cared for to an object, but the reduction of the nurse to that level as well (Gadow, 1984).

When including the metaphysical components of the spiritual experience in the intersubjective caring occasion, the nurse is allowed to experience and explain things, yet does not have to concern him- or herself with full prediction; he or she is able, however, to include the mysteries of life and unknowns yet to be discovered.

An actual caring occasion is located not only in the simple physical instance of a given moment, but the event or experience has internal relations to other objects and subjects in the phenomenal field plus internal subjective relations between the past, present, and imagined future for each person and for the whole. An actual caring occasion can be present in the life of both the nurse and the other person beyond the physical instance of the given point in time. Past, present, and future instance merge.

The actual caring occasion in a presenting moment has the potential to influence both the nurse and the other in the future. The caring occasion then becomes part of the subjective, lived reality and the life history and mystery of both. Both are coparticipants in becoming in the now and the future, and both are part of some larger, deeper, complex pattern of life.

SUMMARY

Transpersonal caring in nursing is a moral ideal, a means of communication and intersubjective contact through the coparticipation of one's entire self. Transpersonal caring, therefore, is a means of progress where an individual moves toward a higher sense of self and harmony with his or her mind, body, and soul; with self and others; and with self and nature.

Transpersonal caring allows humanity collectively to move towards greater harmony, spiritual evolution, and perfection. The idea and ideals associated with transpersonal nursing can accommodate art, science, ethics, and spirituality. With its attention to the human process, caring and care activity, the intersubjective feelings, and the individuality of each nurse and recipient of care, the process allows for combinations of expressions of human caring in different moments and contexts, and with different outcomes, that can never be fully explained or predicted.

The emphasis on the human component of caring is consistent with my view of the person. Transpersonal caring not only allows for release of emotions and the evolution of the person's spiritual self or soul, but it promotes congruence between the person's perception and experience, and promotes self as is and ideal self, and harmony within (the person's mind, body, and soul), with others and with nature. The process allows the nurse to reflect the self back upon the self. It can potentiate healing regardless of external circumstances.

The context for viewing the person and the nurse in the theory of transpersonal caring is in the moment-to-moment human encounters. The coming together of the two—the one giving care and the one being cared for— comprise an event. The event connotes an actual caring occasion in which intersubjective caring transactions occur.

Once the person moves toward a higher sense of self with increased harmony, then one's own self-healing processes and capacity for finding meaning in existence are available. One can then better choose between health and illness and inner healing, regardless of any disease or bodily or human condition.

The ideas expressed here allow nurses to call on the inner depth of their own humanness, consciousness, and personal creativity as they realize the conditions of a person's inner self and their own. The intersubjective process of human caring is infinite and will continue to expand as knowledge and approaches expand and as humanity evolves.

ENDNOTES

1. Special recognition and thanks to Marilyn Stiles, R.N., M.S., doctoral candidate and research assistant at the University of Colorado School of Nursing, who assisted with editing and bibliographic reference citations throughout.
2. This chapter draws heavily from two earlier works (Watson, 1979, 1985).
3. Causal past derives from Whitehead (1953) and involves collective but unique past experiences and events that each person brings to the present moment. Each person's causal past and presentational immediacy has the potential to influence the future.
4. Acknowledgments to Glenn Webster for the notion of increasing diversity.
5. Please see Watson (1979) for a more complete description of each carative factor.
6. Transpersonal refers to an intersubjective human-to-human relationship in which the person of the nurse affects and is affected by the person of the other. Both are fully present in the moment and feel a union with the other. They share a phenomenal field that becomes part of the life history of both and both are coparticipants in becoming in the now and in the future. Such an ideal of caring entails an ideal of intersubjectivity, in which both persons are involved.
7. Based on Whitehead's (1953) notion of *event* as an actual occasion.

REFERENCES

American Nurses' Association. (1980). *Social policy statement.* Kansas City, MO: Author.
De Chardin, T. (1967). *On love.* New York: Harper & Row.

Emerson, R. W. (1982). Essay on nature. In L. Ziff (Ed.), *Selected essays*. Middlesex, England: Penguin.

Gadow, S. (1984, March). *Existential advocacy as a form of caring: Technology, truth, and touch*. Paper presented to the research seminar series on the development of nursing as a human science. School of Nursing, University of Colorado Health Sciences Center, Denver.

Gaut, D. (1983). Development of a theoretically adequate description of caring. *Western Journal of Nursing Research, 5*(4).

Jung, C. J. (1968). Pyschology and alchemy. In H. Read, M. Fordham, & A. Adder (Eds.), *The collected works of C. J. Jung* (Vol. 12, pp. 99–101). Princeton, NJ: Princeton University Press.

Leininger, M. (1981). *Caring: An essential human need*. Thorofare, NJ: Slack.

Smith, J. (1983). *The idea of health*. New York: Teachers College.

Watson, J. (1979). *Nursing: The philosophy and science of caring*. Boston: Little, Brown. Reprinted by Colorado Associated University Press, Boulder, CO.

Watson, J. (1985). *Nursing: Human science and human care*. East Norwalk, CT: Appleton-Century-Crofts.

Whitehead, A. N. (1953). *Science and the modern world*. Cambridge, England: Cambridge University Press.

A Critique of Nursing: Human Science and Human Care

Lynn G. Ryan

This chapter critiques the nursing theory developed by Jean Watson (1985). Her theory of nursing is metaphysical and proposes for human care a moral ideal that has important consequences for human civilization. Although the theory is innovative, it has its roots in Florence Nightingale's original premises that include an art and science of nursing.

Stevens' (1984) criteria for the internal and external evaluation of a theory is used as a guideline for assembling and presenting the information.

INTERNAL EVALUATION

Commonplaces

Stevens (1984) identifies *commonplaces* as "common topics addressed by most theorists (p. 11)." The topics that follow are those identified as commonplaces in Watson's theory. Each term is followed by a description of Watson's interpretation of that commonplace.

GLOSSARY

NURSE: This role is based on human caring for one who is ill. It demands of the nurse a knowledge of health-illness, environmental-personal interactions, the nurse caring process, self-knowledge, and knowledge of one's power and transaction limitations.

NURSING ACTS: Through nursing acts, Watson (1985) states, "emphasis is placed upon helping a person gain more self-knowledge, self-control and readiness for self-healing, regardless of the external health condition (p. 35)." It is a nursing art and nursing science directed toward the protection, enhancement, and preservation of human dignity.

HEALTH: Health is a process that Watson (1985) describes as involving "unity and harmony within the mind, body and soul (p. 48)." Her model of health is "eudaimonistic," which is described by Smith (1983) and consists of the I and me concept in harmony. Watson (1985) summarizes the eudaimonistic model of health as follows: I = Me: Health (harmony, with the world and open to increased diversity); and I ≠ Me: Illness (in varying degrees and person less open to increased diversity) (p. 48).

ILLNESS: Illness is subjective turmoil or disharmony within the spheres of the person. These spheres consist of the mind, body, and soul.

PERSON: A person exists as more than the sum and total of the parts and consists of mind, body, and soul in unification. They are the experiencing subjects, with an interconnected evolution to the world. This interconnection encompasses relationships with other beings and a feeling of a place within nature. A disruption in this interconnection results in a diminishing harmony.

PATIENT: A patient is a person or groups with a need for assistance in the promotion of self-control, choice, and self-determination with health-illness decisions.

RELATIONSHIP OF NURSE TO PATIENT: The two are coparticipants in the human care process. All of human caring is related to intersubjective human responses to health-illness conditions.

RELATIONSHIP OF PATIENT TO HEALTH: Patient determines health or illness in response to the harmony or disharmony that exists. Prolonged disharmony causes decreased openness to diversity whether related to genetic constitutional vulnerability or not.

Clarity

The components of this theory are in general clearly presented. Much information is provided about the author's philosophical perspective and this information allows the reader to more clearly understand the developing theory. Watson's metaphysical position is explained throughout the theory and in particular in the chapter "Nursing and Metaphysics (1985)." Comprehension is enhanced with a knowledge of metaphysical concepts, but even without such a background the concept is well illustrated through the use of an excerpt from Taylor's (1974) book on metaphysics.

Consistency

The next five sections refer to Watson's consistent use of her model's structure and function.

Terms

Human care. Human care, at times, appears to be used interchangeably with *nursing care* in this theory. Caring for others who inhabit our society is a standard by which civilization is measured. It is a moral responsibility not limited to the nursing profession. Nursing's place in the human care process needs definition beyond Watson's explanation of its commitment to this process. In other words, how can we delineate nursing's function in human care as different from other efforts at human care?

Human science. Watson and others have proposed a "new science" for nursing study, which includes the concepts that:

- Humans are the experiencing subjects.
- Interconnected evolution exists between humans and the world.
- Health is a process and change is ongoing.
- The nurse and the patient are coparticipants in the process.

Watson acknowledges nursing as a relatively new discipline and as such many aspects are under continuing development. This, combined with a scientific world view that is open, has many advantages and some disadvantages. An ever-developing body of knowledge provides new enlightenment but can also lead to confusion in definition and application.

Phenomenal field. This consists of the individual's frame of reference, unique to the individual, known only to him- or herself. It is used consistently throughout Watson's text (1985).

Causal past. This term refers to an individual's unique past experiences that are brought to the present moment. It has been formed by the collective past experiences and is continuously undergoing change as the individual experiences and absorbs each new life experience. Each new sensation or exchange becomes a part of the causal past and forms a well of information that the individual constantly consults or enhances. The causal past is a component of the phenomenal field and is used with consistency.

Carative factors. These factors have been described in depth by Watson (1979, 1985). They provide guidelines for nurse-patient interactions that are based upon a sensitivity to self and others. The consistent expansion of these factors is evident in her model, with her emphasis on humanism and the transpersonal caring relationship.

Transpersonal caring. Watson (1985) describes a caring relationship as "a union with another [with a] high regard for the whole person and their being-in-the-world (p. 63)." This caring is the moral ideal of nursing. Some confusion exists with regard to the domain of nursing and its delineation from other caring professions. This type of caring would not be the exclusive domain of nursing, and a more clear explanation of the boundaries of the profession is needed.

Interpretation

Watson describes this theory as metaphysical in nature. She states that "it goes beyond the rapidly emerging existential-phenomenological approaches in nursing . . . to a higher level of abstraction and a higher sense of personhood, which incorporates the concept of the soul and transcendence (1985, p.49)." It is an important distinction that the concept of soul is added to the traditional existentialist perspective of a mind-body whole. It adds a new dimension of spirituality. She accepts the concept of intersubjectivity and the ability of the mind-soul to transcend time and space.

Principle

Watson (1985) includes the following as the primary principles of her theory:

- Nursing is viewed within a human science and art context.
- Mutuality of the person or self of both the nurse and patient exhibits mind-body-soul gestalt, within a context of intersubjectivity.
- Human care relationship in nursing is a moral ideal that includes concepts such as phenomenal field, actual caring occasion, and transpersonal caring. (p. 73)

Her synopsis of major ideas assumes a knowledge of the complex interpretation and personal philosophical perspective this theory presents. To the reader familiar with the theory and its underlying structure she does succinctly describe the major premises.

Method

Stevens (1984) proposes four categories for method of theory development: dialectic, logistic, problematic, and operational. Although Watson (1985) describes in a chapter on methodology a "qualitative-phenomenological-naturalistic" approach, she seems to be describing a research methodology for the accumulation of information and not her theory construction technique. She is suggesting research methodology for further study of human care and the art and science of nursing.

To classify Watson's theory in one of Stevens' categories, it appears to most closely follow the dialectic method. In the theory, reasoning builds by assimilation and the components are seen as part of a whole, a whole that is greater than the sum of the parts. This is a philosophical perspective to which Watson subscribes as well as a method for assembling the theory.

Approach

Watson proposes that nursing be both art and science. Nursing at its highest level would include a physical, procedural function and a relationship with the patient that transcends the material world and makes contact with the inner self. The theory develops the human care and human science components into the transpersonal caring relationship Watson believes nursing should have as an ideal. She is consistent in the belief that a moral commitment to human care is integral to nursing at its highest level.

Logical Development

The components of this theory are discussed and developed and Watson's (1985) perspective is well-presented. However, one may question the organization of the chapters and want to rearrange them to provide a better flow. Perhaps the chapter on theory components and definitions could be placed as an introduction or review at the end. It breaks the flow of construction as the chapters proceed from background information on human science and human care to the development of the transpersonal caring concept.

Level of Theory Development

Watson describes her model as a descriptive theory and acknowledges the newness of it, expressing the hope that it will stimulate additional theory development. This author agrees with her assessment. The theory does present new ideas and concepts that hold great potential for further development.

Nursing Domain

Stevens (1984) describes an enhancement theory of nursing as one that "sees nursing as a means of improving the quality of the patient's existence, either in total, in relation to health, or in relation to some specified aspect of his being (p. 259)." In Watson's (1985) theory, emphasis is placed on helping a person gain more "self-knowledge, self-control and readiness for self-healing regardless of the external health condition (p. 49)." This comprises enhancement of the quality of the patient's existence and falls within the category of the enhancement domain.

EXTERNAL EVALUATION

Stevens (1984) states that an external criticism, "evaluates a nursing theory as it relates to the real world of man, of nursing and of health (p. 65)." Under the subheadings reality convergence, utility, significance, capacity for discrimination, scope, and complexity, information will be offered regarding the applicability of Watson's theory to the "real world."

Reality Convergence

Under this subheading the applicability of the theory is evaluated from three perspectives: principle, interpretation, and method.

Principle

Using Stevens' (1984) external evaluation criteria, reality convergence for principle depends upon whether or not the basic premises are rejected or accepted. Watson's principles relate to the complex individual, with human dignity whose inner resources and composition constitute the self and determine the response to the health insult. Although her principles contain important new concepts such as the need for a moral commitment to human caring and the mind-body-soul composition of the inner self, this author finds no difficulty accepting her principles as an idealistic view of the nursing role.

Interpretation

Watson's interpretation of nursing is idealistic. It does not seem that the nursing profession is currently prepared to fulfill the functions she describes. However, as previously acknowledged this is a relatively new theory, and one that proposes a new direction for nursing. Changes in nursing education and service may yet provide the type of preparation necessary to implement Watson's model.

The expectations for the caring relationship are also idealistic. The transpersonal caring relationship demands a commitment from both participants in the exchange. The problems that arise when one of the individuals does not have that commitment needs to be addressed with more depth.

This does not mean that there is no need for idealism in nursing—far from it. Watson's desire for a caring relationship that acknowledges the importance of the human spirit and promotes human dignity is important. However, clarification of the domain of the proposed nursing function, and additional information about the potential problems with interaction in the caring relationship, are needed.

Method

This theory does not lend itself to research by the traditional scientific method. Watson (1985) acknowledges this in a chapter on methodology and suggests some alternate methods. Although this is a theory that proposes much enhancement of the nursing role and has excellent research potential, determination of an appropriate research method presents some problems. If this theory is to survive, acceptable research techniques must be found and those techniques must be acceptable for this theory and its development.

Utility

The ideas and ideals presented provide a generalized perspective with which to view patients. The implementation of this art and science of nursing does not confine itself to a specific type of patient with a particular need but would lend itself to the individualized situation.

The profession is not currently being educated to fulfill the nurse role as Watson presents it, nor is nursing practice, in general, ready to implement these ideals. The current trends in nursing do seem to be interested in expanding and enhancing the nurse-patient relationship and the significance of patients' involvement in their own state of health has received much attention and acceptance. These trends seem to encourage the study of this concept, and the evolutionary nature of the profession provides fertile ground for new ideas.

Significance

The health field is ever-changing. Health care costs are rising and there is a trend toward shorter hospital stays. Efficiency and maximum value for each health care experience are essential. With these trends in mind this theory's emphasis on maximizing the interaction experience is especially appropriate.

In addition, the theory addresses significant issues in nursing. Two such issues are the nurse-patient interaction and the need to give definition to the role of nursing as a separate entity in health care. The increased necessity for understanding the individual's perspective in care that has ever-increasing moral implications is especially relevant because of today's medical advances.

Capacity for Discrimination

In her earlier book Watson (1979) addressed the difference between nursing and the traditional medical role. Nursing's domain was described as carative and the medical role as curative. Although this theory continues to define this distinction by explaining the carative function of nursing, it still leaves confusion about the boundaries of that carative role. It has established the desire for all nursing to be committed to human caring, but all human caring is not nursing. This aspect of the caring process needs further explanation.

Scope

The scope of this proposed nursing role is not limited by anything but time. It would initially take time to establish the relationship defined, but the effort and time involved would provide maximum potential for effective interaction. This interaction is basic to the nursing role, of which the ultimate goal is the protection, preservation, and enhancement of human dignity without which there can be no health.

Complexity

Although this theory proposes a complex role for nursing practice and possesses an abstract philosophy as its foundation, it is not prohibitively complex in explanation. A knowledge of metaphysics and existentialism, and a familiarity with Watson's previous works, does aid comprehension, but the lack of such would not make the material indecipherable.

SUMMARY

Watson (1979, 1985) proposes for nursing an art and science that is directed toward the protection, enhancement, and preservation of human dignity. The ultimate goal of her proposed nursing function is not so radically different from current nursing trends. The method, however, by which this ultimate goal is achieved and the moral commitment she has determined as essential present a new perspective for that role. She proposes a complex role for nursing that, not unlike her philosophical concept of person, is more than the sum and total of its parts. It is a concept worthy of further study and it is currently undergoing such study on an international basis. Through further research and development and as a perspective through which a conceptual framework for education may be developed, it holds great future potential.

REFERENCES

Smith, J. A. (1983, April). The idea of health: A philosophical inquiry, *Advances in Nursing Science, 3*, 43–50.

Stevens, B. J. (1984). *Nursing theory: Analysis, application, evaluation.* Boston: Little, Brown.

Taylor, R. (1974). *Metaphysics* (2nd ed.). Englewood Cliffs, NJ: Prentice-Hall.

Watson, J. (1979). *Nursing: The philosophy and science of care.* Boston: Little, Brown.

Watson, J. (1985). *Nursing: Human science and human care, a theory of nursing.* East Norwalk, CT: Appleton-Century-Crofts.

Research Testing Watson's Theory
The Phenomena of Caring in an Elderly Population

Gloria M. Clayton

> Pure logical thinking cannot yield us
> any knowledge of the empirical world;
> all knowledge of reality starts from
> experience and ends in it. Propositions
> arrived at by purely logical means are
> completely empty of reality.
>
> *Einstein (1973)*

Albert Einstein's view of generating knowledge from experience supports Watson's theme of intersubjective caring. Each caring episode between a nurse and patient is unique based on the nurse, the patient, and the experience itself. Study of the phenomena of intersubjective caring requires in-depth study of individual cases. Through the process of describing and analyzing individual caring episodes researchers may discover a central, complex process that explains the interactions. Although this discovery would not prescibe behavior patterns for nurses, it might highlight ways for nurses to increase their sensitivity to patients' experiencs. This sensitivity and the process of conveying it to the patient are critical to the success of nursing care. Each patient understands only his or her unique experience. The nurse is either a part of the experience or not. Kastenbaum (1982) explains the importance of the experience by maintaining that the experience is reality.

To understand the caring needs of the elderly, a starting point is investigating caring transactions between patients and nurses that stand out or are highlights in the lives of elder persons. The purpose of this study was three-fold:

1. To investigate the phenomena of transpersonal caring interactions between elderly individuals and nurses.
2. To determine the caring needs of the institutionalized elderly.
3. To determine congruence of results with Watson's theory.

Nursing and Caring

Transpersonal caring is the intersubjective human-to-human relationship in
which the person of the nurse affects and is affected by the person of the other.
They share a phenomenal field that becomes part of the "life history of both and
are coparticipants in becoming in the now and the future (Watson, 1985, p.
58)." In Watson's theory the nurse uses her- or himself to detect, appreciate,
and feel at union with the here and now of the other person. The nurse is present in the relationship in her or his uniqueness and personal life history. This
uniqueness of the nurse enhances the creativity of nursing and of the relationship. While preserving and valuing the dignity of the individual, the nurse
feels morally committed to protect the right of the person to determine his or
her own meaning. This view does not discount traditional cognitive and psychomotor activities of nursing; rather, they are incorporated into a transcended
and intimate caring relationship that is the basis of nursing. As Leininger
(1977) states, "it is caring that is the most essential and critical ingredient to any
curative process (p. 2)."

Although nontraditional, this view of nursing is part of a broader view of
nursing science that focuses on personhood rather than sickness, behavior, or
predicated nursing actions. In the mid-1960s Travelbee (1966) wrote "the role
of the nurse must be transcended in order to relate as human being to human
being (p. 49)." Patterson and Zderad (1976) defined nursing as a "lived
dialogue" between the nurse and the nursed that is directed toward "nurturing
well-being and more-being." In the early 1980s Gadow helped clarify the ideal
of nursing:

> If nursing is distinguished by its philosophy of care and not by its care
> functions, and if nurses themselves formulate that philosophy, they transcend
> a particular concept of nursing only in order to realize a more developed con-
> cept, an ideal: a philosophy of nursing which unifies and enhances the experi-
> ence of the individuals involved rather than devaluing and alienating that expe-
> rience. (p. 80)

Perhaps Benner (1984) most clearly describes the person-to-person encounters: "The nurse-patient relationship is not a uniform, professionalized
blue print but rather a kaleidoscope of intimacy and distance in some of the
most dramatic, poignant and mundane moments of life (p. xxi)."

Concomitant to the focus on personhood, caring has been recognized by a
number of nursing leaders in addition to Watson as a critical topic in nursing
scholarship. Leininger's work as a pioneer in caring has received international
recognition. She has been instrumental in the development of an annual con-

ference on caring research. In Leininger's nursing theory human care is the central component. Gaut has developed (1983, 1986) a theoretical definition of caring and in later work developed categories for evaluating caring behavior. Carper (1979) indicates the critical need for caring in a society that places such high value on technology. In addition to the research reported in this chapter, nursing research has focused on caring, caring needs, and caring behaviors. Swanson-Kauffman (1983) identified the caring needs of women who miscarried. Larson (1981) developed caring behavior themes based on her analysis of cancer patients' perceptions of nurse behavior. Clayton and Murray (1987) have studied the caring component of the student faculty interaction. Wolf (1986) has surveyed nurses to determine nurse-identified caring behaviors, and Mayer (1986) investigated the perceptions of nurse caring behaviors held by cancer patients and their families. Although additional research is needed, the body of knowledge to date supports Watson's value of the nurse as a vehicle of caring.

The nurse is clearly a coparticipant in the human caring transaction. To understand what occurs for the patient in the caring occasion, it is necessary to understand what occurs for the nurse. As Watson (1985) explains, "The art of caring in nursing begins when the nurse, with the object of joining another (or others) to oneself with a certain feeling of care and concern, expresses that feeling by certain external indications (p. 4)." She further clarifies, "the nurse enters into the experience (phenomenal field) of another and the other person enters into the nurse's experience. This shared experience creates its own phenomenal field and becomes part of a larger, deeper, complex pattern of life (p. 4)." The two coparticipants cannot be artificially separated as they are the phenomena unfolding in the relationship. Thus it was necessary in this study to explore with nurses the caring occasions and not limit the investigation to elderly persons alone. The focus of the study became the person-nurse dyad.

Methodology

Watson's theory influences the design of research testing her theory. Fawcett and Downs (1986) describe the relationship between theory and research.

> Research is neither more nor less than the vehicle for theory development. It is the method used to gather the data needed for the theory. This is true whether the purpose of the research is to generate a theory or test one. When the purpose is theory generation, the phenomena of interest suggests things to look for. (p. 4)

Because transpersonal caring is the gestalt of the relationship, it requires nontraditional methodologies for investigation.

Others support the value of nontraditional methods in nursing research. "Pragmatic activity, human concerns, and meanings call for investigative strategies that do not require the kind of decontextualization of strict operationalism (Benner, 1985, p. 5)." Duffy (1986) supports the use of qualitative research by describing its purpose, "to gain knowledge and understanding of people, events, conditions, historical factors and other phenomena of concern to humans (p. 5)." Silva and Rothbart (1984) speak to "the inadequacy of logical empiricism to deal with certain phenomena in nursing, in particular, those phenomena dealing with humanism and holism (p. 2)." In her second book Watson (1985) includes a chapter on methodology in which she indicates her theory is best studied "within the framework of qualitative-phenomenological-naturalistic approach (p. 79)." She also anticipates and invites the development of new methods for investigating the phenomena of nursing.

The design for this study evolved as a result of discussions with Watson and coinvestigators. The elderly study is one part of a collaborative investigation to study caring across the life span. Three colleagues, Broome, Kemp, and Murray, are conducting similar work with children, pregnant women, and women in their middle years, respectively. We struggled to design studies that could use the same methods for these diverse groups. Grounded theory and phenomenological interviews emerged as the approach to the study of caring across the life span.

Phenomenology provided the goal for the interviews and observations: to describe the caring interaction as it was lived by the coparticipants. As Lynch-Sauer (1985) states, "the purpose of phenomenology is to understand a human experience" with the goal being "to systematically examine human experience and from this examination derive consensually validated knowledge (p. 95)." Watson (1985) indicates in defining the concepts of her theory that "the phenomenal field is the individual's frame of reference that can be known only to the person (p. 55)." Thus to test some understanding of the phenomena of the caring interaction we chose the phenomenological interview. By having the coparticipants describe their experience and then validating with them what we heard and interpreted, we hoped to achieve a systematic explication of the caring occasions.

Grounded theory provided the mechanism for recording and analyzing the data. Wilson (1985) described grounded theory as "the most highly evolved and explicitly codified method for developing categories and propositions about their relationships (p. 415)." This constant comparative method developed by Glaser and Strauss triggered a comparison between participant and participant, participant and category, category and category, and category and literature throughout the study. Swanson-Kauffman (1986) described this experience as living the research, and that description certainly pertains to this study.

CARING OCCASIONS FOR ELDERS

Four elderly person-nurse dyads provided caring transactions for exploration. The elderly were nursing home residents over the age of 65. Two males and two females were included in the study. The elderly person member of the dyad was contacted first. In an early interview the person was asked to describe an experience with a nurse that stood out as a "peak" or "highlight" experience. It was necessary to meet with each elder subject four to six times to establish a level of comfort and trust in which they were willing to discuss experiences with nurses. Because they resided in a nursing home, the elders perceived nurses as having power over them.

Once the subject articulated a peak experience, the occasion was explored with them in depth. A short list of questions was used to partly structure the interview, but they allowed the interview to be conversational and to establish a flow of its own. Lofland (1971) supports this technique. Each interview was taped and then transcribed, which proved to be a very valuable source of information. When each elderly subject had identified the nurse involved in the experience, the first of two interviews with the nurse was scheduled. As background the nurse was reminded of the patient and the occasion highlighted by the patient was briefly described. The nurse's perception of the event was then explored. Again the interview was partly structured by a list of questions and taped.

Following the interviews the transcribed notes and the tapes were studied for a sense of the individual's perception of the occasion. The visual and auditory forms were complementary and both provided insight into the experience. Each subject then received a final interview. By this time the first interview had been coded and a list of questions made up about any unclear points in the first interview. At this time the understanding of the previous communication was described. Validation was requested that what was heard and then interpreted was an accurate representation of what the person had said. Additionally, the person was questioned for any additional thoughts about the event that may have been forgotten or for some reason not reported in the previous interview. Finally, the emerging categories of data were presented for validation.

After the first interview and simultaneously as other interviews occurred, the data were analyzed. As soon as a transcript was received, which had been typed in a three column format as suggested by Chenitz and Swanson (1986), the tape was played while the author read the transcript. In this way any significant nonverbal information such as pauses in the conversation or emotional charges, and so on, could be noted. Then began the process of coding. This process was ongoing and dynamic throughout data collection. The category development emerged as a result of study of the data and my constant reflection on the notes and interviews and constant comparison of all information sources.

During data collection a great deal of time was also spent with the dyad. Each dyad was observed at least twice. This served to validate the information shared by the subjects. Because the two members of each dyad were interviewed individually, an opportunity to see them together and to watch their interactions was required. Because these were participant observation sessions observations could not be recorded at the time they occurred; rather, field notes were made immediately following each session. These notes were transcribed in the same format as the taped sessions and included in the data analysis.

Preliminary data analysis revealed four recurring themes consistent with Watson's carative factors. Both the elders and nurses related feelings of heightened sensitivity to their own feelings prior to and following the caring interaction. One nurse reported an inability, early in her relationship with the elder, to accept his religious view of life after death. She cut off any attempt on his part to discuss this belief. As he was elderly, frail, and ill, he considered death an imminent experience and frequently discussed his belief about what happens after the death of the body. This nurse repressed her own unresolved belief about death, and this caused her unwillingness to hear his conversation and need to express his views. The caring event described by this dyad did not occur until the nurse worked through her own views about death and thus could allow the gentleman's expression of his belief even though it did not concur with her view.

The elder reported to me his awareness of the nurse's struggle to reconcile this feeling, although the two of them had never discussed it. The caring experience occurred when each member of the dyad was sensitive to the self and to the other. This dyad and others reported increased sensitivity after the caring experience. There seemed to be a follow-through phenomenon that permitted increased tolerance and understanding of others in the environment. Successful caring occasions decreased the risk of participating in caring relationships.

The dyads also indicated the existence of a helping-trusting relationship. Elders reported behaviors of nurses that opened the possibility for trust. These included eye contact, patience in allowing the elders time to do things for themselves where possible, a calm attitude and voice tone, and the general impression of liking the work or of wanting to be with older people. One characteristic from the nurses that fits this category is a sense of nonpossession and the lack of a need to control. The nurses recognized that although the nursing home residents were aged, many were ill, and most were frail, they needed independence, individuality, and respect. As one nurse explained, old people are not children, they do not seek pet names, structure, or lack of privacy. The dyads again reported an increased ability to develop a helping-trusting relationship after the first successful experience.

The environment surrounding the relationship was described as supportive, protective, and permissive. The view of the elders that the nurse in the dyad recognized the need for these three factors to be pervasive in the environment was essential for the caring occasions to occur. This relates to Watson's original premise of the uniqueness of each individual. Elders wanted to feel that the environment adapted to their particular needs. One participant had a history of falls, and she wanted the security of feeling protected from future falls; however, she did not want or need constant attendance and support.

Finally, existential forces pervaded the four relationships studied. Although behaviors could not be described that conveyed this force, the elders expressed a recognition that the nurses understood and appreciated residents' situations.

Each of the four elderly participants struggled in a unique way with institutionalization. The nurse in the caring encounter appreciated the predicament and the individual's need to find meaning or resolution to the problem. The elderly in the study felt free to be their "honest selves" with the nurses in the dyads and strongly voiced appreciation for this freedom.

The carative factors described occurred in all of the dyads studied. Another pervasive variable was the carryover effect. The nurses and the elders seemed more able or more willing to engage in caring relationships and occasions with others after the event described for this study.

Additional findings included three caring needs for the elderly subjects. While feeling the need for varying degrees of protection, the older persons simultaneously needed to feel that their environment permitted independence. The elderly subjects expressed the need to share their life events, to talk over with another occasions from their past. Finally, the elderly needed reinforcement of their current status. All of these persons had some physical problems. They feared further impairment and thus more dependence. They wanted the nurses to provide feedback regarding their status, to let them know that they were not worse today than yesterday.

The findings from this study are congruent with Watson's theory of caring, but additional research is needed. Key philosophical and moral ideals associated with the human-to-human caring process need to be further delineated. Additional exemplar cases need to be explored wherein events preceeding and following caring transactions can be investigated. Caring needs of diverse populations and caring behaviors of nurses need study to determine goodness of fit. The spiritual dimension, a foundation to Watson's theory, has been scantily studied in nursing. Watson's ten carative factors need to be examined. In addition to topics for study that test the theory, new methodologies must be explored. Multiple methods will expand our understanding of the caring phenomena. Creative approaches such as Watson's own study of an aboriginal tribe in western Australia will enhance our understanding. The process of human-to-human caring is infinite in its creativity and will never be stagnant; thus, the research opportunities are limitless and will continue to evolve.

REFERENCES

Benner, P. (1984). *From novice to expert.* Menlo Park, CA: Addison-Wesley.

Benner, P. (1985). Quality of life: A phenomenological perspective on explanation, prediction, and understanding in nursing science. *Advances in Nursing Science, 8*(1), 1–14.

Carper, B. (1979). The ethics of caring. *Advances in Nursing Science, 1*(3).

Chenitz, C., & Swanson, J. (1986). *From practice to grounded theory.* Menlo Park, CA: Addison-Wesley.

Clayton, G., & Murray, J. (1987, January). *Caring experiences of student/faculty dyads.* Presented at the Fifth Annual Research in Nursing Education Conference, San Francisco.

Duffy, M. (1986). Qualitative research: An approach whose time has come. *Nursing and Health Care, 1*(5), 237–239.

Einstein, A. (1973). In P. Schilpp (Ed.), *Albert Einstein: Philosopher-scientist*. LaSalle, IL: Open Court.

Fawcett, J., & Downs, F. (1986). *The relationship of theory and research*. East Norwalk, CT: Appleton-Century-Crofts.

Gadow, S. (1980). Existential advocacy. In S. Spicker & S. Gadow (Eds.), *Nursing images and ideals* (p. 80). New York: Springer.

Gaut, D. (1983). Development of a theoretically adequate description of caring. *Western Journal of Nursing Research, 5*(4), 313–324.

Gaut, D. (1986). Evaluating caring competencies in nursing practice. *Topics in Clinical Nursing, 8*(2), 77–83.

Kastenbaum, V. (1982). *The humanity of the ill.* Knoxville, TN: University of Tennessee Press.

Larson, P. (1981). *Perceptions of important nurse caring behaviors.* Unpublished D.N.S. dissertation, University of California, San Francisco.

Leininger, M. (1977). The phenomena of caring. *Nursing Research Report, 12* (2, Pt. 5), 2.

Leininger, M. (1981). *Care: An essential human need.* Thorofare, NJ: Slack.

Leininger, M. (1984). *Care: The essence of nursing and health.* Thorofare, NJ: Slack.

Leininger, M. (1985). Transcultural nursing care diversity and universality: A theory of nursing. *Nursing and Health Care, 6*(4), 208–212.

Leininger, M. (1986, July). Care facilitation and resistence factors in the culture of nursing. *Topics in Clinical Nursing, 8*(2), 1–12.

Lofland, J. (1971). *Analyzing social settings.* Belmont, CA: Wadsworth.

Lynch-Sauer, J. (1985). Using a phenomenological research method to study nursing phenomena. In M. Leininger (Ed.), *Qualitative research methods in nursing* (pp. 95–97). Orlando: Grune & Stratton.

Mayer, D. (1986). Cancer patients' and families' perceptions of nurse caring behaviors. *Topics in Clinical Nursing, 8*(2), 63–69.

Patterson, J., & Zderad, L. (1976). *Humanistic nursing.* New York: Wiley.

Silva, M., & Rothbart, D. (1984). An analysis of changing trends in philosophies of science. *Advances in Nursing Science, 6*(2), 1–13.

Swanson-Kauffman, K. (1983). *The unborn one: A profile of the human experience of miscarriage.* Unpublished Ph.D. dissertation, Boulder, CO: University of Colorado.

Swanson-Kauffman, K. (1986). A combined qualitative methodology for nursing research. *Advances in Nursing Science, 8*(3), 63.

Travelbee, J. (1966). *Interpersonal aspects of nursing.* Philadelphia: Davis.

Watson, J. (1985). *Nursing: Human science and human care.* East Norwalk, CT: Appleton-Century-Crofts.

Wilson, H. (1985). *Research in nursing.* Menlo Park, CA: Addison-Wesley.

Wolf, Z. (1986). The caring concept and nurse identified caring behaviors. *Topics in Clinical Nursing, 8*(2), 84–93.

23

Man-Living-Health
A Theory of Nursing

Rosemarie Rizzo Parse

Nursing is a scientific discipline with unique ontologies and methodologies. As with other scientific disciplines, nursing encompasses diverse beliefs, practice, and research methodologies. The major paradigms in the science of nursing are the person-environment totality paradigm and the person-environment simultaneity paradigm (Parse, Coyne, & Smith, 1985). These paradigms are distinguished by their beliefs about human beings and health. In the totality paradigm people are viewed as a bio-psycho-socio-spiritual organism, a total human being made up of parts. Humans are considered an organism adapting to the environment, and health is a state of physical, mental, social, and spiritual well-being. The beliefs of the paradigm are congruent with linear causality; thus the research and practice methodologies focus on cause-effect and associative relationships.

In the simultaneity paradigm, person is viewed as a synergistic being in mutual and simultaneous interchange with the environment, and health is a process of becoming. The beliefs of this paradigm are consistent with mutual and simultaneous human and environmental change, and thus research and practice methodologies focus on energy interchange and experiences as humanly lived.

Man-Living-Health is a theory of nursing evolving from the simultaneity paradigm. People are thus viewed as synergistic and health as becoming. The language of the theory is abstract, as is required in science. The use of the "ing" ending reflects the process orientation of the theory. The hyphens in Man-Living-Health are intended to demonstrate a conceptual bond among the words that posit human health as ongoing participation with the world (Parse, 1981). Positing health as ongoing participation with the world grounds this theory in the human sciences, which emphasize the connectedness of life events and focus on human participation in experiences. Lived experience is health, and the cocreation of health occurs through human connectedness

253

with others and the environment. Health unfolds in intersubjective inter-relationships as people live the personal meaning of situations in rhythmical patterns while moving beyond the moment to the not-yet. Health is the person's self-emergence and cannot be described as good, bad, more, or less. It is not a state, but a continuously changing process (Parse, 1981).

ASSUMPTIONS OF THE MAN-LIVING-HEALTH THEORY

The assumptions grounding the theory evolve from the works of Rogers, Heidegger, Sartre, and Merleau-Ponty. Rogers' work is rooted in ideas from von Bertalanffy, de Chardin, Polanyi, and Lewin. The works of Heidegger, Sartre, and Merleau-Ponty—contemporary existential phenomenologists—are rooted in ideas from Kierkegaard and Husserl. The four building blocks and three principles from Rogers are synthesized with tenets and concepts from existential phenomenology to form the assumptions of the Man-Living-Health theory (Parse, 1981). The nine assumptions are written at the philosophical level of discourse. There are four about person and five about health. These assumptions (Parse, 1981) specify the beliefs about people and health that led to the creation of the principles. The assumptions emphasize choosing meaning, experiencing multidimensionally, rhythmically coconstituting patterns, living value priorities, transcending with possibles, and negentropic unfolding. From the nine assumptions, three on Man-Living-Health were synthesized (Parse, Coyne, & Smith, 1985). These three make more explicit the themes of meaning, rhythmicity, and cotranscendence apparent in the nine basic assumptions.

PRINCIPLES OF THE MAN-LIVING-HEALTH THEORY

The three principles of the theory evolve from the assumptions and are written at the theoretical level of discourse (Parse, 1981). Each principle includes three concepts. These nine concepts are the main concepts of the theory and from these, theoretical structures are created that guide research and practice. The principles explain (1) structuring meaning multidimensionally; (2) cocreating rhythmical patterns; and (3) cotranscending with the possibles.

The first principle, related to structuring meaning multidimensionally (Parse, 1981, pp. 42–50), refers to creating a personal reality through living the many levels of the universe all at once. To say that people create a personal reality is to make explicit human participation in health. People cocreate lived experiences. Health is human lived experiences, and thus people cocreate health. Personal reality is created through the concepts of imaging, valuing, and languaging. *Imaging* is prereflective or reflective picturing of the world through a frame of reference. Prereflective-reflective imaging is shaping personal knowledge explicitly or tacitly all at once. Explicit knowing is that which is reflected upon critically; tacit knowing is unreasoned and acritical. *Valuing* is choosing cherished beliefs from multidimensional experiences. A cherished belief is recognized by its consistent presence in everyday choices. *Languaging* is expressing cherished beliefs through speaking and moving. Imaging, valuing, and languaging are processes in the cocreation of human reality, which is structuring meaning multidimensionally.

The second principle, which specifies cocreating rhythmical patterns of relating (Parse, 1981) refers to coconstituting a personal way of being by living the paradoxes of "everydayness." People cocreate patterns in cadence with the environment. Patterns distinguish people from the environment. Patterns of relating distinguish one person from another and are recognized in living the conceptual paradoxes of revealing-concealing, enabling-limiting, and connecting-separating. A paradox is an apparent opposite. Apparent opposites reflect both sides of an experience. Both sides of the paradox constitute the lived experience that is health. The paradox *revealing-concealing* is the simultaneous telling and not telling about self to self and others. In revealing a particular view other views are concealed. One cannot tell all that one knows about a situation, nor can one conceal all. The notion of not being able to share all that one knows gives rise to the nature of person as an unfolding mystery.

Enabling-limiting is the simultaneous living of opportunities and limitations in a situation. Every choice has both opportunities and limitations and the outcomes of choosing are not completely known.

Connecting-separating is moving with some phenomena and away from other phenomena all at once. Within the connecting, there is a separating, and within the separating there is connecting. Revealing-concealing, enabling-limiting, and connecting-separating are the paradoxical processes lived in cocreating rhythmical patterns of relating.

The third principle, related to cotranscending with the possibilities (Parse, 1981) refers to continuously reaching toward what is not-yet. The idea of continuously reaching toward the not-yet posits change as the fundamental nature of humanity. People are always changing as lived experiences reflect the chosen priorities of the moment. This everchanging process is becoming. Reaching toward the not-yet happens through the concepts of powering, originating, and transforming. *Powering* is the propelling force of pushing-resisting in interhuman encounters. It is the process of intentionally moving toward different possibilities. *Originating* is creating anew through living the paradoxes of conformity-nonconformity and certainty-uncertainty. People strive to be unique and like others at the same time. Uniqueness flows from human relationships and works of art. The ways in which one is irreplaceable to others, and one's creative endeavors, are manifestations of one's uniqueness. With the sureness in decisions there is also the unsureness in relation to the outcomes. Originating is one's particular way of self-emergence. *Transforming* is the changing of change, or viewing the familiar in a different way. It is people witnessing and living a shift in world view. (Parse, 1981). Discovering a different view reveals new possibles that enhance the changing of change. Powering, originating, and transforming are processes in cotranscending with the possibles.

Together, the nine concepts of the Man-Living-Health theory flowing from the three principles are imaging, valuing, languaging, revealing-concealing, enabling-limiting, connecting-separating, powering, originating, and transforming (Parse, 1981).

THEORETICAL STRUCTURES

Theoretical structures or propositions stated in nondirectional terms may be invented from the nine concepts of the theory. One concept from each principle may be joined to constitute a theoretical structure (Parse, 1981). For example, *transforming* is the enabling-limiting of valuing. These propositions or theoretical structures are written at the theoretical level of discourse and require that the researcher and practitioner move these to a lower level of discourse in a more concrete statement to guide research and practice (Parse, 1987).

MAN-LIVING-HEALTH RESEARCH METHODOLOGY

Since the Man-Living-Health theory is rooted in the human sciences, human science research methodologies are appropriate for inquiry. In a young science like nursing, research methods may be borrowed from congruent disciplines until unique methodologies are developed. Research enhancing the Man-Living-Health theory has been implemented utilizing the borrowed qualitative, descriptive, phenomenological, and ethnographic research methods. The focus of all of these methods is to uncover the meaning of experiences as humanly lived. The experiences of health, reaching out, persisting in change, retiring, aging, and being exposed to toxic chemicals, have been studied and the results related to the Man-Living-Health theory (Parse, Coyne, & Smith, 1985).

A new research methodology unique to nursing has recently been developed for inquiry related to the Man-Living-Health theory. The Man-Living-Health research methodology evolves directly from the ontology. It was designed in adherence to the principles of methodology construction (Parse, 1987). This new methodology is to be utilized for the study of lived experiences as related to health as defined in the Man-Living-Health theory. The entities for study are lived experiences related to being and becoming, value priorities, negentropic unfolding, and quality of life.

A critical element in the processes of the method is dialogical engagement. Dialogical engagement is the researcher-participant encounter, the purpose of which is to uncover the meaning of the lived experience being studied. Extraction-synthesis is the name given to the process that moves the participant's description up the ladder of abstraction to a proposition in the language of the Man-Living-Health theory. Although there are similarities between the new method and other qualitative methods, there are explicit differences that point to the uniqueness of the new method for nursing (Parse, 1987).

MAN-LIVING-HEALTH PRACTICE METHODOLOGY

Practice methodologies in nursing have been based on the nursing process. The nursing process is really the problem-solving process derived from logic and used by all persons in all disciplines. It does not flow from the ontological bases in the discipline of nursing. The development of nursing practice method-ologies consistent with the ontological bases of the discipline is necessary in the evolution of nursing science. The practice of nursing will vary dramatically depending on its theory base. Theory-based practice is a growing movement in nursing today. It is a way of making explicit nursing's unique contribution to the health care system.

A practice methodology unique to the theory of Man-Living-Health has been developed (Parse, 1987). The methodology evolves directly from the ontol-ogy; the dimensions and processes flow from the principles of the theory. The dimensions of practice are illuminating meaning from principle one, syn-chronizing rhythms from principle two, and mobilizing transcendence from principle three. The coordinate processes are explicating, dwelling with, and moving beyond.

The nurse practicing the Man-Living-Health theory is *illuminating meaning* through *explicating* with persons and families. The family members, with the nurse present, share the what was, is, and will be as it is appearing now in dis-cussing a particular situation. The family interchange has a rhythmic flow. The nurse moves in *synchrony* with the rhythm set by the family by *dwelling with* the family's way of living the situation. In *dwelling with* the family rhythm new in-sights arise and the meaning of a situation becomes more clear. The new in-sights shift the rhythm and all participants *move beyond* the moment toward what is not-yet. This is *mobilizing transcendence* (Parse, 1987).

The Man-Living-Health theory has its own unique research and practice methodologies. These methodologies are congruent with the ontology and are presently being tested and refined through research and practice. The con-tinuous testing and refining of the research and practice methodologies of a theory enhance that theory, thus contributing to nursing science by expanding the boundaries of the discipline.

REFERENCES

Parse, R. R. (1981). *Man-Living-Health: A theory of nursing.* New York: Wiley.

Parse, R. R., Coyne, A. B., & Smith, M. J. (1985). *Nursing research: Qualitative methods.* Bowie, MD: Brady.

Parse, R. R. (1987). *Nursing science: Major paradigms, theories and critiques.* Phila-delphia: Saunders.

The Theory of Man-Living-Health: An Analysis

Louise Pugliese

The Man-Living-Health theory evolves from the concept that human beings are a whole, different from and more than their parts. People are open beings who have an energy interchange with the environment to cocreate their constantly changing health. Parse (1987) stresses that the whole of a person determines his or her quality of life. The nurse and the patient mutually derive "meaning" of a situation for that patient. Techniques by the nurse foster making the implicit, explicit. Through the nurse's structuring skills the individual shares, in his or her unique rhythmical pattern, thoughts and feelings concerning the meaning of the lived experience.

Phillips (1987) views Parse as having a new and different insight into human beings that is different from the scholarly works that spurred her scientific inquiry. By utilizing Stevens' (1984) analysis of nursing models, Parse's theory adheres to the logical order and scientific design necessary in guiding nursing research and nursing practice. This author differs with Phillips' comment that "Parse uses the process of deduction to create each of the assumptions (1987, p. 184)." The high level of abstraction required by existential phenomena creates an all-at-once process of both deductive and inductive reasoning for theory development.

Parse reaffirms that nursing is a distinct discipline from medicine. The theoretical structure of Man-Living-Health assists nursing in becoming an independent scientific discipline in the caring for and healing of people. Nursing problems have been tested. Parse welcomes further testing of problems utilizing her theory of Man-Living-Health in determining potential outcomes of a person's health pattern. As Kaplan (1964) stated, "A theory is validated, not by showing it to be invulnerable to criticism, but by putting it to good use (1964, p. 322)."

INTERNAL EVALUATION

Theorist

In 1981, Parse published the book *Man-Living-Health: A Theory of Nursing*. This theoretical structure evolved from a synthesis of existential phenomenological thought from Heidegger (1962, 1972), Kierkegaard (1941), Husserl (1962, 1965, 1970), Sartre (1963, 1964, 1966), Merleau-Ponty (1963, 1973, 1974), and Rogers (1970). Ideas were enhanced by the works of von Bertalanffy (1968), de Chardin (1965, 1966), Polanyi (1958, 1959, 1966, 1969), and others.

Parse received a masters degree in nursing from the University of Pittsburgh. She has been actively engaged in various positions in nursing service, research, education, and family nursing practice. She obtained a doctorate of philosophy from the University of Pittsburgh. Parse has published three other works entitled *Nursing Fundamentals, Nursing Research: Qualitative Methods,* and *Nursing Science: Major Paradigms, Theories, and Critiques.* She presently is a professor of graduate nursing and coordinator of the center for nursing research at Hunter College in New York City. Parse acts as a consultant in nursing education, research, and nursing science. She fosters nursing research studies using qualitative methodology. Parse is the founder of Discovery International, Inc., which provides programs oriented toward advancing the scientific discipline in nursing.

Commonplaces

Nursing

From the perspective of the Man-Living-Health theory, nursing is a scientific discipline concerned with understanding people and health. The major focus of the practice of nursing is the caring and healing of unitary human beings through illuminating meaning, synchronizing rhythms, and mobilizing transcendence (Parse, 1987). The nursing focus is on health from a human science view rather than a medical model of illness. The scientific discipline of nursing for Parse (1981) is structuring meaning multidimensionally, cocreating rhythmical patterns of relating while cotranscending with possibles. The nurse in the human-to-human interrelationship with persons focuses on the lived experience of health rather than on predictive aspects of medical science.

Patient

Parse sees person as the key to all aspects of her theoretical assumptions. Person is characterized as living unit that is more than and different from the sum of his or her parts. The whole of a human is characterized by his or her own unique patterns. Parse states that people are an intentional being in the world. From creation to death, humans grow in complexity and diversity through interrelationships, choosing, becoming, and risking. Parse differs from other existential phenomenologists in stating that choosing begins before birth, at the moment of conception, or perhaps before that, and that choices are made at multidimensional levels of the person's universe. Death does not mean the end. In death, humans evolve at another level of the universe. Parse believes death is a transformation and the individual gives personal meaning to dying based on values.

Health

In the Man-Living-Health theory, health is viewed as a continuously changing process of becoming that people experience in the energy interchange with the environment. Health can only be identified by a person's own description. Health is based on human valuing and uniqueness, and is cocreated through a person's relationship with others. Health is relative to human attitude and potential. It is not a static point on a linear continuum of good and bad. Through the freedom of choice human health is derived by risk-taking. The outcome of choices are not always known, but humans assume responsibility for personal decision making.

Relationship Between Nursing Acts and the Patient

Nursing acts center on the person's qualitative participation in experienced situations. There is an open relationship whereby the nurse participates with the person uncovering the meaning of the situation as experienced by the person. This is an essential part of the nursing practice of Man-Living-Health. Cocreating the rhythms of revealing-concealing, connecting-separating, and enabling-limiting, points to an interrelatedness between humanity and self, humanity and others, and humanity and the environment. It is through this interrelatedness that health is cocreated. The meaning of health to each individual and the dreamed possibles are uncovered in the nurse-person interrelationships.

Relationship Between Nursing Acts and Health

Because nursing activity is open interchange at many levels of the universe, the nurse illuminates with the person's choices of health. The responsibility in the nursing act is illuminating the meaning of the choices of possibles related to health. The nurse illuminates the power of people in transcending with the possibles to reach beyond the actual, in the unfolding of human health. Both the nurse and the person grow, yet are separate, and health is learned by both from the suffering and joy present in everydayness.

Relationship of Patient to Health

Each person is responsible for personal choices related to health. These choices surface in energy interchange with the environment. As people grow in life, interchanging energy with the environment and others, human health becomes more complex. The health status of the individual is reflective of his or her valued choices.

Clarity

In 1987, Parse specified the priorities and research methodologies for the Man-Living-Health theory for nursing practice. Parse has clearly outlined the relationship of the assumptions, principles, concepts, and theoretical structures of the Man-Living-Health theory. Examples are offered to enhance clarification of the philosophical vocabulary of existential terminology. Nurses are for the most part unfamiliar with existential phenomenology, which results in unwarranted criticism about the clarity of the Man-Living-Health theory.

Consistency

Parse developed existential terms in her theory such as imaging, valuing, languaging, revealing-concealing, enabling-limiting, connecting-separating, powering, originating, and transforming. The terms described are consistent threads that weave the structure of nursing in the Man-Living-Health theory. The relationship of terms is compatible with the existential view of the person being and becoming all at once. The highly abstract terms are weighted equally and there is consistent use of the meaning of terms throughout the theory.

Adequacy

Through the theory Man-Living-Health, nursing is defined as a scientific discipline, different from other health related professions. The scope is adequately defined as the care of people with their families. The structure of Man-Living-Health meets the definition of a theory by Kaplan (1964), as a symbolic construction, abstract, and conceptually based on the scope of discovery, laws, and pragmatic norms. Parse's theoretical structures are nondirected propositions that guide nursing research and practice in a probablistic manner.

Logical Development

Through both deductive and inductive reasoning Man-Living-Health unfolded. The premise grew naturally that people live health by freely making valued choices with the environment.

The assumptions were synthesized from Rogers' (1970) concepts of energy field, openness, pattern and organization, and four-dimensionality, and from the existential phenomenological concepts of intentionality and human subjectivity. The assumptions lead to the principles in a logically constructive fashion. The nine concepts are explained in the principles. There are three concepts in each principle. The concepts and principles follow from the assumptions.

Level of Theory Development

The ultimate aim of Man-Living-Health is toward the coming to know, which allows for purposeful nursing practice. Parse began relating her thoughts about the delivery of nursing care to nursing students. In her approach to helping them understand nursing theory as a human science, she evolved the abstract nature of the Man-Living-Health theory.

Parse's theory level has reached beyond the descriptive level and has been tested through qualitative studies. Parse, Coyne, and Smith (1985) published *Nursing Research: Qualitative Methods,* which provides descriptive verification of the Man-Living-Health theory. Other studies have been presented at seminars by Parse's Discovery International, Inc. In *Nursing Science: Major Paradigms, Theories, and Critiques* (1987) Parse specifies unique research and practice methodologies for the theory of Man-Living-Health. With this, theoretical probabilities have begun to be suggested.

EXTERNAL EVALUATION

Reality Covergence

Parse's approach is consistent with the view of existential phenomenology. The art of nursing is rooted in the human sciences more than the natural sciences. Parse clearly deals with the perceived values of people as essential in nursing care. Her concept is that people are a whole, different from and more than the sum of their parts, who through energy interchange with the environment are in constantly changing health.

Parse's *Man-Living-Health: A Theory of Nursing* (1981) was written in a descriptive manner with many examples provided for the reader to grasp the theoretical structure and the focus of nursing. Parse's theory lends itself to the growing trend of studying nursing questions by the utilization of qualitative methods, one of which she has specifically devised consistent with Man-Living-Health (1987).

Utility

Parse provides a role reference for the nurse practitioner, educator, administrator, and researcher. Parse invites nurses to utilize and test the Man-Living-Health theory in the delivery of nursing care.

Parse believes that in all levels of nursing practice there is an open interchange between nurse, patient, and family. The nurse, with the patient and family, cocreate health with the environment. The outcome is change. The nurse and the patient will unfold the meaning of health for the individual.

Significance

In any situation where a patient interrelates with a nurse the Man-Living-Health theory can be practiced. Man-Living-Health is a perspective for utilizing qualitative methodologies in nursing research to gain an understanding of the meaning of the lived experiences of health. Parse's theory seems complex at times but then, so is the concept of nursing. Because the research testing of Man-Living-Health has been done only recently, the significance of Parse's essential aspects of nursing are still being tested.

Discrimination

The Man-Living-Health theory has the potential to separate nursing as a scientific discipline, the basis of an autonomous profession, from nursing as a vocation. The process of illuminating, synchronizing, and mobilizing describes the practice dimensions of nursing as unique in providing health care.

Scope

The broad scope of the Man-Living-Health theory is comprehensive, as is evidenced in the description of the principles. Parse's theory can be utilized in all nursing domains. It is an asset to the profession of nursing that Parse's theory can be utilized by all nurses in the caring and healing of people.

Complexity

The advantage of the theory is that nurses can easily perceive and understand the scientific discipline of nursing as a caring art. There is succinctness in the presentation of Man-Living-Health. It is set forth in three principles, nine concepts, and three theoretical structures. These all flow from the nine assumptions. Man-Living-Health is written at an abstract level as theories should be. It offers nurses the opportunities to derive practice and research propositions.

SUMMARY

Man-Living-Health is a new paradigm of nursing rooted in the human sciences. "It identifies man as one who coparticipates with the environment in creating and becoming, and who is whole, open and free to choose ways of living health (Parse, 1981)."

REFERENCES

de Chardin, T. (1965). *The phenomenon of man.* New York: Harper & Row.
de Chardin, T. (1966). *On love and suffering.* New York: Paulist Press.

Heidegger, M. (1962). *Being and time: A translation of Sein and Zeit.* J. MacQuarrie & E. Robinson (Trans.). New York: Harper & Row.

Heidegger, M. (1972). *On time and being.* New York: Harper & Row.

Husserl, E. (1962). *Ideas: General introduction to pure phenomonology.* New York: Collier-MacMillan. (Originally published in 1931.)

Husserl, E. (1965). *Phenomenology and the crisis of philosophy.* New York: Harper & Row.

Husserl, E. (1970). *The crisis of European sciences and transcendental philosophy.* Evanston, IL: Northwestern University Press.

Kaplan, A. (1964). *The conduct of inquiring; Methodology for behavioral science.* San Francisco: Chandler.

Kierkegaard, S. (1941). *Sickness into death.* (W. Laurie Trans.). Princeton, NJ: Princeton University press. (Originally published 1849.)

Merleau-Ponty, M. (1963). *The structure of behavior.* Boston: Beacon.

Merleau-Ponty, M. (1973). *The prose of the world.* Evanston, IL: Northwestern University Press.

Merleau-Ponty, M. (1974). *Phenomenology of perception.* (C. Smith Trans.). New York: Humanities Press.

Parse, R. R. (1981). *Man-Living-Health: A theory of nursing.* New York: Wiley.

Parse, R. R., Coyne, A., & Smith, M. J. (1985). *Nursing research: Qualitative methods.* Bowie, MD: Brady.

Parse, R. R. (1987). *Nursing science: Major paradigms, theories, and critiques.* Philadelphia: Saunders.

Phillips, J. (1987). A critique of Parse's Man-Living-Health theory. In R. R. Parse, *Nursing science: Major paradigms, theories, and critiques.* Philadelphia: Saunders.

Polanyi, M. (1958). *Personal knowledge.* Chicago: University of Chicago Press.

Polanyi, M. (1959). *The study of man.* Chicago: University of Chicago Press.

Polanyi, M. (1966). *The tacit dimension.* Garden City, NY: Doubleday.

Rogers, E. (1970). *An introduction to the theoretical basis of nursing.* Philadelphia: Davis.

Sartre, J.-P. (1963). *Search for a method.* New York: Knopf.

Sartre, J.-P. (1964). *Nausea.* New York: New Dimensions.

Sartre, J.-P. (1966). *Being and nothingness: A principles text of modern existentialism.* (H. Barnes Trans.). New York: Philosophical Library.

Stevens, J. (1984). *Nursing theory: Analysis, application, and evaluation.* (2nd ed.). Boston: Little, Brown.

von Bertanlanffy, L. (1968). *General systems theory: Foundations, development, applications.* New York: Braziller.

25

Research and Practice Application Related to Man-Living-Health

Mary Jane Smith

This chapter presents two examples, one in research and one in practice, of the testing and application of nursing knowledge, namely the Man-Living-Health theory. The methodologies for research testing and practice application are congruent with the ontological base described by Parse (1981), as discussed in Chapter 23. Both examples focus on the phenomenon of rest-unrest. The research study uncovers the meaning of the lived experience of rest for subjects confined to bed, and the practice application relates to a situation of unrest in the family.

RESEARCH STUDY

Rest is thought to be associated with health and healing. It has been and still is a ubiquitous thread weaving throughout the fabric of the nursing literature. Nightingale (1860) believed that the reparative process was facilitated by rest. Narrow (1967) suggests that rest is related to a feeling of control, understanding, and purpose so that the person experiences acceptance and freedom from irritation. Norris (1975) was interested in the phenomenon of restlessness. She defined restlessness as, "non-specific, repetitive, unorganized, diffuse, apparently nonpurposeful motor activity that is subject to limited control (p. 107)." The American Nurses Association Social Policy Statement (1980) includes rest as an illustrative example of a human response that is a focus for nursing intervention.

The purpose of this inquiry was to uncover a structure of meaning for the lived experience of rest. In keeping with this intent, the phenomenological method was chosen. The phenomenological method is congruent with the Man-Living-Health theory (Parse, Coyne & Smith, 1985). *Phenomenological* means the study of that which appears. The phenomenological method is a qualitative method that identifies the characteristics and the significance of human experiences as described by subjects. In qualitative research the researcher's interpretations are intersubjective. That is, given the researcher's frame of reference, another person can come to a similar interpretation. Qualitative data are processed through the creative abstractions of the researcher as the subject's descriptions are studied to uncover the meaning of human experience.

> The phenomenological method explicitly takes into account the human being's participation with a situation by using descriptions written or orally presented by the subjects as the raw data. It is through the analysis of the descriptions that the nature of a phenomenon is revealed and the meaning of the experience for the subject understood. And it is the major task of phenomenology to elucidate the essences of the phenomenon under investigation. This includes not only the phenomenon in itself but also the context of the situation in which it manifests itself. Phenomenology is particularly appropriate for the sciences in which Man's humanness and connection with the world, is the point of inquiry. (Parse, Coyne, & Smith, 1985, p. 16)

Research Question

The research question was "What is the structural definition of rest for subjects confined to bed?"

Researcher's Perspective

The phenomenological method does not begin with a conceptual framework. The researcher's beliefs about the phenomenon being studied are, however, made explicit in the phenomenological method. For this researcher, rest is a lived experience of health. It is an experience that can be described by the person who is living it. Rest is a way of being in tune with the world, a gentle feeling of harmony. It is a quiet connecting and separating with one's world. There is a flow of easiness in rest that calls one to image a variety of options in the unfolding process of becoming.

Sample

The sample for this study consisted of 60 men and women between the ages of 18 and 35 years recruited from a university setting. These subjects participated by writing descriptions of their experience of rest.

Protection of Subjects' Rights

The nature of the study, time commitment, and option to withdraw from the study were described to the subjects in a consent form. Confidentiality and anonymity were assured. All participating subjects read and signed the consent form.

Data Gathering

Sixty subjects rested in bed for 2½ hours in a room where quietness was maintained. The subjects were told that they could move about freely in bed but were told not to talk or smoke and that they must remain awake. They were assured that if at any time they wished to terminate their participation they could get up and leave the room. In addition, subjects were told that they would be paid $10 when they had completed the study. At the end of 2½ hours of bed rest, the subjects were asked to describe in writing their experience of rest.

Data Analysis

Van Kaam's (1969) application of the phenomenological method involves six operations of scientific explication:

1. A listing of descriptive expressions.
2. Identification of common elements.
3. Elimination of those expressions not related to the phenomenon.
4. Hypothetical definition of the phenomenon.
5. Application of the hypothetical definition to the original descriptions.
6. Final identification of the structural definition.

The researcher dwelled with the descriptions through the intuiting, analyzing, and describing processes, and elicited the descriptive expressions and common elements. A descriptive expression is a statement that completes an idea about the lived experiences. A common element is an abstract statement naming a major theme that surfaces from the descriptive expressions. To be considered a common element, a statement must be explicitly or implicitly found in the majority of descriptions and compatible with all. There are usually several common elements in any phenomenological study using the Van Kaam method (1969). The common elements were synthesized into a hypothetical definition of the phenomenon, which is applied to all descriptions. Through final analysis and synthesis, a description of the phenomenon surfaced. Judges were used to verify the descriptive expressions, common elements, and structural definitions. These judges are experienced researchers familiar with the phenomenological method. Using judges for testing and retesting the researcher's intuiting provides verification for assertions derived from the data.

Presentation of Data

A total of 124 descriptive expressions in the subjects' words were listed. The listed expressions required little reduction or elimination because the subjects were all relating to a similarly structured situation. The three common elements of the lived experience arising from the descriptions were deliberate picturing, paradoxical swinging, and easy drifting. These were the common elements of the lived experience.

These common elements were viewed as major constituents of the experience of rest. A major constituent is a moment of the experience that is explicitly or implicitly expressed in a significant majority of the descriptions.

Some examples of subject's descriptions under each major constituent follow:

Deliberate Picturing	*Paradoxical Swinging*	*Easy Drifting*
I started thinking of things that would make time go faster like a T.V. game show and a volleyball game.	I don't like lying in bed and not doing anything. But I found myself thinking about the future and how I would live my life.	I would float off to a time past, dream and then come back and forget where I was.
I did some fantasizing about a boy I have recently gotten to know.	It was pretty boring but after a while I thought about last weekend.	I allowed myself to move in and out of touch with the sounds of the activities around me.
I spent most of the time pondering the feasibility of making a move to Nantucket.	I was really uneasy at first but then I tried to see patterns in the ceiling.	I was relaxed enough to fall asleep but I was not sleeping. I was just out there dreaming.
Being Monday, my thoughts were of the past weekend with my boyfriend.		

The next step in the analysis phase was the identification of a hypothesis. The hypothetical definition can be viewed as a synthetic description that incorporates a structure of meaning. This is the essence of the study. For this study the synthetic description was as follows: Rest for persons confined to bed in a structured situation is easy drifting with paradoxical swinging surfacing in deliberate picturing.

The last step of the analysis process was application of the hypothesis to the descriptions. It was found that the hypothesis was compatible with every description. All of the analysis processes were validated by two other persons.

Findings

The findings show that rest for persons in a structured confined situation, is easy drifting through paradoxical swinging surfacing in deliberate picturing.

The first element, easy drifting, relates to the spontaneous wavelike flow of being with self and being with others, in the past and in the present, in the present and in the future, and with time passing both quickly and slowly. This was revealed as a patterned continuous movement and flow of experiences. Subjects described an effortless movement in multidimensional space-time. The movement was light and airy, unbounded and wistful.

The second element, paradoxical swinging, was related to the experience of being confined and not really being confined all at once. The subjects were at rest (in bed) and not at rest (not feeling rested) at one and the same time. The subjects in this study described rest in the context of a structured 2½ hour period of confinement. In the midst of restriction and freedom the subject was both enabled and limited in the situation. This struggle with freedom and confinement energized a spiraling out of the situation. And finally, in deliberative picturing, the third element, subjects went beyond the actual limits of the situation to concentrating on specific life events. Subjects imagined themselves in places and with people different from the confined situation. In creating a representation of a different situation subjects experienced the situation differently.

Discussion

The description elucidated in this study of being at rest for persons confined to bed is clearly related to the theory of Man-Living-Health (Parse, 1981). Indeed, the description is a way of living health, incorporating the principles of cocreating rhythmical patterns, structuring meaning multidimensionally, and cotranscending with the possibles (Parse, 1981).

Cocreating rhythmical patterns of relating is an essential element of the description and is readily apparent in the subjects' descriptions. Struggling with paradoxical swinging is living the opportunities and limitations of the situation. The subjects described being confined as limiting yet also described experiencing opportunities surfacing in the situation. This is an example of living the enabling limiting paradox. The subjects chose a way in which to live with this paradox. Resting was an experience of enabling limiting in that both the opportunities and limitations in the situations were present all at once. Both sides of the lived experience were present in the context of the situation. The situation in which the subjects described rest was structured confinement, and rest surfacing in this context enabled and limited the subjects all at once.

The principle of structuring meaning multidimensionally can be seen in deliberate picturing. Deliberate picturing is a way of imaging. Subjects' descriptions showed specific detailed imaging of life events. This picturing of life events was the subjects' structuring of meaning in the context of the confined situation. Deliberate picturing is the critical pondering of rest; a very specific way of imaging and making real multidimensional experience. The reality being lived as rest is at several levels all at once.

The principle of cotranscending with the possibles is related to the common element, easy drifting. The drifting experience described by the subjects showed the moving to a dream state for undetermined periods of time. The dream state was experienced as floating above the situation and reflected a moving beyond the moment. The Man-Living-Health theory posits that moving beyond the moment is transcending and that this happens through powering. Powering is propelling from one vantage point to another. Propelling from one vantage point to another is a way of easy drifting. This easy drifting is expressed as an element of the lived experience of rest.

It can be concluded that the common elements emerging from the subjects' descriptions of rest corresponds with the principles of Man-Living-Health. This study supports the proposition that rest is imaging the enabling-limiting of transforming.

Implications for practice relate to promoting rest with individuals who are in confined situations. Some examples of confined situations are restricted living environments, being confined to bed, and living with constricting family relationships. Based on the findings of this study, actively participating in illuminating meaning-synchronizing rhythms and mobilizing transcendence may lead to rest. This happens through the nurse being truly present to the person in a way that acknowledges the opportunities and limitations in the paradoxical swinging of the rest experience, which all at once leads the person to image another dimension of the situation through deliberate picturing, thus mobilizing transcendence. Transcendence can be viewed as a vehicle for promoting reframing of the confined situation so that new meanings can surface.

For example, asking a person in a confined situation to describe their daydreams and trancelike state may make explicit a mode of transcendence and shed a new light on daydreaming in the confined situation. Transcendent states tend to be ignored as topics of discussion because of the peculiar way in which they are perceived. Calling a person to reflect on these states making them explicit and acceptable may mobilize rest.

If rest in a confined situation is drifting off through paradoxical swinging, surfacing in deliberate picturing, then the nurse could promote easy drifting through inviting the person to wonder with music. Drifting to music and moving toward the picturing of life events may enhance rest.

Additional phenomenological studies of the experience of rest in confined situations are indicated. For example, asking prisoners to describe their experience of rest might illuminate yet another side of the lived experience of rest. In addition, obtaining descriptions of rest from persons who are not confined would also explicate the phenomenon of restfulness.

Further research on being at rest using the synthetic description as the focus for an exploratory study would further verify the description. Exploring with confined subjects their experience of deliberate picturing of events in space-time, swinging with paradox, and easy drifting, using a descriptive methodology is meant by this.

PRACTICE APPLICATION

Theory guides practice as the nurse thinks and acts with clients in relation to a theoretical proposition. The proposition that rest is imaging the enabling-limiting of transforming was supported in the research study. This proposition is the foundation for the practice proposition that rest is signifying meaning through choosing the opportunities and limitations in the situation while easing with change.

In cocreating situations with others, the significant meaning given to the situation becomes apparent. The meaning given to a situation is the person's personal picturing, which is how one sees the self living an event. This picture is a view from a particular frame of reference, which can be expanded or narrowed depending on choices. Choosing the opportunities and limitations in a situation is related to the flow of options surfacing for the person. The options are known both explicitly and tacitly. Thus not all options are in one's reflective choosing. In each situation, options offer both opportunities and limitations from which one freely chooses. Choosing occurs within the context of a situation including prior choosings cocreated with others.

Easing with change evolves from the concept of transforming. This refers to the changing of change in interhuman encounters that moves a person beyond the actual to the possible. The movement of transforming is rhythmical. The flow of this rhythm is uplifting and calming. For example, in the ebb and flow of the tides, there is the rising up of the wave to higher and higher peaks, as well as the relaxation of tension in the current. This rhythmical process of tension-relaxation shifts as the current changes continuously, developing different patterns of flow. The practice proposition that rest is signifying meaning through choosing the opportunities and limitations in the situation while easing with change, guides the nurse in practice with a family who is confronting a situation of unrest.

Family Situation

The Oak family consists of a couple (Peter and Martha) in their mid-50s whose two children are married and living out of state. The couple lived by themselves for 5 years. Within the past 6 months, Mr. Oak's mother (Clara), a spry, energetic 83-year-old woman, moved in with the couple.

As the family patterns unfolded, various conflicts arose among the family members. In discussing the situation with a friend, Martha was moved to call a nurse with whom she could discuss the situation further. In the course of the conversation Martha told the nurse about the situation and described a persistent skin rash she had developed. The nurse referred her to a physician in the area and then made arrangements to meet with her. The nurse met with the family shortly after Martha called. Martha had seen the physician, who told her that she was having trouble with her nerves. Martha took the medicine the physician had ordered. In the nurse-family discussion patterns were illuminated, rhythms synchronized, and energies mobilized in expanding the meaning moment for each member of the family. Each member of the family in the presence of the other signified what living together as a family meant, what advantages and disadvantages each saw in the situation, and how each wanted to change the situation. A family health profile included the pespective of each member of the family. This was discussed with the family.

Family Health Profile

Peter thought things were going fairly well. His mother was well-taken care of, seemed happy, and was adjusting well to her new living arrangements. She helped in daily management of the household and was very open and giving to him. He recognized that Martha was upset at times but believed that occasional conflicts are a normal part of everyday living. When Martha talked with him about his mother, Peter defended his mother and told Martha to relax and give the situation time. He believed that given time, things would work out. Martha and Peter did not spend much time together anymore because Clara was included in most activities.

Martha viewed herself as being burdened by Clara's constant pursuit of taking on household tasks that she could not manage and therefore did not complete. She loved Clara and agreed that Clara could be a help with the cooking, cleaning, and washing if she would stop trying to do so much. Clara constantly told Martha what she should do in relation to household activities. Martha got upset and usually left the room or went shopping, when the "shoulds get too much for me to handle." Martha left because she did not wish to hurt Clara's feelings. Martha viewed her husband as hard working, busy, and not involved in the conflicts associated with managing the house. Martha believed Peter did not realize how his mother was a source of unsettlement to her.

Clara viewed herself as a help to Martha and did not understand why Martha was so upset and not appreciative of her help around the house. Clara loved Martha and treated her as the daughter she never had. Clara knew that she liked to keep busy with many things and that she was a help to Martha. She thought Martha should do things the way she suggested and should be more attentive to Peter's desires. Clara missed her friends from back home and wished she could get out of the house once in a while.

Family Health Pattern

Upon dwelling with the nurse-family discussion and the family health profile, the nurse synthesizes a family health pattern that will focus the nurse-family discussions. The family health pattern for the Oak family was, "Escalating unrest surfaces with loving relationships in striving for family harmony."

Nurse-Family Activities

Nurse-family discussion centered on the health pattern. The family decided to work toward changing the health pattern by focusing on ways to bring about family harmony. Through nurse-family discussion Clara, Martha, and Peter all agreed on the following:

1. The strong love and caring among them would be a focus of their attention. Each person would find ways to clearly show that love.
2. Peter would spend special time alone with Martha once a week.
3. Martha would tell Clara when she was getting upset with her so Clara could be more aware of how she was relating to Martha.
4. Clara would attempt to take on more encompassible household chores so that she could complete them, and would encourage Martha to do things the way she wishes.
5. Clara would begin playing cards with the community bridge club that met twice a week.

The nurse-family interchange that led to the above agreement happened through illuminating meaning, sychronizing rhythms, and mobilizing transcendence. The nurse lived true presence with the Oak family. True presence is an intersubjective way of being with, that intensively focuses on the family so that the significant meaning each gives to the situation becomes apparent. In a climate of being truly present, the family saw and chose the opportunities and limitations in their changing situation.

The nurse met with the family regarding the activities once every 2 weeks. During these sessions each family member shared their perspective and feelings related to moving toward family harmony. At the end of 2 months, the family believed that great strides had been made and that the unrest was no longer escalating. Clara, Martha, and Peter appeared more comfortable with one another, and a deeper understanding of creating family harmony was apparent. During the last visit the family agreed that although unrest would always arise now and then, it no longer was a predominant feature of their family relationships.

The nurse in this situation was guided by the proposition that rest is signifying meaning through choosing the opportunities and limitations in the situation while easing with change. Each member of the family lived and stated explicitly the meaning of being together. Choosing to be together in ways that confirmed their love and caring for each other required imaging the enabling-limiting ways in transforming their relationship. The family members' relationships with each other changed according to their own desires.

CONCLUSION

The research study and practice situation reported centered on the rest-unrest rhythm. This rhythm is related to imaging the enabling-limiting of transforming that flows from the principles of the Man-Living-Health theory. Rooting research and practice in a knowledge base that explicates a unique perspective of nursing is the process that stretches the boundaries of nursing science.

REFERENCES

American Nurses Association (1980). *Nursing: A social policy statement.* Kansas City, MO: Author.

Narrow, B. W. (1967). Rest is . . . *American Journal of Nursing, 67,* 1646–1649.

Nightingale, F. (1860). *Notes on nursing.* London: Harrison.

Norris, C. M. (1975). Restlessness: A nursing phenomenon in search of meaning. *Nursing Outlook, 23,* 103–107.

Parse, R. R. (1981). *Man-Living-Health: A theory of Nursing.* New York: Wiley.

Parse, R. R., Coyne, A. B., & Smith, M. J. (1985). *Nursing research: Qualitative methods.* Bowie, MD: Brady.

van Kaam, A. (1969). *Existential foundations of psychology.* New York: Doubleday.

The Systems-Developmental-Stress Model

Marilyn Chrisman
Joan Riehl-Sisca

Applying current nursing models to nursing practice is not an easy task. Direct technical and nontechnical patient care requires an organized frame of reference that can be operationalized succinctly through the nursing process. Those models we had knowledge of did not completely suit this purpose. There were two major areas that compromised their utility: (1) applicability to clinical practice and (2) comprehensiveness and flexibility. In an attempt to overcome these obstacles, we developed a model for use in nursing practice that we believe can be applied to the entire spectrum of nursing activities.

The model that emerged from our endeavors is called the Systems-Developmental-Stress (SDS) Model. The purpose of this model is to provide a framework for practice and a conceptual approach for the nursing process. Both structure and process are emphasized. The structure refers to systems development and encompasses a broad philosophical base that incorporates assumptions, values, and ethical principles that are pertinent to nursing. It conceptualizes a schematic description of how person and health can be viewed from a nursing perspective. The process, on the other hand, refers to stress and provides an approach for analyzing human problems within the structure. The patient problems that are identified can be explored and can suggest definitive implications for nursing intervention. The structural framework, the application of the stress process to a variety of nursing activities, and implementation of the Systems-Developmental Stress model are discussed in the following sections.

STRUCTURE

The structure in Figure 26-1 describes two major aspects of human life. First, people exist within a framework of change. Birth, growth and development, maturation, and death are integral parts of living. Second, at any point in time, a person can be viewed as a unit of interlocking biological, interpersonal, and intrapersonal systems that are open to the environment and subject to change.

The framework of this model incorporates aspects of human beings in the form of systems and developmental theory. Although both concepts are congruent with reality, both are required; one is not a real description of life without the other. For the purposes of analyzing human problems, the person can be conceptualized as a system moving through time and developmental stages.

This structure provides an orientation for nursing practice. The nurse deals with the patient anywhere along the life continuum. The patient's present always consists of a past and a potential future. The patient exists in an environment and as a part of changing time. His or her development is natural, genetically directed change that affects all systems. And stages of active development extend beyond the attainment of adulthood. However, a comprehensive description of the total human developmental sequence is elusive and needs continued nursing research and study.

Because nursing has an impact on the lives of individuals and society, the professional beliefs and ethics that underlie this nursing perspective of people as a system in change should be reviewed. The following statements describe the underlying nursing attitudes in the model:

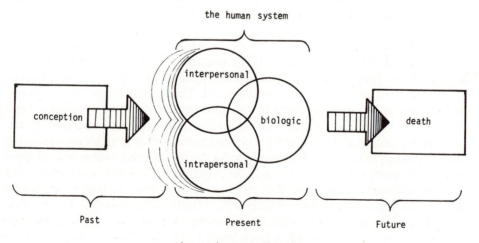

Figure 26-1. The structural framework of the SDS model.

1. Professional nursing intercedes in the systems-developmental continuum with a therapeutic purpose.
2. Underlying all nursing activity is a caring (concern for the welfare) for the individual.
3. The nurse is the patient's advocate.
4. The nurse supports life and the quality of life.
5. Critical analysis of the patient and his or her condition is accompanied by respect for the patient as an individual.
6. The patient is an integral part of planning and decision making.
7. The nurse supports and promotes health. Health has been identified by the World Health Organization as physical, mental, and social well-being.

In clinical practice, the nurse focuses on aspects of the total person, analyzing the patient's (1) biological, interpersonal, and intrapersonal systems; (2) interactions of these systems; and (3) relationships among the systems, time, and the environment. In this model, the systems approach is utilized for two reasons. First, it is an organized way to analyze interdependent aspects of a given condition. Second, the systems can easily be broken up into areas that traditionally have been studied and written about in the literature. We will now examine these systems in detail.

The human biological system may be analyzed according to the following categories:

  I. Cardiovascular
 II. Gastrointestinal
III. Genitourinary
 IV. Integumentary
  V. Motor-skeletal
 VI. Neurologic
VII. Respiratory
VIII. Endocrinologic
 IX. Immunologic
  X. Other

Of course such a differentiation has built-in limitations, such as arbitrary anatomic and functional divisions, but it can provide a useful guide to physiological problems as well as medical diagnostic categories. In addition, the biological subsystems are congruent with many major health system specialties.

The interpersonal subsystems identify social variables and their interplay with biological and intrapersonal systems. They include the following areas:

 I. Cultural
II. Socioeconomic

III. Interactional
  A. Space (e.g., territoriality)
  B. Patterns (e.g., play, dependency-independency)
  C. Roles
    1. Sexual
    2. Occupational
    3. Familial
    4. Affiliative
    5. Communal

The intrapersonal subsystems relate to the personal self. They are never seen, but are always felt and reacting. Subsystems include:

  I. World-life view (e.g., optimism, fatalism)
  II. Self-concept
    A. Body image
    B. Self-awareness
    C. Self-esteem
  III. Ego controls (e.g., emotional self-control)
  IV. Emotional pattern (e.g., passive-aggressive)
  V. Religio-spiritual view (e.g., religious beliefs)
  VI. Intelligence

In summary, the model structure includes the following assumptions:

1. Human beings can be viewed as a set of dynamic systems interacting within an environment and along a developmental continuum.
2. Development includes biological, interpersonal, and intrapersonal change; each perspective interrelates with every other and influences health.
3. An individual moves along the continuum by a gradual mediation from one developmental state to another. Information and effects from the past are stored, incorporated into the present, and projected into the future. (Cultural determinants affect the temperal preoccupation of societies and their members.)
4. Change is inherent to life. The systems attempt to maintain stability within change.
5. The patient's situation can be described as the interface between the human system and time-environment.

The purpose of the model structure is to provide a broad theory base to the understanding of humans and life. It should encourage the nurse to examine the multitude of variables that may affect the patient at any point in time. Systems can be studied in the present while at the same time considering the input of the patient's past and the potential of his or her future. Also, the structure should motivate analysis of patient behavior and facilitate predictions and projections of the consequences of nursing intervention. Hence, study of systems theory, development, and behavior is necessary for optimal utilization of the structure of this model.

THE STRESS PROCESS

The stress process is discussed as it relates to the patient and as it relates to the clinical situation. The stress process approach is a comprehensive way of identifying patient problems. And in practice it can be applied to technical and nontechnical nursing therapy such as monitoring or interpersonal problem solving. The stress process is thus universal in its relevance and applicability to nursing.

The Systems-Developmental Stress model, like all models, has its own terminology. To utilize this model effectively, one must be familiar with the following definitions of the stress process.

GLOSSARY

STRESSOR: The precipitating or initiating agent that actives the stress process.

STRESS: The dynamic force that produces strain or tension within the organism.

STRESS STATE: The reactive condition of an organism that occurs as a result of stress.

ADAPTATION: The coping response of the organism to the stress state, the stress, or both.

STRESSED CHANGE: The difference in the organism as a result of the stress process and not directly related to the change due to normal development.

STRESS PROCESS: The sequence of reactions that occur in response to a stressor.

The stress process can be diagrammed as shown in Figure 26-2.

The Patient and the Stress Process

It is important to distinguish the components of the stress process. The term *stressor* is useful to identify the agent that provokes the stress state. It is not a cause, although it may be a catalyst or a crucial aspect of the cause. The *stress*, or force that produces the stress state, may originate from the stressor or from the organism (patient) itself. For example, a child may panic at the sight of a harmless animal. Although the animal is the stressor, it is the child's psyche that

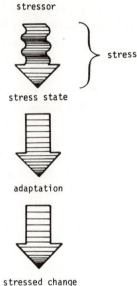

Figure 26-2. Representation of the stress process.

produces the stress. In another example, if a man is hit by an automobile, the auto may be the stressor, but its velocity and mass applies the stress. The distinction here is helpful in planning intervention in patient problems.

Therapeutic intervention by the nurse may include the manipulation of stress. Depending on the situation and the patient, the nurse may plan to reduce, eliminate, or resolve the stress. In some cases, the nurse may plan to increase or introduce stress.

Stress state describes the turmoil within the organism that results from stress. For example, damaged tissues, bleeding, and hypotension may be part of the stress state of the body after an accident. Decreased cognitive function may be the psychological stress state in the same situation. In short, the stress state describes the impact of the stress.

Adaptation is the crux of the stress process because it guides and directs the resulting change. Adaptation may be positive or negative, but it is more likely to fall somewhere between the two extremes. For example, a fever may be a positive adaptation to infection, but if the fever rises to damaging levels it becomes a negative adaptation. Psychological shock after an accident may be a positive adaptation, but if it persists and prevents the individual from successfully interacting with the environment it is negative adaptation. In coping with stress, individuals may adapt in several ways. They may avoid or prevent exposure to the stressor, or eliminate, reduce, or resolve the stress. Frequently individuals seek out stress as a lifestyle, a challenge, or a path to self-awareness. The nurse assists the patient in positive adaptation to stress. Positive adaptation culminates in active survival with a sense of well-being, promoting individual growth and strength.

The term *stressed change* refers to the change in the individual brought about by the introduction of stress and adaptation to the stress. Stressed change can be differentiated from the expected, predetermined change of normal development. Indeed, deviation from normal development may be a stressor. And the subjective or objective impact of that deviation may introduce stress along with the stressed change that results. But the normal human developmental pattern creates change also, which may or may not relate to stress. The two types of change should be distinguished to clarify the clinical situation.

Stress is the source of adaptation. The change that results may either be desirable and an advantage to the organism or undesirable and a disadvantage. Stressed change may either decrease or increase the successful functioning of the organism. This depends upon the integrity of the organism, the nature and severity of the stress, and the mode of adaptation.

The stressor and the stress may impinge on the organism from either the internal or external environment, or both. Stress, as the force that produces strain, has at least six characteristics (Fig. 26-3).

1. The *stress quotient* is the current, specific stress divided by the total stress that the organism experiences at a point in time. Total stress implies simply the residual stress accumulated from past experiences and

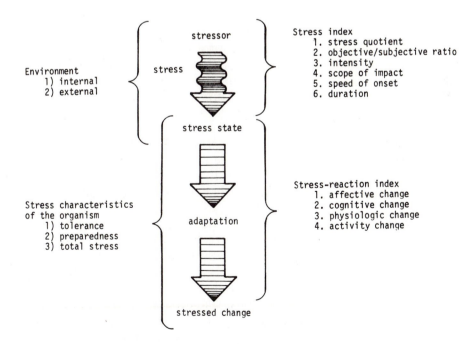

Figure 26–3. Characteristics of the components of the stress process.

the variety of stress that affects the individual at this time. For example, total stress includes a person's history of fears, anxieties, failures, physical handicaps, immune status, and so forth, as well as the possible stress of pain, sounds, smells, temperature, and similar stimuli that affect him or her at the moment.

2. The *objective/subjective ratio* is the quantitative relationship between stress that can be measured by discrete objective data and stress that is interpretative or subjective.

3. The *intensity of stress* may be roughly divided into severe, moderate, or slight levels. Stress of severe intensity always requires reduction. Moderate stress may be therapeutically supported or decreased. In stress of slight intensity, the level should be supported or increased. The therapeutic approach depends upon: (1) the organism's tolerance to stress; (2) how prepared the organism is to cope with stress; (3) the stress quotient; (4) the potential direction of the stressed change.

4. *Scope of impact* refers to the spread of the stress force on the organism. Scope may include the percept of area damaged (for example, a 40 percent burn) or the variety of ways the stress affects the organism. An illness, for instance, might not only cause physical suffering but also loneliness, financial burden, and loss of self-esteem.

5,6. The *speed of onset* and *duration* of the stress may also have specific effects not only on the stress state but on the adaptation.

The *stress reaction index* may apply both to the stress state and the adaptation. In many cases one is an essential part of the other, because the reaction to stress may be the beginning of an adaptation mechanism. The four categories of the index are rough descriptions of the types of reactions that may occur. They are useful in assessing the effect of the stress on the organism, the subjective impact, and the initial and late adaptive responses. The stress reaction index includes:

1. *Affective change*—observations or reports of disturbed or altered affect, which can vary among a wide range of emotions and feeling tones.

2. *Cognitive change*—changes in cognitive function that may include perception, thought, judgment, problem solving, or consonance-dissonance.

3. *Physiological change*—reactions to stress that cover the range of endocrine, neurologic, cellular, and varied chemical responses and manifestations to biological and psychological stress states.

4. *Activity change*—patterns of whole-body response. Byrne and Thompson (1972) discuss six categories of behaviors that are useful in assessing reactions to stress. An adapted version presented here involves the accentuated use of one mode or pattern of behavior, alteration in activities, disorganization or a change in the organization of behavior, change in sensitivity to the environment, behaviors that reflect altered

THE STRESS PROCESS

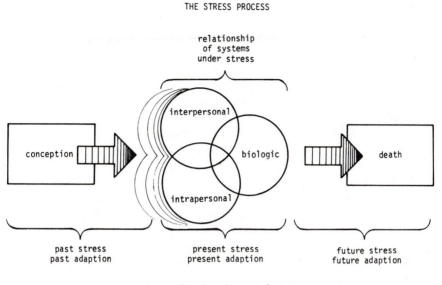

relationship
of systems
under stress

conception   interpersonal   biologic   intrapersonal   death

past stress
past adaption

present stress
present adaption

future stress
future adaption

temporal and environmental stress

Figure 26-4. Application of the stress process to the systems development continuum.

physiological activity, and behaviors based on a distorted perception of reality.

In summary, the systems-development continuum describes a structure. The stress process identifies the problems that can arise in both the function and form of the structure. Problems in function refer to system equilibrium and developmental progress. Problems in form refer to the effect of temporal dimensions and environment on the organism. Figure 26–4 relates the stress process to the systems-development continuum.

The synthesis of the stress process and the systems-developmental continuum provides direction and guidelines to the nursing role, goals, modes of action, and application of the model to clinical practice.

THE CLINICAL SITUATION

An applied model should be congruent with the variety of nursing activities that make up nursing practice. What does the nurse do? Most nurses who deal in direct nursing care to patients are engaged in both technical and nontechnical activities. These activities are relevant to the stress process and can be compared in the following manner:

1. Monitoring and detecting signs and symptoms of physical and psychological stability or instability is a major nursing function. As related to the stress process, monitoring can help to identify the stressor, the nature and indices of the stress, the characteristics of the stress state, the patient's mode of adaptation and the mode's effectiveness, and descriptive aspects of the stressed change. Viewed in this manner, monitoring is no longer just a task, but part of a process in which the nurse is an active participant.
2. Preventive activities encompass a wide range of nursing actions. Viewed from the perspective of the SDS model, prevention can be focused on any aspect of the stress process, within any one or group of systems, and within any developmental stage. For example, safety and comfort measures avoid and reduce potential stressors and stresses.
3. Coordination of therapy consumes a large part of nursing time. Coordination can be perceived as balancing the introduction of stress and maximizing the therapeutic effect through organization of the treatment regimen. Coordination is focused on the stressor and adaptation phases of the stress process.
4. Most nurses who give direct care are involved in the administration of medical therapy. Incorporation of nursing therapy into medical therapy multiplies the effectiveness of both. The nurse can utilize the stress process by planning appropriate stress interception, and assist adaptation as medical therapy is administered.
5. Nurse leadership includes the guiding and directing of interventions in the stress process of patients. As a leader, the nurse also recognizes and intervenes in the stress process of the health care organization and among its staff.
6. Finally, nursing therapy can intervene directly and indirectly in the stress process of patients. Use of technique and technical skills can prevent, reduce, remove, or balance the stress that a patient encounters.

Incorporating the concept of stress process into nursing practice can increase the relevance and effectiveness of nursing care. An important aspect of this model is that it helps to reduce the difficulty that has frustrated many nurses who try to apply theory in a situation that often expects only the performance of tasks. Tasks are a part, but only one part, of applied theory and total nursing care.

Because nursing has evolved a division of labor among levels of nursing personnel, it is important to question how the model can relate to different nursing positions. Some suggestions follow.

The Nursing Assistant. The nursing focus here is on monitoring and detecting major signs of physical problems and patient feelings. The nursing assistant's actions are aimed at implementing directed safety and comfort measures. Temporal reference is present-oriented, and the surrounding physical environment is considered in giving care. To the nursing assistant, therefore, the stress process can be a way to achieve a sense of purpose in caring for the patient.

The Licensed Vocational/Practical Nurse. The LVN helps to plan, effect, and direct safety and comfort measures. She administers directed medical and nursing therapy. Temporal reference is oriented to past and present and the surrounding physical space is considered in giving care. To the licensed vocational nurse, the stress process is a method to examine physical and prominent psychosocial problems and to apply appropriate knowledge and skill.

The Registered Nurse. The nursing focus is the interplay of biological, intrapersonal, and interpersonal systems in relation to time and the developmental continuum. Temporal reference includes the patient's past, present, and future. The surrounding environment is considered in relation to the patient's former environment and the environment(s) that he or she will yet encounter. To the registered nurse, the stress process is a way to operationalize the knowledge base of systems development.

Nurse educators, researchers, and administrators can also apply the model in determining how their various perspectives affect nursing practice.

THE NURSING PROCESS

Since the SDS model is based on a description of human reality, it is pertinent to all situations that deal with human life. The stress process is a framework that not only identifies problems but also points up the strengths of individuals, groups, or organizations. Psychiatric, public health, pediatrics, community mental health, obstetrics, industrial, medical-surgical, and other nursing specialties can apply the model effectively through the nursing process.

The systems-development structure of the model should only provide guidelines for considering pertinent major variables. If the structure is incorporated into basic nursing education, it is not necessary to transfer the model intact to the nursing care plan. What is important, however, is that the model should influence each step of the nursing process, described as follows.

Assessment

Nursing assessment is organized information gathering with a therapeutic purpose. Any mode of data collection is appropriate, such as records, observations, interaction, interviews, self-reactions, and physical, physiological, or psychological measurements.

Nursing assessment should include examination of the patient's:

1. Developmental variables.
2. Temporal-environmental impact.

3. Systems analysis—a review of the function and adaptability of the biological, interpersonal, and intrapersonal subsystems.
4. Stress process as related to systems-development.

Nursing Diagnosis

A nursing diagnosis is a descriptive statement of real or potential problems inherent in the stress process. The diagnosis should refer to any component of the stress process, such as identification of the stressor, statement about the stress, description of the stress state, problems in adaptation, or problems with anticipated or actual stressed change. The diagnosis should focus on the patient, especially on reactions at any phase in the stress process. Diagnoses can be drawn from the rich variety in nursing literature, which includes a diversity of subjects—for example, anxiety, sleep deprivation, and decubiti.

Objectives

A nursing objective is a statement of the therapeutic goal. The objective may be to support an optimum stress level, to help the patient cope with real or potential stress, or to reduce or eliminate stress. In all these cases, the objective is to achieve a predicted or desired end behavior or functioning (stressed change). Nursing objectives identify short- and long-term priorities.

Intervention

Nursing intervention involves the choice of an interception for the stress process based on knowledge of systems development. Intervention necessarily implies a projection and prediction of consequences. The mode of intervention includes therapeutic use of self, others, techniques, or the environment.

Evaluation

Evaluation of the nursing process can be directed toward any or all of the following conditions: (1) occurrence of the stressor; (2) effect of the stress; (3) successful adaptation; and (4) the patient's functioning level after stressed change.

In summary, the nursing process is a problem-solving guide. The stress process helps to identify the problems within the context of systems and development.

A SAMPLE ASSESSMENT TOOL FOR THE SDS MODEL

The nurse can vary the assessment plan technique according to the patient and the patient situation. Assessment tools such as that given in Table 26–1

TABLE 26-1. INITIAL NURSING ASSESSMENT

Name: Mann, Thomas (fictitious); 12 Main Street, Capital City, Calif., no phone.
ID No. 4-22-835

Admitted:	1-24-89
Discharged:	1-24-89
Age	52
Race	Black
Sex	M
Birthplace, area raised	Georgia, came to Calif. in 1968
Parent's birthplace	Georgia
Marital status	M
Children	One son, 17
Income	Not employed, wife makes about $13,000/year as waitress
Religious preference	Baptist
Would you like a minister/ priest to visit?	No
Medical diagnosis	Severe chronic lung disease with diplococcal pneumonia
Previous hospitalizations	1965—right lobectomy
	Ten hospitalizations since 1978 associated with lung disease

1. Physical Review

Cardiovascular:

Bilateral pulses in extremities	Strong, even bilateral pulse
Color, blanching, edema in extremities	Fair color, good filling, no edema
Neck veins on sitting	Slight distension at 45°

Gastrointestinal:

Problems	No problems
Last B.M.	Today

Genitourinary:

Problems	None

Integument:

Decubiti, location and description	Quarter size, pink area between buttocks
Skin turgor, coloring	Fair turgor, fair overall coloring

Motor Skeletal:

Range of motion, strength, and muscle tone	Full ROM, good strength
Posture	Stoops when stands, shoulder slightly abducted

Neurologic:

Level of consciousness	Alert, oriented to person, place, time, and purpose

Respiratory:

Cough	Fair, moderate strength
Breath sounds	Clear upper lobe, bronchi over lower base
Respiratory pattern	Shallow and rapid, little use of diaphragm
Sputum	Sputum thick white
Tidal volume	400 cc
Blood gases	PaO_2 61
	$PaCO_2$ 49
	pH 7.40
	HCO_3 30
	O_2 sat. 92%
	Hypoxia, compensated respiratory acidosis

(cont.)

289

TABLE 26-1. (CONTINUED)

Endocrine:
Signs of imbalance   None outstanding

Immunologic:
Signs of imbalance   None outstanding

Other physiochemical values   Within normal limits

Vital signs   Pulse, 88
                                                                    Blood pressure, 110/80
                                                                    Respiration rate, 28
                                                                    Temperature, 98.2 oral

Notes from physician's exam   Patient has had a 20-lb weight loss in last month.
                                                                        Quit smoking 4 years ago. Allergic to penicillin

Medications at home   *Digoxin* 0.25 mg every day
                                                                        KCL, one tablespoon twice a day

Medication   *Diazepam* 5 mg three times a day
                                                                    Oxytriphylline 200 mg three or four times a day
                                                                        as needed

2. Interview with patient; activities of daily living

Diet:
Describe your usual breakfast, lunch, dinner,   No breakfast, coffee at ten, sandwich for lunch,
   and snacks you eat at home.   chops and greens for dinner
Any food allergies?   None
What foods or fluids do you dislike?   Milk
How is your appetite: Here____ At home____?   Improving here, good at home

Sleep and Relaxation:
Do you have any trouble sleeping   None
   here____ at home____?
What helps when you can't go to sleep?   Watching a nightshow on TV
What helps relieve tension?   "Don't let myself get tense."
What do you do to relax?   Ride around in a car

Elimination:
How often do you have a B.M.?   Every day, after coffee
How often do you urinate/pass water?   3–4 times a day
Any difficulties?   "No"

Activity:
What kinds of jobs have you had?   Dishwasher, bartender
What do you do for exercise?   "Nothing"
How many people do you meet in an   About 10 or 15
   average day?
Who lives with you?   Wife and son

Normal Health:
Describe a normal day.   Up in the morn, wash up, help tidy the house, eat
                                                            lunch, go to the park, visit friends, dinner, TV
Describe your normal health.   No usual trouble, except for lungs
How is your vision?   "OK"
   hearing?   "OK"

(cont.)

TABLE 26–1. *(CONTINUED)*

breathing?	"Better"
walking?	"OK"
Any recent change?	"No"
Do you require any care that we should know about?	"No"

Medication:

Do you take medicines or drugs at home?	"A little yellow pill and a heart pill and some red liquid"
What do you take them for?	"To keep well"
Do you have any reactions or allergies or medicines?	"No"
What helps relieve pain or discomfort at home?	"Aspirin"

Perceptions on Health:

What are you in the hospital?	"I'm not sure."
What has your doctor told you?	"He says I'm doing better."
What does this mean to you?	"I'll be glad to go home."
Has your illness caused any problems with your wife/husband, friends? family? finances? employment?	My wife is spending too much money at home. I haven't worked for a while since I've been feeling poorly."
Do you feel that what happens to you can be controlled or is it just a matter of luck?	"Part of it is up to me and part of it is up to God."
Have you ever been in a hospital before?	"Yes"
What did you like or dislike that you remember?	Liked nothing special, disliked having to be cared for

Perceptions of Self:

What kind of person are you? How would you describe yourself, Mr. Mann?	"I'm a decent, sociable kind of person."
How would you describe your body?	"It's OK."
What is the worst part?	(points to throat, and healing tracheostomy stoma)
What is the best part?	(points to head and smiles)
Of all the things you do, what are you best at doing?	"Nothing"
Who is the most important person to you right now?	"My doctor"
What worries you most right now?	"Nothing"
How do you solve your problems?	"Just think about them and then go ahead and do what has to be done."
Do you have any pain or discomfort now?	"No"
What do you hope for most in the world?	"To get back on my feet"
Any questions about your care?	"No"
Is there anything we can do to make you more comfortable?	"I'd like a backrub."

3. Interview of Family & Friends

Is Mr. Mann usually in good health?	(Wife, 45 years old, neatly dressed) "Pretty good, except in the winter"
Does he need any help at home?	"Not really"

(cont.)

TABLE 26-1. (*CONTINUED*)

What was your reaction to his condition and hospitalization?	"It will be good to have him home again."
Do you have any questions about the care or his condition?	"How long will he be here?"
Who will assist at home if transportation, finances, activity, equipment, diet, medications necessary?	"He does most of it, but my son and I are there if he needs help."

Nurse's Observations

(1) Appearance	Disheveled, but clean; thin and tall; 140 lbs, 6 feet, 1 inch; slightly graying hair
(2) Communication pattern	a) quiet voice, speaks in halting sentences between deep breaths b) occasional eye contact c) body stance is tense and close and limbs are close to torso
(3) Interaction pattern/feeling tone	a) appropriate, if tense b) primarily passive, but initiates interaction at times c) intent but friendly with occasional appropriate humor
(4) Environment	a) four-bed ward room with two other patients. Corners filled with respirator equipment. Door open to noisy hallway. Windows face hills
(5) Patient's activity-rest schedule	Although not confined to bed rest, Mr. Mann remains in bed most of the day; rest interrupted by inhalation therapy, medications, meals and evening visitors

Developmental Stage:

Expected: middle-aged adult, appropriate biological, intrapersonal, and interpersonal systems	Observed: same

Situation Analysis (the interface between systems and environment)

Mr. Mann has one lung and it is affected with chronic bronchitis and emphysema. Usually he manages his limited activities well, but every year for the last 10 years he's been hospitalized for a pulmonary-associated disorder. He has never received training or education in pulmonary rehabilitation! He will probably have recurrent pneumonia and congestive heart failure, but there is a real possibility that through education and training:

1. He will have fewer respiratory problems
2. Hospitalizations will decrease as home management improves
3. General health will improve with an increase in subjective well-being

Stress Analysis

Analysis of the stress process is helpful in learning this model's type of approach to patient problems. It is necessary to transfer the complete analysis to the nursing care plan. However, to clarify difficult, complicated problems, it can be a useful tool. Two examples of how a patient problem may be analyzed are as follows:

(*cont.*)

TABLE 26-1. (*CONTINUED*)

I. **A.** (Stressor) Hospitalization
   B. (Stress) Isolation from family, restricted activity, forced dependency
   C. (Stress state) Loneliness, frustration
   D. (Adaptation) Contains feelings, complies with therapy
   E. (Stressed change) Not observed at this time
II. **A.** (Stressor) Chronic obstructed airways
   B. (Stress) Retention of CO_2, underventilation
   C. (Stress state) Respiratory acidosis and hypoxemia
   D. (Adaptation) Actual:
      1. Metabolic compensation to raise pH
      2. Increased respiratory rate
      Potential, long-term and short-term:
      3. IPPB respiratory therapy
      4. Breathing exercises and retraining
      5. Postural drainage
      6. Hydration
      7. Medications
   E. (Stressed change) Potential:
      1. Improved ventilation
      2. Increased activity
      3. Decreased hospitalizations

The nursing care plan for Mr. Mann should include the nursing diagnosis and intervention plan. A permanent copy of the entire nursing process should be recorded in the chart for reference and progressive evaluation of the patient's progress. An outline of the nursing process for Mr. Mann is given in Table 26–2.

---

have several distinctive characteristics. As with any direct interaction with the patient, the assessment is also an initial nursing intervention. The patient becomes alerted to the kind of information the nurse is interested in and becomes aware of the nurse's concern for him or her as an individual. Usually the questions only serve as an impetus for the patient to air thoughts and uppermost concerns. This experiential nature of the tool allows for a great deal of flexibility and the tone and content of each patient interview is individualized. Further individualization is possible by supplements to the tool that focus on specific problems. Assessment is ongoing, but a thorough initial study provides an important baseline and direction for further inquiry and therapy.

Nurses have two major responsibilities in incorporating interviews into the assessment plan. First, they should be familiar with the principles and techniques of interviewing and counseling before using a similar approach. Second, they should be very aware of their reactions and interpersonal approach during the interview in order to use its therapeutic effect to the maximum.

The specific tool presented in Table 26–1 assesses only portions of the patient's developmental status, systems review, and stress history. Four major sections of the assessment examine the patient from four perspectives. The physical review, chart review, interviews, and nurse's observations all provide relevant information. This assessment analysis applied to the nursing process

TABLE 26–2. THE NURSING PROCESS APPLIED TO A CLINICAL SITUATION

Nursing Diagnosis	Objective	Intervention	Evaluation
1. Lack of knowledge and understanding of disease and therapy	1. Provide information while supporting acceptance of therapy	1. (a) Teach lung function, disease status, therapies (b) Coordinate and support teaching program for health team (c) Nondirective counseling (Rogers, 1951) to assist patient to assimilate information and its impact on his life	1. Pretest–posttest Return demonstration Follow readmissions
2. Chronic CO_2 retention	2. Increase patient's ability to effectively ventilate	2. Home management training (refer to training manual)	2. Follow in clinic and home
3. Potential poor compliance due to complexity of home therapy	3. Follow through with clinic appointments and home therapy by patient	3. (a) Visiting nurse (b) Interdisciplinary team discharge conference with patient and family	3. (a) Phone follow-up with visiting nurse (b) Clinic follow-up
4. Healing decubitus between buttocks	4. Complete healing	4. Keep clean, dry, and relieved of pressure. Teach patient self-care and supervise positioning	4. Daily assessment

helps to order the information into a therapeutic plan. The abbreviated case that is presented shows how the tool can be applied to clinical situations.

The chart review serves to provide factual background information, the benefit of information from other disciplines, and a check on information provided by the patient. It can include data relevant to all systems, and to development and stress.

The physical review may utilize as sophisticated an approach as the nurse feels is necessary with each patient. It gathers information that may or may not be included by the physician or other members of the health team. The examination also provides an introductory rapport and relationship between the nurse and the patient.

The interview with the patient includes three sections: activities of daily living, perceptions on health, and perceptions on self. Assessment of the interpersonal system is obtained through the patient-nurse interaction during the interview. Answers to such questions as "How many people do you meet in a day?" and "Has your illness caused any problems with your family?" increase the nurse's understanding of the patient's interpersonal system. The section on perceptions provides the nurse with important qualitative information on the patient's intrapersonal system. Interestingly, patients do not object to these types of questions, but answer thoughtfully and sometimes poignantly.

The nurse's observations are both objective and subjective. They cover different systems, the environment, and the interaction between systems and environment. And all four major sections provide information on the patient's developmental status.

From this assessment tool it should be clear that the nursing process can be utilized in an efficient and brief manner with a minimum introduction of new words and unwieldy organization. The concept of stress process *can* be operationalized concisely while providing a theoretically sound, comprehensive, and consistent approach to nursing care.

SUMMARY

Nursing practice is complex. Nursing functions include an assortment of technical and interpersonal skills, often finely intermeshed with one another. Out of this rich variety has come challenge and real, valuable service to individuals and society. However, a great deal of role confusion, uncertainty, and questions about responsibility and accountability have been raised both within and outside the nursing profession. To clarify our rationales and therapeutic purpose, an organized approach to nursing care is imperative.

The SDS model has been presented as a comprehensive and flexible approach to identify and solve nursing problems related to patient care. The patient or client is, after all, the reason for being and the purpose of nursing practice. And the nurse who deals directly with the patient requires a coherent and practical guideline for nursing care.

The model presented in this paper represents a synthesis of structure and process that can be activated through a problem-solving approach to nursing care. It is relevant to nursing education, research, and practice. The purpose of the model is to begin to apply theory in the pragmatic world of patients and organizations.

REFERENCES

Byrne, M. L., & Thompson, L. F. (1972). *Key concepts for the study and practice of nursing*. St. Louis: Mosby.
Rogers, C. R. (1951). *Client-centered therapy*. Boston: Houghton.

The Systems-Developmental-Stress Model in Psychiatric Nursing

John English

This chapter presents a paradigm adapted from the Systems-Developmental-Stress (SDS) model designed by Chrisman and Riehl (1974). The adaptations were done in the interests of making the model specific for psychiatric nursing. However, care was taken to keep the model generalizable enough so that it could apply to all the conditions likely to be encountered in psychiatric nursing practice.

Essentially, the model was intended to provide students and practitioners with a way to look at and think about the condition of clients' lives and their problems, and to give a framework to plan psychiatric nursing intervention. For this reason we referred to the model as a paradigm. *Paradigm* is defined in Webster's New Collegiate Dictionary (1983) as an outstandingly clear example or a pattern. In the literature a paradigm has been described as a map or a world view. The map or the view is not the world itself, but a representation of it.

It has been noted by Flynn (1980) that paradigms have a habit of changing as our perception of the world changes. These perceptual changes are the result of advances in knowledge and awareness of the human condition in the real world.

Since first tentatively introducing the model to students in the School of Psychiatiric Nursing in Selkirk, Manitoba, Canada, as one of several which could be used by psychiatric nurses, the faculty has increasingly appreciated its relevance and applicability. As a result of this enhanced appreciation the faculty has adopted this model, as modified as a paradigm, upon which to base the curriculum.

This step was not an easy one to take. The faculty has had to relearn a vocabulary and make a conscious effort to apply the terminology of the paradigm when discussing clients with students. The students seem to learn the material with more ease; indeed, they contributed greatly to the faculty's learning by helping to clarify points by questioning areas where ambiguity existed. As a result of this reciprocal learning process, the original model has undergone further adaptations. These changes are most noticeable in the tools presented as examples in the original. Some terminology has also been changed so that it more accurately reflects our particular perception of the mental health care environment.

Inviolate in this whole process has been the structure and the process of the original model. Apart from the changes in language these remain as originally conceived by the authors. The underlying theories are almost considered as verities and are treated with respect and unchallenged by this faculty.

STRUCTURE OF THE PARADIGM

The structure contains two viewpoints of human life—people as a system and people as a developing organism. These viewpoints are considered within a framework of change, because change accounts for human development from conception to death. Both the viewpoint of people as a system and of people developing over time are realistic and necessary to adequately describe real life.

As a system, human beings are described as having psychological (intrapersonal), social (interpersonal), and biological (physical) subsystems. These subsystems are seen as having strong interrelationships within the entire system and are of equal importance (see Fig. 27-1).

The system is perceived as growing or developing through time as people go through life's stages. Diagramatically this development may very simply be represented as an unidirectional flow from conception to death (see Fig. 27-2). Combining these two viewpoints gives us the structure of this paradigm (see Fig. 27-3).

This framework—indeed the entire paradigm—is consistent with Adolph Meyer's (Mora, 1980) concept of psychiatric disorders, which he saw as reactions of the personality to psychological, social, and biological factors.

PROCESS OF THE PARADIGM

Specifically, the process of this paradigm refers to the stress process, which is universal in its relevance and applicability. Because of this, it provides a comprehensive method for perceiving a client's life situation and problems.

For the purposes of this paradigm the stress process is, again simplistically, perceived as a unidirectional flow (see Fig. 27-4).

To be able to understand the paradigm one must know the meanings of the following terms.

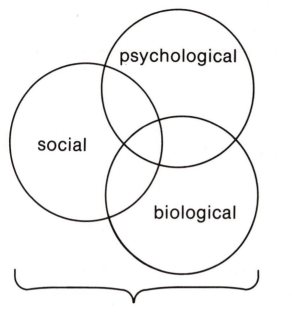

Figure 27-1. The human system.

STRESSOR: The causative agent that initiates the stress process.

STRESS: The dynamic tension that produces strain or tension within the human system.

STRESS STATE: The condition of the human system when it reacts to stress.

ADAPTATION: The response of the human system that enables it to better cope with the stress state or the stress.

CHANGED STATE: The difference in the human system when it has reestablished equilibrium following the stress process; as distinguished from change due to normal development.

STRESS PROCESS: The sequence of reactions that occur in response to a stressor.

STRUCTURE AND PROCESS

Succinctly, the SDS paradigm considers the human system as comprised of mutually interactive psychological, social, and biological subsystems. The system is in a continuous state of development as it moves through time; it is also subjected to stressors, which initiate the stress process. Both the structure and the process are diagramatically represented in Figure 27-5.

The paradigm now leads us inevitably to a definition of health. Using the language of this model, *health* is manifested, as the individual evolves and matures, as a dynamic state of equilibrium derived from the synergistic interac-

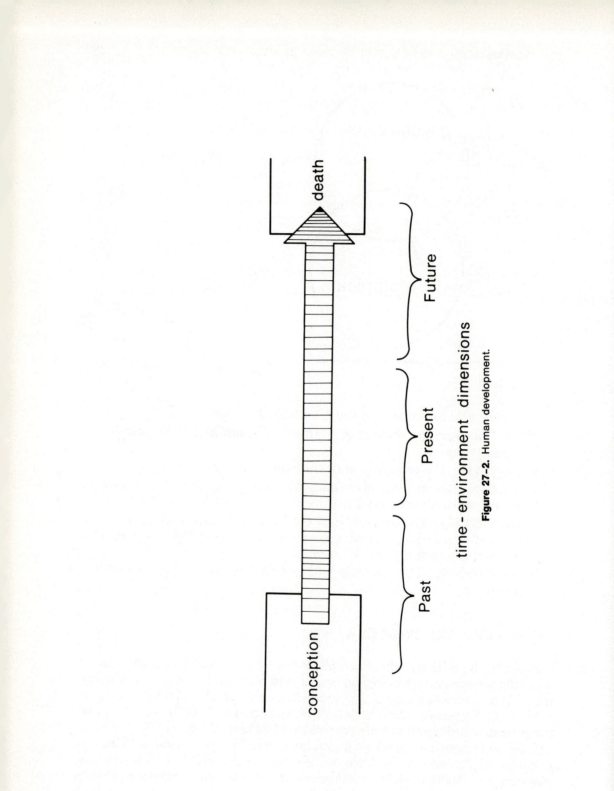

Figure 27-2. Human development.

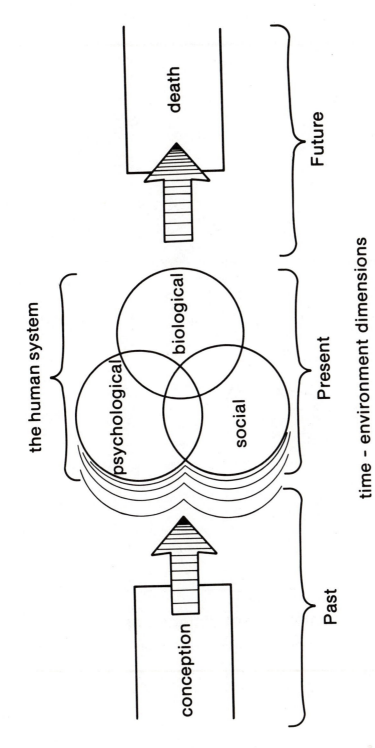

Figure 27–3. The structural framework of the SDS paradigm.

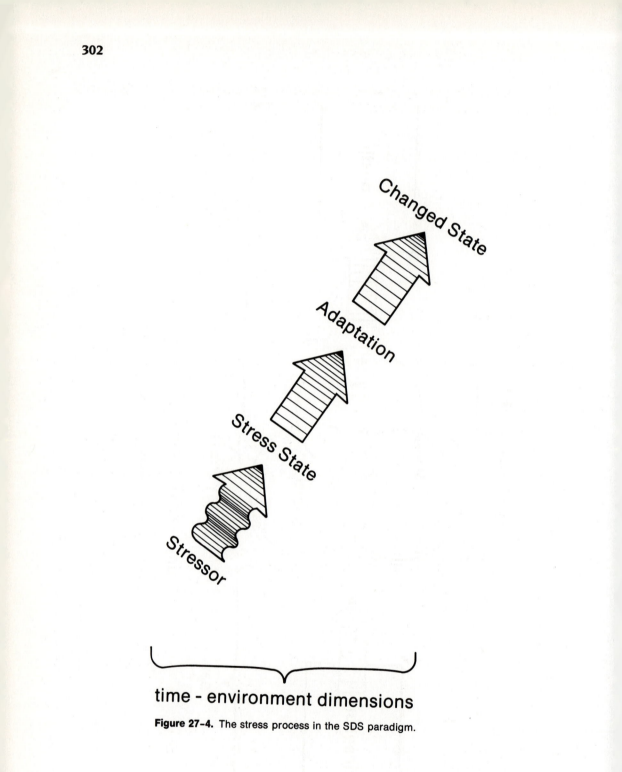

Figure 27–4. The stress process in the SDS paradigm.

tion of psychological, social, and biological positive adaptations to stressors arising from changes in internal or external environments.

USING THE PARADIGM

To use this paradigm psychiatric nurses must hold certain values, which are reflected in the attitudes they adopt. In turn, these attitudes influence the psychiatric nurse's professional behavior. Behaviors indicative of values held should include:

- Supporting and promoting health.
- Demonstrating caring concern for the welfare of the client.
- Acting as an advocate for the client when necessary.
- Supporting life and the quality of life.
- Assessing and formulating the client's life and problems is accompanied by respecting the client as an individual.
- Including the client, whenever possible, in the planning and decision-making processes around issues concerning his or her welfare.
- Interceding in the human system with therapeutic purpose.

In clinical practice the psychiatric nurse focuses on the total human system. This holistic approach means that not only must all the subsystems be considered but also the interactions of the subsystems and the relationships of the human system to time and to the environment (interfacing with other systems and suprasystems).

By using a systems approach it is possible to think in an organized way about interdependent components in the human condition. The human system described here has been divided into subsystems, which have been extensively studied and described in the literature (Berkow, 1982).

SUBSYSTEMS

Psychological Subsystem

This subsystem relates to the personal self. Elements in this subsystem are always felt and interacting. These elements include:

- Thought processes.
- Self-concept (body image, self-awareness, and self-esteem).
- Affective responses.
- Ego controls (e.g., emotional self-control, impulse control).
- World view (e.g., optimism, pessimism, fatalism).

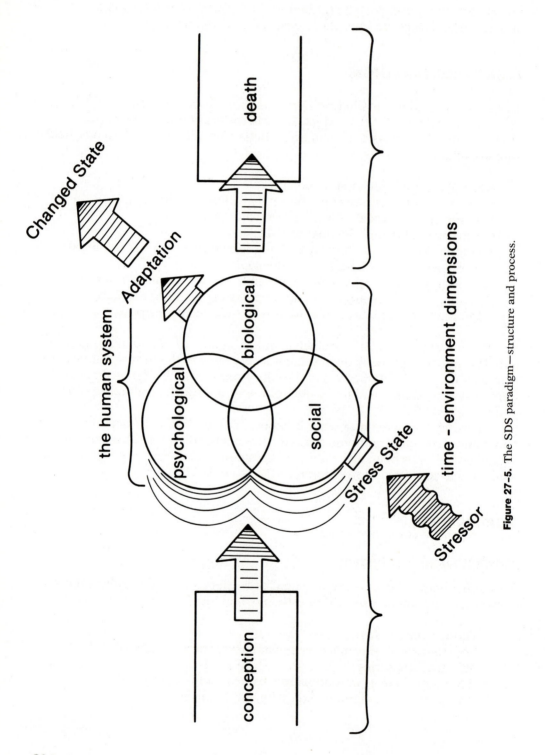

Figure 27-5. The SDS paradigm—structure and process.

- Intelligence.
- Religious beliefs.

Social Subsystem

This subsystem concerns interpersonal variables. Elements from both the other subsystems interact with elements from this subsystem. The elements in the social subsystem include:

- Cultural factors.
- Socioeconomic considerations.
- Transactional factors, including (1) patterns (e.g., play, dependancy-independancy); and (2) roles—occupational, communal (e.g., neighborhood, community), affiliative (e.g., friends, clubs), familial, and sexual.

Biological Subsystem

The body is the concern of this subsystem. By making arbitrary anatomical and physiological divisions (elements) it is possible to organize thinking, knowledge, and communication about physical functions and problems. The divisions are consistent with major medical specialities.

The elements of this subsystem are:

- Neurologic.
- Endocrine.
- Immunologic.
- Reproductive.
- Muscular-skeletal.
- Cardiovascular.
- Respiratory.
- Lymphatic.
- Reticuloendothelial.
- Gastrointestinal.
- Integumentary.
- Genitourinary.
- Other.

Consideration of these subsystems and their interactions provides a structure for assessment. This approach is consistant with that used in DSM III (APA, 1980) where multiple types of mental disorders are described. The basis for the approach used by the authors in this work was also derived from Adolph Meyer's thinking (Mora, 1980).

TERMINOLOGY

Full use of the paradigm involves the assessment of the stress process on the human system. Here, consideration must be given not only to the distant and recent history of the stress process experienced by the client, but also to how the stress process effects the therapeutic relationship between the client and his or her psychiatric nurse therapist. It is therefore necessary that users of the paradigm be very familiar with the terms' meanings; for this reason the terms are repeated below with further explanation.

Stressor is the term used to identify the agent that provokes the stress state. It is not meant to be the cause itself, although it may act as a catalyst. The stress that gives rise to the stress state may start with the stressor or from the client. For instance, a person may panic at the thought of having to cross a high bridge. The bridge can be thought of as the stressor; however, it is the person's psyche that produced the stress. Chrisman and Riehl (1989) cite the following physical example: "If a man is hit by an automobile, the auto may be the stressor, but its velocity and mass applied the stress. The distinction here is a help in planning intervention (p. 282)."

Psychiatric nursing intervention includes the management of stress. Such management would be tailored to the individual's adaptation and could include the elimination, reduction, or resolution of stress, or even the introduction of increased stress.

Stress state portrays the upset within the person as a result of stress—for example, the feeling of unreality and disconnectedness with the world by a person undergoing severe psychological shock. Physically damaged tissues, lowered blood pressure, and bleeding comprise the stress state of a person after having suffered an accident. Stress state, then, simply describes the impact of the stress on the person.

Adaptation is the real issue of the stress process because it influences the change outcome. Adaptation can have positive or negative results. For instance, the psychological shock following a traumatic event can have positive aspects because it allows the person to bring defenses into play that can help in psychological readjustment. However, if the state of shock continues over an extended period of time, then it is negative in its effects and leads to maladaptation. Physiologically, Chrisman and Riehl (1989) cite fever as a positive adaptation and go on to point out that if the fever is so high as to cause damage, then that illustrates negative adaptation.

A person may adapt to cope with stress by avoiding stressors (taking another route to avoid a high bridge) or by eliminating, reducing, or resolving the stress. Many people seek out stress as a way of life that provides a challenge or acts as a stimulus for growth.

The role of the psychiatric nurse is to help the client adapt to stress so that the stressed change outcome is positive rather than negative. Of course, positive adaptation promotes active survival, a sense of well-being and individual growth and strength.

Changed state is the term used in this paradigm to refer to the change that occurs as a result of the stress and the person's adaptation to the stress, as distinct from change that comes from normal development. Normal development produces its own particular types of stresses. These stresses should be distinguished during assessment to clarify a formulation of the client's problems.

Adaptation occurs as a result of stress. The resulting changes may be desirable (positive) or undesirable (negative). Changed state then may increase or decrease the favorable performance of the human organism depending on the wholeness of the organism, the nature and severity of the stress, and the form of the adaptation.

STRESS ASSESSMENT AND REACTIONS

It should be recognized that we all need some stress in our lives to act as a motivating agent. However, sometimes too much stress can produce turmoil in a person. This type of stress can be assessed by considering the following questions:

- What is the source of the stress? Stress can arise from either internal (psychological or physiological) or external (social or physical) environments.
- What is the intensity of the stress? Here intensity may be roughly divided into severe, moderate, or slight levels. Severe stress would always require intervention to reduce it. Moderate stress may need to be decreased, or the client may need support through the stress process. Slight stress may need to be increased, with support given to the client. The therapeutic approach depends on the person's residual stress, tolerance to stress, and preparedness to cope with the stress, and the potential direction of the change state.
- What is the scope of impact? This refers to impact of the stress on the human system. Biologically, it may include percent of an area damaged—for example, a 40 percent burn—or the variety of ways the stress affects all the subsystems of the person. An illness, for instance, may not only cause physical suffering but also loneliness, financial burden, and loss of self-esteem.
- What was the speed of onset—sudden, quick, gradual, slow, or insidious?
- How long has the stress been endured?
- What residual stress does the client have? This refers to stress accumulated from past experiences that are currently affecting the client. For example, the person's history of fears, anxieties and failures, physical handicaps, immune states, and so forth.

In addition to the necessity of assessing the stress, the reaction to the stress also needs to be appraised. The most convenient way to do this is to consider its effects on the subsystems and in the systems interaction with the environment (*see* Fig. 27–6).

Reactions of the Psychological Subsystem

These include changes in affect and changes in cognition. Changes in this area may be expected to effect mood, perception, thought, judgment, problem solving, and even sensorium.

Reactions of the Social Subsystem

Changes in this subsystem could include socioeconomic factors as well as alterations in role relationships in important areas of a client's life.

Reactions of the Biological Subsystem

Considered here are alterations in the functioning of any of the elements that comprise this subsystem—from cellular changes to effects on whole body systems.

Reactions of the human system with the environment may also alter. Interface relationships with other systems or suprasystems may undergo a change in their intensity or nature. These changes are usually detected through alterations in communication between the effective systems.

Chrisman and Riehl (1989) summarize as follows:

> The systems developmental continuum describes a structure. The stress process identifies the problems that can arise in both the functions and form of the structure. Problems in function refer to system equilibrium and developmental progress. Problems in form refer to the effect of temporal dimensions and the environment on the organism. (p. 285)

ROLE OF THE PSYCHIATRIC NURSE

We have defined a paradigm as a map or a world view. With this in mind it is appropriate to read our map in relation to the real world of patient care. To do this we need to consider the role of the psychiatric nurse in relation to clients. By doing this, we follow the tradition of more conventional map makers who always keep the user in mind when designing and constructing a map.

Psychiatric nursing requires that its practitioners engage in a wide range of functions. These functions can encompass various therapeutic modalities through the use of self, or they can involve physical nursing care or application of technology. In addition to the use of the nursing process, psychiatric nurses need to work with other health care professions. These functions are described below using the language of this paradigm.

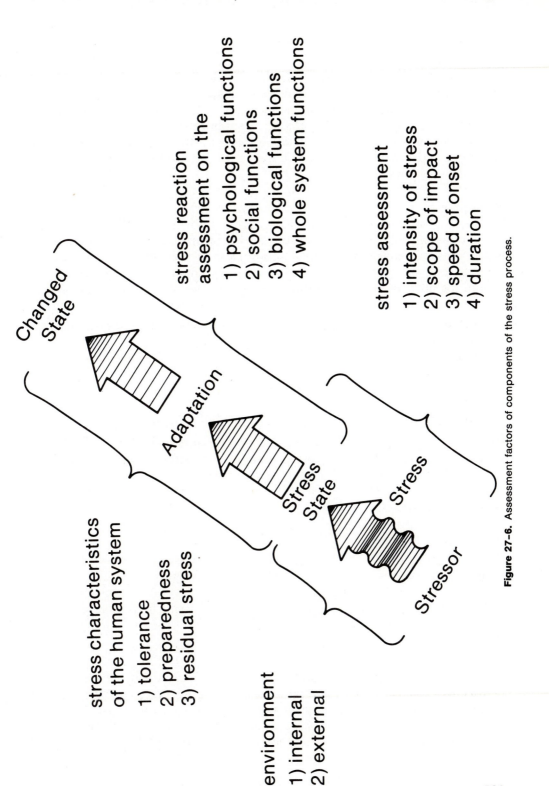

stress characteristics
of the human system

1) tolerance
2) preparedness
3) residual stress

environment

1) internal
2) external

Changed
State

Adaptation

Stress
State

Stress

Stressor

stress reaction
assessment on the

1) psychological functions
2) social functions
3) biological functions
4) whole system functions

stress assessment

1) intensity of stress
2) scope of impact
3) speed of onset
4) duration

Figure 27–6. Assessment factors of components of the stress process.

Use of the Nursing Process

Psychiatric nurses use the scientific method, or the problem-solving process termed the *nursing process*. This paradigm is particularly apt for use with the nursing process because it is holistic in its scope.

Through use of the stress process it is possible to identify a client's problems and in addition identify strengths or supports that may help in problem solving. Areas for consideration are guided by the structural part of the paradigm and the relationships (interfaces) of the human system with other systems or suprasystems.

Assessment

Psychiatric nursing assessment is organized information gathering with a therapeutic purpose. Appropriate sources for information may include interviews; physical, physiological, or psychological measurements; observations; records; and interactions or self-reactions. Psychiatric nursing assessment should include examination of the:

- System—analysis of the function of the psychological, social, and biological subsystems.
- Development—developmental variables and temporal-environmental impact.
- Stress—the stress process as it relates to systems and development.

Monitoring and detecting signs and symptoms of psychological, social, and biological stability or instability are major assessment functions of the psychiatric nurse. The relationship of assessment to the stress process is illustrated in Figure 27–6. Viewed from this perspective, assessment can no longer be seen as just a task, but must be perceived as a process in which the psychiatric nurse is an active participant with the client and with other health disciplines.

Psychiatric Nursing Diagnosis

This is a statement of a real or potential problem inherent in the system or the development as a result of the stress process. The diagnosis should refer to the effect of stress on the subsystem(s) or their interface(s). Diagnoses can be drawn from the rich diversity of subjects found in nursing literature—for example, compliance, sleeplessness, and decubiti.

Objectives

These are statements of goals for therapy. For instance, an objective may be to help a client avoid a real or potential stressor; it might focus on a particular psychiatric nursing activity to change the intensity, scope, or duration of the stress; or it may even be designed to support an optimum stress level. In all these cases, the objective is to achieve a predicted or desired end behavior or level of functioning (changed state). Objectives for psychiatric nursing care may be stated as short- or long-term priorities.

Objectives may also be stated to reflect activities necessary to prevent deterioration of a client's condition due to unmitigated stress. For example, safety and comfort measures avoid or reduce potential stressors and stresses.

Implementation

This involves choice of psychiatric nursing action directed toward any part of the stress process. Each action is always based on knowledge of the client's system and development with a projection or prediction of consequences. Use of technique, therapeutic use of self or others, and technical skills can prevent, reduce, remove, or balance the stress encountered by a client. Most psychiatric nurses who give direct care are also involved in the administration of physicians' therapy; thus they can multiply the effectiveness of both. The psychiatric nurse can use this paradigm to assist clients' adaptation as the physicians' therapy is administered.

Evaluation

In the nursing process, evaluation refers to the progress of the client as related to the objectives for care. Thus the focus of the evaluation would be on the particular part of the stress process addressed in the objective. Evaluation data provide a framework for communication to other psychiatric nurses and health team members about the progress of the client.

Embodying the concept of the stress process in the psychiatric nursing process can effect the insight with which care is planned and the effectiveness of the psychiatric nursing intervention.

Coordination of Care

Coordination of therapy can consume a large part of a psychiatric nurse's time. Essentially, coordination can be perceived as balancing the introduction of stress and maximizing the therapeutic effect through organization of the overall plan of care. Coordination focuses on the stressor and adaptation phases of the stress process.

Psychiatric Nursing Leadership

Leadership means providing guidance and direction to providers of direct care as they intervene in the stress process of clients. At the level of the suprasystem, the psychiatric nurse leader provides intervention in the stress process in the health care organization and among its staff.

Because institutions have evolved divisions of labor among various levels of nursing personnel, it is important to identify how this paradigm relates to other members of the nursing team. For instance, the nursing aide or attendant primarily focuses on identifying major signs of physical or social problems of patients; their implementation is under direction and supervision and is aimed at providing comfort and safety measures. They work in a "here and now" orientation. The psychiatric nursing assistant helps with the planning and implementation of nursing actions that promote comfort and safety for clients. Under direction, they administer nursing and medical therapies. They work in the "here and now," and in addition refer to the past in their orientation to client care. The stress process provides a framework for examination of overt psychological, social, and biological problems.

Registered psychiatric nurses focus on the interplay of the psychological, social, and biological subsystems in relation to the continuum of development of the client. They relate their activities to the client's past, present, and future and consider the past, present, and future environment of the client. The stress process is a means of practically applying their knowledge of systems and human development.

Sample Assessment Instrument

This assessment (Appendices 27–A through 27–C) has been developed using the structure and process elements of the model. The data to be gathered and considered are organized around the three subsystems of the model. Special emphasis has been placed on the psychological subsystem, and an outline for performing a mental status examination (Appendix 27–B) has been included. The inclusion of this material is for the benefit of students who generally need a specific guideline until they are sufficiently comfortable with the process to effectively perform the examination more covertly.

The assessment guide (*see* Appendix 27–A) is not meant to be a nursing history to be used in residential institutions. Many such institutions have developed means whereby important initial information can be quickly gathered and incorporated into an initial plan for the safety and comfort of the client. Rather, this assessment instrument is intended to act as a guide to an in-depth assessment so that treatment planning for a longer period of time can occur.

Section 7 of the tool (Appendix 27–A), the interpersonal transactions within the interview context, has been included so that the psychiatric nurse has an opportunity to illustrate a client's problems or difficulties by providing anecdotes of interactions within the therapeutic relationship.

The formulation schema (*see* Appendix 27–C) has been provided to help the psychiatric nurse sort through and think about the data collected. A written formulation should be fairly brief and should attempt to explain the stress process experienced by the client. It should be no more complex than the data warrant.

CONCLUSION

A recent follow-up study of 1 year graduates included a question on the value of the SDS paradigm to the graduates practice. A 5-point semantic differential scale was provided and an invitation to comment on the rating was made. A hearteningly positive response was received—on the 5-point scale (with 1 representing low value and 5 representing high value) we found a mode of 4.0, a mean of 3.6, and a median of 3.6. All the comments on the rating were positive, although one respondent noted that psychiatric nurses tended to place insufficient evidence on assessing the biological subsystem. Another respondent reported that the interdisciplinary team on which she worked did not use the model, making her feel somewhat isolated. There are also indications in the comments that lead the faculty to appreciate the need to further help students understand the value of introducing selected stressors into the environment of clients with chronic psychiatric disorders who have long been housed in institutional settings.

Over the past few years of teaching and using the SDS paradigm, the faculty has learned that it is best to introduce it early in this 2-year program. Yet it is important that students have an introduction to the theories contained in the model prior to its introduction. Thus, systems theory, the concept of health and illness, stress theory, and adaptation are all taught prior to expounding on the SDS paradigm itself. We have also found that it is important that all nursing courses use the paradigm as an integral way of presenting the course objectives and in teaching the course content. Of prime importance, however, is the use of the paradigm in clinical practice situations and in pre- and postclinical conferences. It is here that students struggle with and learn the importance of thinking in an organized way about their clients' lives and problems. Thus they are better enabled to provide insightful empathic individualized care to a clientele that continually presents us with one of the greatest challenges in health care today.

REFERENCES

American Psychiatric Association. (1980). *Diagnostic and statistical manual of mental disorders* (3rd ed.). Washington, DC: Author.

Berkow, R. (Ed.). (1982). *The Merck manual of diagnoses and therapy* (14th ed.). Rahway, NJ: Merck.

Chrisman, M., & Riehl, J. (1989). The systems-developmental stress model. In J. Riehl (Ed.), *Conceptual models for nursing practice* (3rd ed.) (pp. 277–295). Norwalk, CT: Appleton & Lange.

Flynn, P. (1980). *Holistic health: The art and science of care.* Bowie, MD: Brady.

Mora, G. (1980). Adolph Meyer. In H. I. Kaplan, A. M. Freedman, & B. J. Sadock (Eds.), *Comprehensive textbook of psychiatry* (3rd ed.). Baltimore: Williams & Wilkins.

Websters new collegiate dictionary. (1983). Springfield, MA: Merriam-Webster.

Appendix 27–A _____

Assessment Summary Guide

1. IDENTIFYING DATA

Name, address, age, phone, date of birth, marital status.

2. REFERRAL SOURCE AND REASON

    A. Include relevant details of routes of referral to the unit, including name and phone numbers of referring persons or agencies.
    B. *PRESENTING PROBLEM*—Include, where possible, verbatim quotes by patient about the nature of the problem.

3. HISTORY OF PRESENTING PROBLEM

    A. Sequence of events that led to present condition.
    B. Note precipitating stressors and circumstances surrounding breakdown.
    C. Include sketch of *present life situation* and patient's current functioning r.e.: Interpersonal sphere (family, work/school, social life).

4. BIOLOGICAL HISTORY

    A. Health history—physical.
    B. Significant illness in the family.
    C. Functional enquiry:
        Appetite.
        Sleep.
        Weight.
        Medication being taken.

5. HISTORY OF SOCIAL FUNCTIONING

A. Composition of family, parental and marital, with ages.
B. Social, economic, ethnic, and religious background and legal infractions.
C. Education.
D. Employment.
E. Sexual and marital history and present functioning.

6. PSYCHOLOGICAL FUNCTIONING

A. Developmental history.
B. Psychiatric history.
C. Mental status examination.
　　Appearance and behavior.
　　Talk.
　　Thought.
　　Mood.
　　Sensorium functioning, level of consciousness, orientation, memory, and intelligence.
　　Judgment and insight.

7. INTERPERSONAL TRANSACTIONS WITHIN THE INTERVIEW CONTEXT

8. FORMULATION AND IDENTIFICATION OF PROBLEMS IN ADAPTATION

9. PLAN FOR INTERVENTION

To effect adaptive process.

Appendix 27-B _____

Mental Status

1. APPEARANCE AND BEHAVIOR

This should include a short description of what nurses, students, physician and others in contact with the patient have observed, including a brief statement of the patient's physical condition.

General Description

A. Dress: neat, untidy, eccentric, etc
B. Posture: relaxed, rigid, tense, erect, recumbent, etc
C. Facial expression: mobile, fixed, ecstatic, depressed, angry, etc
D. Attitude: friendly, aggressive, cooperative, resistive, negativistic, etc
E. General mood: objective statements from observation, calm, elated, anxious, irritable, depressed, tearful, listless. (Note: variations and discrepancies between mood and thought content and changes of mood at different times of the day)
F. Motor activity: under or over restless, dystonia, graceful movements

2. STREAM OF TALK

A. Rate, quality, amount, and form—under pressure, retarded, blocked, relevant, logical, coherent, concise, illogical, flight of ideas, neologisms, word salad, circumstantial, rhyming, punning, loud, whispered, screaming, etc

3. SUBJECTIVE EMOTIONAL REACTION AND MOOD

In contrast to observed mood, data on subjective mood are obtained by answers to questions such as:

How do you feel?

What part of the day is most pleasant? Most difficult?

Do you become angry, depressed, irritable, frightened, panicky? When? Why?

At times, do you feel you'd rather die than continue this way?

4. CONTENT OF THOUGHT

Note:—Here, more than anywhere else, care must be taken to avoid direct questioning or slavishly following the outline. Many patients will not answer or will get angry if asked, "Do you hear voices?" or "Do you see people who you know aren't there?" Yet these same patients may have hallucinations and be much relieved if they are allowed tactfully to share these disturbing experiences with someone. At one point or another they may need reassurance. They may ask for it, saying "Nurse, this sounds crazy." They should be reassured, told that such things happen quite frequently to people under emotional stress.

A. Obsessions, Compulsions, and Phobic Thoughts

Do you have thoughts that you are unable to control or rid yourself of?

Do you fear storms, heights, crowds, traffic?

Are you compelled to follow a certain ritual while dressing, eating, walking, etc?

Do you feel tense if the above are not done?

B. Feelings of Unreality and Depersonalization

Do you feel as if you were in a fog?

Do things look dim or distant to you?

Do things look as if you were in a dream?

Do things that happen to you feel unreal?

Do you feel unnatural?

C. Delusions (Gradual Approach)

Have you had any unusual, unpleasant, or perplexing experiences?

Have you had any peculiar thoughts, dreams, imaginations?

D. Persecutory Trends

Are you considered friendly and popular?

Do people like you? Treat you well?

Do they talk about you?
Are you suspicious of others?
Do you feel annoyed, wronged, poisoned? How do you explain?

E. Passivity Feelings

Do you think others may be able to influence you? How?
Do you think that some people can read minds? Can they read yours?
  Control you? How?

F. Somatic Trends

Has any part of your body changed? Reference to elimination, senses,
  digestion, pain, sweat, genitals, sexual powers.

G. Illusions

(Important in the examination of delirious patients although usually the
  presence of illusions is established on objective evidence.)
Have you misinterpreted shadows or noises?
Do body sensations lead you to think you are being touched?

H. Hallucinations (Gradual Approach)

1. *Auditory:*
  Do you hear buzzing in your ears? Noises?
  Do you know of anybody who ever heard noises?
  Did anything like that ever happen to you?
2. *Visual:*
  Flashes of light?
  Did you ever imagine you saw things as if in a dream?
  Did you imagine that you saw things and people, and wondered
    whether you were dreaming or awake?
3. *If any hallucinations, ask:*
Auditory What do they say? Pleasant, unpleasant? Whose voice? Man?
          Woman? In both ears? What does it mean? Are they talking to
          you? About you?
Visual   At night or day? Eyes open or shut? Where? What or whom
          do you see? What does it mean?
4. *Gustatory:*
  Things taste the same? Peculiar?
5. *Olfactory:*
  Queer odors?

5. SENSORIUM EXAMINATION

This test is most important in delirium and dementia. It addresses attention, memory, grasp of general information, and capacity for logical thought. Frequently this part of the examination may annoy or provoke the patient, as the patient is apt to equate direct questioning in areas of attention, memory, and information as tests of intelligence. As a matter of fact, much of what follows may be obtained casually and indirectly in eliciting the historical data in the conventional manner. Information concerning orientation and memory can be obtained through inquiry of when the patient came to the hospital, events that have transpired since, etc. It is best when possible to avoid direct questioning and to obtain as much information through indirect and casual means.

A. *Orientation* as to time (day, month, year), place, person, and situation. Does patient recognize doctors, nurses?

B. *Memory*

Remote past: Use questions that can be checked, such as: How old are you? When were you born? When married? How old? Date of birth of children?

Recent past: Home address? Telephone number? When and how did you come to the hospital? Events in past 24 hours? What happened when first arrived in hospital?

Retention and recall: Repeat forward 31759 or 43285 (7th year). Repeat reversed 6528 or 4937 (9th year). Repeat reversed 15286 or 69482 (14th year). Recall 375 Vine Street after five minutes, one hour, next day.

C. *Grasp of general information:*   Name governor, mayor, last five presidents (three is average), four large cities, wars, current events, etc

D. *Calculations:* Multiplication, addition, count coins, simple arithmetical problems. (May have been obtained from asking patient his or her age, ages of children, etc)

E. *Reading, writing, and speech:* (Test phrases). Describe speech and writing. Have patient read cowboy story and note if patient gets meaning and can tell story. Note character of reading, memory lapses, errors, and confabulation.

> A cowboy from Arizona went to San Francisco and took his dog, which he left at a friend's while he purchased a new suit of clothes. Dressed finely, he went back to the dog, whistled to him, called him by name, and patted him. However, the dog would have nothing to do with him in his new hat and coat and gave a mournful howl. Coaxing was of no avail, so the cowboy went away and donned his old garments, whereupon the dog immediately showed his wild joy on seeing his master as he thought he ought to be.

F. *Level of awareness:* Serial subtraction of 7's and 3's from 100. (This test is dependent on at least a grammar school education.) Attention should be paid to the manner in which the test is performed. It is not only a test of arithmetic ability. Serial subtraction, which taxes continuously and repeatedly the ability to attend and to concentrate, is one of the most valuable tests in detecting slight changes in attention produced by delirium. Long before arithmetic errors may be manifested, the client may betray decreasing ability to perform the task by heightened effort, perserveration, increase in total time of the test, frequent hesitation or questioning, requesting a new start, or becoming irritable, deprecating the test and the examiner.

G. *Judgment:* Does the client show good or poor judgment in his or her general activities? Does the client give due value to practical considera- tion? Difference between lie and mistake, dwarf and child, idleness and laziness, poverty and misery, character and reputation. Plans for the fu- ture; is judgment better on impersonal than on personal matters?

H. *Abstractions:* Proverbs such as: "Squeaking wheel gets the grease." "A rolling stone gathers no moss." "The apple falls near its tree." "The tongue is the enemy of the neck." Note whether interpretation is: (1) literal, (2) the meaning of the proverb is understood, (3) and whether the client sees any relationship to his or her personal situation and whether all proverbs are interpreted in the light of personal problems.

I. *Insight:*   **1.** Verbatim statement—client's formulation of him- or herself in present situation.

   2. Is the client aware of mental or physical defects: Does the client realize that the difficulty is within him- or herself, or does he ascribe it to external sources?

   3. Does the client make any statement as to emotional nature of his or her illness? Insight into etiological or dynamic factors.

Appendix 27–C

Formulation Schema

Prior to considering a formulation of a patient's difficulties or problems, you should have completed the assessment format up to and including the Mental Status examination (Appendix 27–B).

The schema is presented as a series of questions designed to guide your thinking about the material you have gathered using the Assessment Summary Guide (Appendix 27–A).

1. How is the client's stressed state explained?

A. By changes in biological homeostasis:
Neurologic changes.
Biochemical changes.
Body function changes—eating, sleeping, elimination, and exercise.
Physical illness.
B. By changes in social relations:
Family.
Other object relations.
C. By changes in psychological homeostasis:
Appearance and behavior.
Subjective emotional reaction and mood.
Thought content.
Sensorium functioning.
D. Environmental stressors.

2. How is the client's adaptation explained?

A. By considerations of learning theory models:
Operant conditioning.
Classical conditioning.
Modeling.
B. By psychodynamic considerations such as:
Defense mechanisms.
Personality trends.
Interpersonal transactions.

C. By present and recent affective equilibria:
What the client fears.
What the client's needs are as he or she perceives them.
What the client's needs are as you perceive them.
How alone the client is.

3. How is the above state of affairs developed?

A. By psychosocial developmental history.
B. By ongoing functioning and structure of the client's nuclear family.
C. By the client's culture derivation.
D. By the client's genetic endowment.

Part IV

Interaction Models for Nursing Practice

The three conceptual frameworks selected for this section are those by Levine, Orem, and Riehl. Levine's model (Chapter 28) is a new addition with this edition. She first published her model about 20 years ago. In a communication with Levine, she referred to the first sentence in her book, which notes that "nursing is a human interaction." There is no doubt, then, on how to classify her model. Following Levine's model is a critique by Glass (Chapter 29) and an application of Levine's conservation principles in Taylor's nursing diagnosis of neurological patients (Chapter 30).

An interpretation of the Orem model is given in Chapter 31, a reprint by Riehl. In discussing the Orem model, Stevens commented that originally Orem used a systems approach but later shifted to an operational methodology. For the classifications utilized in this book, the latter would more nearly suggest an interaction-type model than either of the other two categories. Also, the focus of Orem's model is on patients' self-care. This infers that a nurse-patient interaction transpires even though it may be primarily nurse determined. Orem's model is critiqued by Feathers (Chapter 32) using Stevens' evaluative guidelines. In Chapter 33, Geden discusses the relationship between self-care theory and empirical research.

The last of the three theoretical frameworks presented in this unit is the Riehl Interaction Model. As the name indicates, it is classified appropriately. This model was first introduced in the second edition of this book. In Chapter 34, Riehl includes an analysis by Stevens that, like a self-report, aims for objectivity. Two chapters were written by authors in England, where the model is popular and extensively used. The first (Chapter 35) is by Aggleton and Chalmers and the second (Chapter 36) by Arumugam; both illustrate the model's application in different clinical settings.

The remaining four chapters describe research studies in clinical settings. In Chapter 37, Knauth and Gross illustrate the effective use of the Riehl Interaction Model by childbirth health educators. Using the guidelines for the assessment tool, they develop it further to meet their requirements. In Chapter 38, Wiegand demonstrates an initial investigation in a nursing service setting to determine the nursing staff's awareness and use of theory-based practice. The model presented in Chapter 39 was used by Stumpf as the theoretical foundation in her master's thesis. She investigated the self-concept of children with diabetes and its relationship to their blood glucose control. The last chapter in this part (Chapter 40) is by Foster. For a long time she has been intrigued by patients' use of space. Using Hall's theory and the Riehl Interaction Model, she studied their related concepts with clients in an outpatient setting.

28

The Conservation Principles of Nursing
Twenty Years Later[1]

Myra Estrin Levine

The invoking of the "wholeness" of the individual has become a ritual certainty in the development of nursing theories, even when the underlying philosophical beliefs are widely disparate. The unity, the integrity, the oneness, the wholeness of human experience is universal. But the theoretical tenets that use wholeness are not always consistent or accurate.

Theory belongs at the cutting edge of practice, and the expression of wholeness, although intellectually gratifying, can be *used* as a starting point of analysis only if it can be converted into manageable parts. The task of dissecting the "multidimensional" factors into acceptable components has created a definition of the whole person as a "bio-psycho-social" being, to which there was later added an acknowledgment of "spirituality." The difficulty presented by this description of wholeness begins with the failure to include many dimensions that influence the well-being and lifecourse of the individual. An argument might be made for the importance of history, economics, cultural and even pathophysiological influences, but none of the isolated aspects of wholeness can have meaning outside of the context within which the individual experiences his or her life. The person cannot be described apart from the specific environment in which he or she is found. The precise environment necessarily completes the wholeness of the individual. Erikson (1968) writes that "wholeness emphasizes a sound, organic progressive mutuality between diversified functions and parts within an entirety, the boundaries of which are open and fluid (pp. 81–82)."

THE ENVIRONMENT

The environment is often seen as a passive backdrop against which the individual "acts out" life experiences. But an individual cannot be understood outside of the context of his or her predicament of time and place. Only then are the "open and fluid" boundaries established. It is useful to adopt an analytical scheme that permits an examination of the environment of the individual in modalities that explain the interaction taking place between living beings and the place they inhabit. Bates (1967) has suggested three aspects of environment that affect the individual. He describes the "operational" environment as that which interacts with living tissues even though the individual does not possess sensory organs that can record the presence of these external factors. All forms of radiation, microorganisms, pollutants that are odorless and colorless—every unseen and unheard aspect of the individual's life space—represents an impingement of the operational environment. Those factors that can be recorded on the sensory system—the energies of light, sound, touch, temperature, and chemical change that is smelled or tasted, as well as position sense and balance—are designated the "perceptual" environment. And finally, because human beings are sentient, thinking, future-oriented and past-aware individuals, the environment of language, ideas, symbols, concepts, and invention is designated the "conceptual" environment. This categorization allows for both the immediate and the historical factors that constitute an essential portion of the "realtity" that the individual recognizes, or indeed that is identified *about* the individual by those who assume the role of caregiver.

THE PROCESS OF ADAPTATION

The interaction at the interface between individual and environment is an orderly, sometimes predictable, but always a limited process. The consequence of the interaction is invariably the product of the characteristics of the living individual *and* the external factors, both historical and current. The *process* of the interaction is *adaptation*. Adaptation is a term that, as Dubos (1966) has pointed out, is used with such colloquial freedom that it is nearly impossible to assign it a precise meaning. And still, it has a precise focus. Even when used in "poetic" ways, the process of adaptation is acknowledged as a process of *change*. Its essential function is emphasized in Cohen's (1968) statement that "The purpose of life is to maintain life: adaptation is life (p. 8)."

If in fact the life process *is* the process of adaptation, the complexity of describing adaptation is readily apparent. To understand a process that is multidimensional, and where several of the dimensions or their interactions are not known, suggests the inherent difficulty in using the adaptation concept to describe the outcomes of a relationship between individuals and the environment, or indeed between individuals sharing a common enterprise. Although it is unlikely that an outcome can be specifically anticipated, knowledge of the major characteristics of the process may make the influence of adaptation potentially meaningful as a source of understanding human behavior in the context of a defined habitat.

The process of adaptation is characterized by attributes that direct change towards environmental "congruence" (Goldstein, 1963). Dubos (1966) says that the only measure of adaptive fitness to a particular environment is the extent to which the organisms of the species under consideration can occupy this environment, make effective use of its resources, and therefore multiply abundantly in it (p. 259)."

Adaptation and History

Such active participation by the individual requires a genetic endowment specific to a specific habitat. Thus the fundamental nature of adaptation is a consequence of a *historical* progression: the evolution of the species through time, reflecting the sequence of change in the genetic patterns that have recorded the change in the historical environments. That history is recorded in living cells and living systems of cells, a history so various that only the most obvious events can be identified. Every living cell is evidence of the symbiotic arrangement in which a prokaryotic cell entered a eukaryotic cell, and found advantage to each, allowing for the astonishing proliferation of living things. The mitochondria—the energy-producing system within the cell—carry the DNA of their prokaryotic ancestor, whereas the cell nucleus, its DNA a descendant of the ancient eukaryotic cell, provides the nourishment, growth, and replication that is the essence of life (Margulis, 1971). The diversity of living things testifies to the *adaptability* of species (Dubos, 1966), but even in the wide variation of species and habitat, some similarities of adaptation are striking. Hochachka and Somero (1984) ask, "What selective factors will favor the curious coincidence of body temperatures near 37°C to 39°C for the large majority of avian and mammalian endotherms (p. 375)?"

Their research reveals that the macromolecules, the "working parts" of metabolism, function best within a constricted temperature range. Thus, adaptation to temperature is based essentially on the behavior of biochemical substances. The narrow range of adaptation to temperature is only one of the environmental factors to which species are adapted (DuBos, 1966). Atmospheric pressure, oxygen tension, and the availability of water, electrolytes, and nutrients create narrow ranges of variability as well.

Adaptation and Specificity

The endowment of the species, for all its richness of possible combinations, becomes in individuals the inheritance of their own lineage, sharing some species-specific traits (which often are narrowly adapted) but also in possession of individual potentials (which reflect the promise of adaptability). Thus, adaptations also have the characteristic of *specificity*. It is this aspect of adaptation that creates the "patterns" that reflect the interacting steps achieving a variety of adaptational goals. The physiological processes that defend oxygen supply to the brain are distinct from those that maintain the appropriate blood glucose levels. Each system is highly specific to its task, with appropriate biochemical changes responding to environmental challenges. But in the living organism, these essential functions are synchronized with each other. Most of the species-specific traits that are in response to the external environment are readily recognized. Hochachka and Somero (1984) point out that "highly conspicuous characteristics of the physiological, morphological, behavioral, and ecological levels of biological organization are typically the types of phenomena that constitute the literatures dealing with organismal adaptations (p. 3)."

But they describe "interiorized" biochemical adaptations that "are important in the interfacing of the organism with its environment (p. 4)." Even at the level of macromolecules, which they describe as "enzymes, contractile proteins and nucleic acids (p. 4)," the specificity of the adaptation is essential for the appropriate "fit" of the individual to the external environment. The interiorized adaptations, however, serve the organism as a whole in absolutely essential regulatory functions. They control the energy resources available to the cell as adenosine triphosphate, as well as the energy stored as intermediate metabolites (such as glycogen) and the synthesis of nucleic acids and proteins. The molecular adaptations regulate metabolic rates, changing the "response to the organism's needs . . . as the environment varies (p. 5)." This emphasizes that specificity is dependent on sequential change, but the common view of a strictly linear pattern is oversimplified and misleading. Increasingly, the path of biochemical change is described as "cascades." The process is one of interacting and evolving effect, and not a completion of each sequence before the next begins. The cascade, like the waterfall it suggests, is characterized by the intermingling of the steps with each other—the precursor is not entirely exhausted when the intermediate forms develop and the final stage is congruent with the steps that precede it. Thus, the process *tests itself* as it progresses, including the capacity to stimulate a back-up process in the event that the original sequence fails to achieve its task.

Adaptation and Redundancy

The cascade of change demonstrates a third essential characteristic of adaptation: redundancy. The Latin root, *redundatio,* suggests the "wave motion" that characterizes the availability of a series of adaptive responses when the stability of the organism is challenged. There are, for example, many corrective potentials in the replicating of a DNA strand, as well as in physiological processes— such as maintenance of the blood pH or adequate oxygenation of the central nervous system where redundant, failsafe systems are placed in operation as the primary systems are compromised by untoward change. Some redundant systems function in a time frame. They have the ability to respond instantly to an impending, threatening shift in a physiological parameter. Some are corrective, taking place in an intermediate mode, when utilizing the time interval provided by the faster reaction, and can go about the business of correcting the imbalances. And finally, there are those redundant systems that permit the reestablishing of a previously failed response. Cannon (1963) called this the "body's wisdom"—a store of redundant systems that have resulted from the adaptations that defend the survival of the individual and the species. From the time of conception through birth and throughout the life span, individuals possess a redundancy of function that allows for choices in their interface with the environment. Survival depends on the adaptive ability to use responses that *cost the least* to the individual in expense of effort and demand on his or her well-being.

CONSERVATION: THE PRODUCT OF ADAPTATION

That is, of course, the essence of *conservation.* Such processes establish a body economy that is precise, frugal, and yet capable of safeguarding the individual in a broad range of impinging environmental events. Conservation is clearly the consequence of the multiple, interacting, and synchronized negative feedback systems that provide for the stability of the living organism. The control of physiological functions by negative feedbacks utilizes energy only when the system is turned "on."

So long as physiological balance is maintained, negative feedback systems sustain their function at minimal cost to the organism. Thus the active use of energy resources is conserved until there is a disturbance in the system, in which case the negative feedback system is activated until the desired norm is once more achieved. Energy utilization is saved for those instances when it is essential that a normal balance be restored. Establishing a stable internal environment establishes an energy-sparing condition—a conservation of organismic resources that equips the individual to confront, and often correct, a wide spectrum of environmental challenges. Such challenges are always a form of energy, and the living system is kept stable in the face of uneven or overwhelming energy input by its ability to channel the total energy into manageable negative feedback loops. Cannon (1963) called this homeostasis.

Although individually the negative feedback loops successfully channel each physiological parameter, it is the collective synchronization of multiple negative feedbacks that creates the "stable state" of the internal environment. Stability, balance, and equilibrium have been attractive ideas, not only for biological science but for sociology, psychology, economics, political science, and nurse theorists. But interpreting homeostasis as a system of balance and quiescence overlooks its essential function. Homeostasis is a state of energy-sparing that also provides the necessary baselines for a multitude of synchronized physiological and psychological factors. Homeostasis might be called the state of conservation.

There is always a *selection* of responses to the onslaught of sensory stimuli present in everyone's environment. The individual, in the process of growth and maturation, learns to be selective of those sensory signals that demand attention and those that may safely be ignored. Indiscriminate response to every environmental signal would quickly exhaust the physiological and behavioral potential of the individual.

Although physiological and behavioral responses are identified and usually described as separate entities, in fact the integration of living processes argues that they are one and the same—not merely parallel and not merely simultaneous, but essential portions of the same activity. Integration is defended by adaptations that create the condition of conservation. Order and meaning are created by the individual's ability to receive selected information from the environment and to use it appropriately. Even here there is redundancy, an ability to react at several levels of behavior, which reflects the richness of adaptations available to each individual.

The most primitive response is the adrenocortical-sympathetic reactions described by Cannon (1963) as "fight or flight." By providing a condition of readiness—both physiological and behavioral—every individual has a swift response available for every sudden and unexplained environmental challenge. At still another level there is the inflammatory-immune response, which assures restoration of physical wholeness and the expectation of complete healing. The "stress" response as described by Selye is a third level of integrated defense of the individual, but one that is recorded over time and is influenced by the accumulated experience of the individual. And finally, there is the ability to select environmental information as described by Gibson (1966) as "perceptual systems." As an integrated individual, the senses are not only capable of providing access to the variety of energy sources in the environment, but of allowing the individual to convert them to meaningful experiences. In Gibson's description of perceptual systems, individuals not merely see, they *look;* they do not merely hear, they *listen.*

Thus equipped with the ability to select information from the environment, the individual is an active, seeking participant in it—not merely reacting but influencing, changing, and creating the parameters of his or her life. These levels of response are redundant; that is, they do not follow one another in a prescribed sequence, but are integrated in individuals by their cognitive abilities, the wealth of their previous experience, their ability to define their relationships to the events, and the strengths of their adaptive capabilities.

The use of the term *adaptation* has been elusive as a basis for nursing activity, chiefly because of its colloquial contamination but also because it is widely misused. From its Latin origin, the word means "to fit." Through historical time, the most successful adaptations are those that best fit the organism in its environment. A "best fit" is accomplished with the least expenditure of effort, and with sufficient protective devices built in so that the goal is achieved in as economic and expeditious a manner as possible. That does not always mean in an uncomplicated fashion, because living processes are extremely complex—but even then the variety of alterations required to achieve the goal have been time tested and have survived because they benefited the organism.

NURSING AS A CONSERVATION FUNCTION

Thus, nursing must view the individual so that the "best fit" available can be sustained. The nurse's role is in the conservation or "keeping together" function that should be the major guideline for all nursing intervention wherever it takes place. In 1965, I suggested that there were four conservation principles that were useful rubrics within which nursing care could be designed. Although I have witnessed many instances in which individuals critiquing the conservation principles have misunderstood or trivialized their intent, I have grown in my conviction that they continue to offer an approach to nursing that is scientific, research oriented, and above all, suitable in daily practice in many environments.

The four conservation principles are:

1. The conservation of energy of the individual.
2. The conservation of structural integrity of the individual.
3. The conservation of personal integrity of the individual.
4. The conservation of social integrity of the individual.

These principles will be discussed in the subsequent sections.

Conservation of Energy

The law of conservation of energy is a natural law that to this date has been found to hold everywhere in the universe for all animate and inanimate entities. A law with such universal implications has to be understood by nurses. Energy is a term that has been used in mystical ways, as if it were a force so burdened with mystery that it can only be understood as possessing an unexplained magic. There is free use of such notions as healing energy, transmitting energy from one individual to another through various rituals, and a sense of energy that has to do with a feeling of buoyancy, well-being, and physical and mental "highs."

But energy is not a hidden entity. It is eminently identifiable, measurable, and manageable. Description of the effects of the range of wavelengths in the electromagnetic energy range alone has permitted the creation of instruments capable not only of generating the waves in their many dimensions but also receivers that allow capture of their information by tuning in to precise wavelengths. Microwave ovens, radios, television receivers, computers, satellite transmitters: each performs because their wave frequency is known. It is also evident that microwave ovens will not receive a television picture.

Nurses measure energy parameters in the ordinary course of patient care. The body temperature, for example, measures the energy of heat generated by the living cells as they perform their work. Changes in the energy of heat production in the individual provide important signals as to how effectively his or her body is functioning. Pulse rate is an energy measure—not only in frequency but also in its "feel"—and so is respiratory rate, measurement of blood gases, metabolic rate, and blood pressure. Data of this kind are used in specific ways, but may be lost in subjective assessments of the individual's energy: estimates based on appraisals of how the individual "behaves."

In 1982, I received with delight an *unsolicited* letter from a researcher who said she had used the conservation principles as a basis for her doctoral study. The abstract she sent me of that paper and an earlier one demonstrated clearly that she was using the concept correctly. She had used a variety of physiological measurements to evaluate the energy utilization by coronary patients in toileting and later in bathing procedures. The paper was published by Winslow in *Nursing Research* in June 1985 (without attribution to the conservation principles), and demonstrates the strength of the kind of clinical research that this idea inspires.

Fifteen years ago, a graduate student of mine tried to design an "exchange list" of allowable activities for coronary patients on discharge, based on the cardiac output of the individual patient as calculated by a series of formulas readily available in every exercise physiology text (Wong, 1967). Instead of saying "take it easy," such patients should be given a graduated list of activities from which they can select those that fit their lifestyle but that remain within safe limits of their body's own demands.

The timing, spacing, and total activity of ambulation should be designed on the basis of physiological parameters of the individual patient. Every person responds to surgical procedures or serious illness—or indeed, participation in some high-tech processes—at his or her own level of tolerance. But the individualization of that level of tolerance is rarely undertaken. Energy conservation is an empiric activity of nursing care. Not only are the individual's activities monitored, but much attention is given to oxygenation, nutrition, fluid and electrolyte intake, as well as the impact of drugs on physiological function.

The individual "conserves" available resources but it must be recognized that even at perfect rest, there is a cost of energy for the incessant activities of life: transport, growth, and biochemical and bioelectrical change. The conservation of energy is clearly evident in the very sick, whose lethargy, withdrawal, and self-concern are manifested while, in its wisdom, the body is spending its energy resources on the processes of healing.

Conservation of Structural Integrity

The conservation of structural integrity is concerned with the process of healing. From earliest childhood, individuals are taught to have confidence in the ability of bodies to heal—to restore wholeness and continuity after injury or illness, to return to their pristine state. The youngster who scrapes a knee is comforted by her or his mother's loving attention, a cookie, and multiple changes of bandages. But when the injury is healed, not a trace of it remains. That expectation of perfect restoration remains a firm mind-set throughout life. For all of the emphasis placed on teaching patients to accept limitations in their life activities following insult or injury, insufficient acknowledgment is made of the power of that faith that the person can be hurt but that healing will be complete.

Weiner (1954) said that structure determines function. Fetal development, growth, and physical change are all regulated by the intricate relationships of functional processes turned off and on, accelerated or slowed, but still dependent on the orderly progress towards the goal for which they are adapted. Even a superficial appraisal of the way the body is defended from the environment emphasizes how structure and function are inherently related.

Healing is the defense of wholeness. There are marvelous capacities to renew tissues lost to injury, insult, or disease, including an adaptation that not only provides fibrous tissue substitution, but as the scar grows to maturity, is capable of aligning it with the body's own lines of stress and mobility. It is for this reason that nursing interventions are designed to limit injury so that in the healing process, the scarring will be minimal and not interfere with function. Healing also is a consequence of an effective immune system. The overwhelming fear created by AIDS emphasizes how confidence in the body's defenses gives courage, and how its failure creates panic. The immunological capability of every individual is a consequence of a lifetime's interaction with the environment. By the time the thymus involutes in late adolescence, every individual has a store of antibodies tailor-made for the places in which he or she lives and moves. Science provides the option of receiving created antibodies in situations where they are unlikely to have been produced in the individual, but the relationship between individuals and their world is clearly inscribed on their immune system.

Nurses have empiric awareness of the necessity to defend the structural integrity of individuals, as in the proper positioning to prevent subluxations and other skeletal deformity, to prevent pressure areas where decubiti might form, and to engage in range of motion to keep joints mobile and muscles toned for subsequent use. Nurses defend the structural need to keep the individual as capable of mobilization as possible. His or her structural integrity depends on it.

Sacks (1985) demonstrated that the sense of structural integrity was more than a physiological requirement. He described the various responses reported by individuals with phantom limbs following amputation of a body part. "All amputees . . . know that a phantom limb is essential if an artificial limb is to be used. . . . No amputee with an artificial lower limb can walk on it satisfactorily until the phantom is incorporated in it (p. 64)." He described some amputees' methods for "waking" their phantom limb when they placed the prosthesis.

Conservation of Personal Integrity

The conservation of personal integrity emphasizes that the sense of "self" is much more than a physical experience of the whole body, although it is unquestionably a part of that awareness. Goldstein (1963) described patients with severe brain injuries, some of them German soldiers in the first World War, who struggled to retain their identity even in the face of their overwhelming motor, perceptual, and sensory disabilities. He called it self-actualization. It was an important neurological and later philosophical concept that was sorely misused by two authors who had an undue influence on nursing curricula.

Maslow (1968) who dedicated his book to Kurt Goldstein, turned self-actualization into some kind of super-reaching, characterized by "metamotivation" and resulting in an exalted state of transcendence. Carl Rogers (1961) used the notion to justify a counseling therapy where the therapist created a nondirective, nonjudgmental milieu in which the individual then could "sound out" his or her own problems, understand them, solve them, and go on to greater things. They both trivialized an important basic idea: The defense of self is not a reaching beyond, but rather a reaching into the person. Everyone seeks to defend his or her identity as a self, in both that hidden, intensely private person that dwells within and in the public faces assumed as individuals move through their relationships with others. Even in those instances where the relationship is intimate and close—between child and parent, husband and wife, lover and beloved—only by analogy is it known that our experience of selfhood is somehow an expression of personal identity. But some portion is always very private, and nothing threatens that pride of self more than the vulnerability of dependence. It is simply impossible for one individual to surrender his or her privacy to another, no matter how much the individual must depend on the good offices of the caregiver.

Recognition of the formal rules of separation include all the culture-ridden rituals of distance behaviors. Individuals are quick to sense when another wishes one to withdraw to a greater distance. But it is much more difficult to articulate the anxiety created by a threat to the self—to share it with another individual, however well disposed the person may be. The emphasis over the years on extracting psycho-social information about patients neglects the inevitable guarding of the privacy of that cherished self. Indeed, it is entirely possible that the use of private information as a component of the nursing care plan may be more damaging to the personal integrity of the individual than respecting a desire to withhold information.

In this era of leaks of confidential information and the public clamor of a right to know, the most generous psycho-social approach would be to limit the recording of confidences to only those generalizations that actually make a difference in the choice of treatment plans. The complex of factors that create the selfhood of the individual are every bit as dependent on the growth and development within a specific environment as is the uniqueness of the individual's immune response. So much is lost in distant history; so much lies fallow until called once more into action by new, or more recent circumstances; so much is tempered by experience and the cascade of personality traits that the individual's previous life experiences have cultivated. It is the particular quality of human life that one participate in the immediate present, but uses a store of options that have historical significance, and a lifetime's collection of ideas, beliefs, values, and goals that shape each person into the intensely private self only that person can know him- or herself to be. All individuals must participate freely in decisions that affect them.

Conservation of Social Integrity

Finally, selfhood needs definition beyond the individual, and this is the message of the conservation of social integrity. Erikson's (1963) table of growth and development has long been a favorite in nursing education, but his important contributions have been overlooked.

His writings (1969) focus on the anthropological differences in childrearing in a variety of social systems. He chooses important leaders of the past, Martin Luther and Ghandi, to illustrate how the individual is created by the environment and in turn creates within it.

There is no more grievous condition than that of a human being who is so withdrawn that he or she is incapable of making contact with the surrounding reality—the pity of the deeply depressed, the autistic child, the life spent in a delusional panic. None know better that the self how essential human and humane contact really is. Individuals define themselves by their relationships. An identity places one in a family, a community, a cultural heritage, a religious belief, a socioeconomic slot, an educational background, a vocational choice. Living successfully within that variety of social environments depends on the development of a repertoire of appropriate behavioral responses, every bit as much a product of interactions as the unique definitions of the immune systems and the life events that create the self.

One of the nebulous although very active areas of nursing research has been the identification of what is meant by "coping." Precise definitions are lacking, although it is generally understood that coping refers to the way in which the individual responds to a given social instant. Unlike physiological parameters, the "coping" processes lack precision and distinction, largely because they arise from pasts that are hidden not only to the observer but to the observed as well.

Coping patterns (they are *not* mechanisms in a holistic sense) are judged by the social acceptance of the behavior that is manifested. Every social group creates its own definitions of what is or is not acceptable just as every social group defines health and illness. It is the tremendous variation in social beliefs that adds to the confusion of "measuring" this kind of response. One way to categorize coping patterns (however inconclusive this may seem) might be the following:

1. Everyday responses that have proven to be adequate and acceptable for the individual in the past.
2. Response to crises situations by testing a variety of coping behaviors that have worked in previous situations.
3. Trial-and-error innovations in situations where coping patterns have failed to resolve the crisis.

It is apparent that the individual best able to confront the behavioral decisions is the one whose repertoire of response is extensive, or at least has provided the individual with the courage to explore the consequences of his or her behavior. Frequently the success of a coping pattern rests on the support and encouragement of a group that shares the concerns of the individual. No diagnosis should be made that does not include the other persons whose lives are entwined with that of the individual.

Ultimately, social integrity is governed by the ethical values of the social system. It is only within the orderly regulating of the relationships of the members of the community that individuals can define their places and with them their responsibilities, privileges, and rights. For all the certainty people may have of that appropriate role in their independent life, the introduction of the dependency of entering the health care system creates issues and conflicts that must bring consonance between the reality that confronts them and the expectations others may have of them. The health care system is a vast social order with its own rules, but it is an instrument of society and must guarantee privacy, personhood, and respect as moral imperatives.

CONCLUSION

The conservation principles do not, of course, operate singly and in isolation from each other. They are joined within the individual as a cascade of life events, churning and changing as the environmental challenge is confronted and resolved in each individual's unique way. The nurse as caregiver becomes part of that environment, bringing to every nursing opportunity his or her own cascading repertoire of skill, knowledge, and compassion. It is a shared enterprise and each participant is rewarded.

As a human relationship, nursing bears special burdens of concern. In sickness or health, permission to enter into the life goals of another human being bears onerous debts of responsibility and choice. Reaching out to find the humanity of another person arises from the willful participation of both. Whatever limitations exist in communication and sharing with another the crises of the moment or the slow evolution of a continuing, cooperative relationship, there is never a substitute for honesty, fairness, and mutual respect. Nursing theory must make a difference in the way in which nursing care is transmitted to patients. It is tested finally in the pragmatic, humble daily exchanges between nurse and patient. Ultimately success must be improved care and wise counsel that equip the individuals with renewed strength to pursue their lives in independence, fulfillment, hope, and promise.

ENDNOTE

[1]This chapter is dedicated to the nurses of 4 North Searle, Evanston Hospital, Evanston, Illinois, July-August, 1986. The general content was presented as a paper at the Nursing Theory Congress in Toronto, Ontario, August 19 to 22, 1986.

REFERENCES

Bates, M. (1967, June/July). Naturalist at large. *Natural History 76,* 10.

Cannon, W. B. (1963). *The wisdom of the body.* New York: Norton.

Cohen, Y. (1968). *Man in adaptation: The biosocial background.* Chicago: Aldine.

Dubos, R. (1966). *Man adapting.* New Haven, CT: Yale University Press.

Erikson, E. (1963). *Childhood and society* (2nd ed.). New York: Norton.

Erikson, E. (1968). *Identity, youth and crisis.* New York: Norton.

Erikson, E. (1969). *Ghandi's truth.* New York: Norton.

Gibson, J. S. (1966). *The senses considered as perceptual systems.* Boston: Houghton-Mifflin.

Goldstein, K. (1963). *Human nature.* New York: Schocken.

Hochachka, P. W., & Somero, G. H. (1984). *Biochemical adaption.* Princeton, NJ: Princeton University Press.

Margulis, L. (1971, August). Symbiosis and evolution. *Scientific American, 225,* 48–57.

Maslow, A. (1968). *Toward a psychology of being* (2nd ed.). Princeton, NJ: Van Nostrand.

Rogers, C. R. (1961). *On becoming a person.* Boston: Houghton-Mifflin.

Sacks, O. (1985). *The man who mistook his wife for a hat.* New York: Summit.

Weiner, N. (1954). *The human use of human beings.* Garden City, NY: Doubleday.

Winslow, E., Lane, L. D., Gaffney, F. A. et al. (1985). Oxygen update and cardiovascular responses in control adults and acute myocardial infarction patients during bathing. *Nursing Research, 34*(3), 164–169.

Wong, S. (1968). *Rehabilitation of a patient following myocardial in/out.* Unpublished master's thesis, Loyola University of Chicago School of Nursing.

Levine's Theory of Nursing
A Critique

Janet L. Glass

Key writings of Myra Levine appeared during the 1960s and 1970s and reflect the three main theory-building efforts of nursing occurring during this time. These efforts included "the use of borrowed theory, an effort to develop practice theory, and development of nursing's conceptual models (Fitzpatrick & Whall, 1983, p. 10)."

Levine used past and present ideas and theories in constructing her own model. Her theory constructions seem to be derived from the areas of past nursing, microbiology, physiology, pathophysiology, sociology, and psychology. Readily apparent is the influence of Nightingale, who focused on the importance of creating a positive environment for healing—one in which the person was not permitted to expend too much energy. The theory of multiple causation of disease was another important influence. This idea emphasized the need to provide care for the total patient. In reality, it emphasized caring for the total of all parts of the person. The multiple causation concept can be seen in some of its later forms in Levine's model. Most notably are Hall's (1964) introduction of the concept of total patient care, and the theory of Maslow (1970). Both Hall and Maslow stressed the importance of viewing people as having physiological and psychological components. This concept of multiple dimensions was stressed as well in Tillich's (1961) article "The Meaning of Health," which also seemed to influence Levine.

This concept, however, is probably best illustrated by Levine in her ideas on holism. Holistic thought itself is exemplified by General Systems theory, which von Bertalanffy (1968) calls a "general science of wholeness (p. 37)." This theory is built on the idea of the whole being greater than the sum of its parts. The person, as an open system, experiences movement through boundaries by means of input and output that allows the system to communicate and react to the environment. This enables people to strive toward homeostasis using the system's self-regulatory feedback processes, which involves energy exchanges.

Adaptation theories are also evident in Levine's theory. Early adaptation influences included Dubos (1966), Cannon (1963), and Selye (1956). Other theories apparent in Levine's model included the work of Erikson (1963), who viewed humans as a whole (open system); Bates (1967) and his work on the three aspects of environment; and Dunn's (1961) concept of an illness-wellness continuum.

INTERNAL EVALUATION

At this point an internal evaluation of Levine's nursing theory will be presented. This includes the areas of commonplaces, clarity, consistency, adequacy, logical development, and level of theory development as identified by Stevens (1984).

Commonplaces

Patient
A patient is defined by Levine as the ill person in the hospital who is the focus of nursing acts. This person consists of physiological, sociological, and psychological components of a whole. Fitzpatrick and Whall (1983) use the term "person" rather than "patient." They define this commonplace of Levine's as a "complex individual in interaction with the internal and external environment who responds to change by means of adaptation (p. 340)."

Nursing Acts
Levine (1973) utilizes conservation principles in her approach to nursing and states "nursing is a human interaction (p. 1)." She views nursing acts as holistic, individualized to meet each person's needs, and supporting adaptation. Nursing acts include the use of scientific principles in employing the nursing process. In this sense, Levine views nursing as a discipline. For Levine the nursing process includes the steps of assessment, intervention, and evaluation. Nursing diagnosis is not included by Levine in her early works but does appear later (1973) as part of nursing acts.

Health
When discussing health, Levine primarily refers to illness or ill health arising in a state of deficiency or in the presence of health problems. Health, as well as disease, is viewed as a pattern of adaptive change and therefore it is never a static condition. "Levine's implied definition of health is the maintenance of the unity and integrity of the patient (Leonard, 1985, p. 186)." Ideally, improved health is the goal of nursing acts. The word health is derived from an Anglo-

Saxon word (hal) that means "whole." For Levine the most accurate description of health is "whole," a concept suggested by Tillich (1961).

Relationship of Nursing Acts to the Patient
The nurse provides care for the patient and hence a dependent, undesirable patient role is implied. This is possibly inconsistent with Levine's principle of personal integrity. The nurse assumes a measure of control over the ill patient whose resources must be conserved, thus compromising autonomy. The nurse performs what Levine calls guardian activities and plans the care *for* the patient. The nurse's control over the patient is illustrated by Levine (1973) when she states that "the nurse acts as the 'banker' for the proper balancing of the patient's energy account. The nurse provides for an adequate deposit of energy resource and cautiously regulates the energy spending (p. 15)." This ideally results in equilibrium. Levine also discusses the nursing role as perceived by the patient. The nurse is seen as belonging to the hospital as well as representing it. Because the nurse is responsible for the actions of other personnel performing nursing tasks, they in turn are seen as extensions of the role of the nurse.

Although Levine describes nursing care as patient-centered, the focus of her theory appears to be on the patient or individual in a universal or generalized sense. Despite this, the potential exists for extending the broad concepts to specific individual patient applications. In this respect patient-centered care may be an example of sloganism typical of this period in nursing.

Relationship of Nursing Acts to Health
Levine identifies this relationship as being governed by the nature of the adaptation taking place. She states

> when nursing intervention influences adaptation favorably, or toward renewed social well-being, then the nurse is acting in a therapeutic sense. When nursing intervention cannot alter the course of the adaptation—when her best efforts can only maintain the status quo or fail to halt a downward course—then the nurse is acting in a supportive sense. (1973, p. 13)

Relationship of the Patient to Health
In Levine's theory, the patient is located at the nonwellness end of the health continuum. Wellness is impaired to some degree and results in the person becoming a patient. As health improves the patient has the potential for returning to a nonpatient role. Lack of improved health or further deterioration, on the other hand, results in maintenance of the patient role.

Environment
For Levine, the environmental setting of the nurse-patient interaction is the hospital, and the nurse comes to represent the image of the hospital to the patient. The environment includes perceptual, operational, and conceptual components. The environment is also evident for each patient. Levine sees each

individual as having both an internal and an external environment. The study of physiology and pathophysiology represents the individual's internal environment (Levine, 1973). Borrowing from Bates (1967), Levine further identifies external environment as composed of factors that impact on and create change in the individual.

Clarity

Clarity is good in reading and understanding Levine's theory. The content is meaningful, easily grasped, and does not employ a needlessly lengthy expansion of topics. In addition, it progresses in a very logical, organized, and well-integrated manner. Levine, however, does not specifically define all her terms, which would be helpful.

Consistency

Terms
Terms are used in the same manner throughout Levine's writings and her world view remains constant. This is important, because shifts from a consistent use and meaning of terms has the effect of impairing other areas of theory consistency.

Interpretation
Levine describes the hospital-based world of nursing of the late 1960s and early 1970s. It is consistent with this author's own past experiences of nursing the ill patient. This world is not, however, entirely consistent with nursing today, because it is confined to a hospital setting and many nurses currently provide patient care in nonacute settings outside the hospital.

Levine's theory is consistently interpreted in an essential way. Her

> concept of nursing . . . is totally context-imbedded; the patient's adaptations involve response to and interaction with the environment. The same is true of the nurse; her environment is the patient himself, and the nature of her conservation measures depends on an accurate reading of his responses—so as to promote his productive adaptations. (Stevens, 1984, p. 34)

Principle
Levine is consistent in initiating her theory by assertion of her comprehensive conservation principle as well as by how she explains it and describes the four components of this principle. Levine believes conservation (a process) is primary and cannot be replaced or altered. This principle is supportive of the patient-based reflexive principle of adaptation, which forms part of the theoretical basis of Levine's theory. She states that "for a nurse to apply the four conservation principles, it is essential that she identify the specific patterns of adaptation of every patient (Levine, 1967, p. 46)." Although conservation addresses the nursing act, adaptation, in a complementary fashion, addresses the patient.

The relationship that results supports Levine's (1973) basic premise that "nursing is a human interaction (p. 1)."

Method

Levine uses a problematic method of reasoning. This method is consistent with nursing trends in both theory and practice that were popular during the 1960s and 1970s. It employs the use of problem solving or scientific method by the nurse who then recognizes, defines, and deals with the factors constituting a given problem. Levine uses the concept of people as an open system in relation to her method of problem solving. Problems are related and solving one leads to solutions of others. This is an ongoing process because a person is not a bound system. Hence her attempt is not toward resolution of a single goal but rather trying to resolve a problematic patient situation.

Levine demonstrates consistency in method in the discussion of her four separate problems (conservation principles). Although she treats each conservation problem as an entirety, she does not separate humans into parts. Rather, she visualizes nursing intervention as a conservation activity and employs this "keeping together" function in approaching each individual patient situation. Hence each conservation problem must be resolved by the nurse for each patient. It is only in this manner that conservation is said to exist.

Approach

The organizing structures (key factors) in Levine's theory are clearly evident and used throughout. This is accomplished through the identification of general scientific principles which are then applied in specific patient problem situations. The principles of the organizing foundation (structure) are implemented by the nursing process. This is accomplished through the formulation of nine factors, which Levine terms "models." These factors establish a general conceptual pattern of related nursing processes. Her model has three major parts. These parts, or organizing components, are employed in a consistent manner to aid in understanding the model and Levine's advocacy of a holistic approach to patient care. The factors represent a historical move because they "substitute broad concepts for the procedural rules and allow for variation in practice which is sound and scientific and, therefore, safe for individualizing the care of every patient (Levine, 1973, p. xi)."

Adequacy

This area of evaluation was initially discussed by Stevens (1979) as an aspect of external evaluation. This accounts for Steven's later statement that "the criterion of adequacy sometimes reflects internal criticism and other times branches into external criticism (1984, p. 60)." It is significant to note that what Stevens terms "adequacy" in the first edition is included under the term "reality convergence" in the second.

Overall, Levine's theory is adequate, for it carefully addresses the subject matter it identifies and also because its principles can be applied beyond the original setting of the hospital into such areas as nursing homes. It is, however, inadequate in the sense that the theory does not incorporate a primary level of health promotion, or preventative health teaching, nor does it concern itself with the aspects of community and family except as they relate to the patient.

Logical Development

Levine's theory is logically developed because it draws valid conclusions based on prior premises and reasoning. This is illustrated by her use of nine descriptive factors. Each factor evolves from previously presented content, which is heavily biophysical in nature, and from the conservation of energy principles for a given patient problem. These factors utilize deductive scientific argument. They also are organismic because they are concerned with open, self-maintaining, and self-adjusting biological systems as illustrated by Levine's (1973) use of both negative and positive feedback pictorial diagrams. The logical development of Levine's argument is further evidenced by conclusions flowing from the given theory without the need to fill in any gaps. The theory seems a natural and logical outgrowth of the principles. The theory also shows a logical historically based development as noted in the introduction.

Level of Theory Development

Levine's theory is descriptive in nature because it uses the phenomenon "conservation" and identifies four constituents of the individual patient (energy, structural integrity, personal integrity, and social integrity) that make up this phenomenon. These four constituents are categorical because they share a structural interrelationship. Although they may be viewed as mutually exclusive, together they comprise the whole that is conservation.

The theory is also developed on the explanatory level because it identifies how the constituents of conservation relate to and with each other. At this level, it is both predictive and situation-producing, because the specific applications involved can also apply to general ones, and vice versa. Hence it can be used in both the assessment and intervention aspects of Levine's nursing process.

Levine's model does not seem to be fully developed at its current level. However, it has certainly formed a strong basis for development of other models that incorporate some of her thoughts on such aspects as holism and environment.

Assumptions

"Underlying assumptions . . . mark the boundary between internal and external criticism of a theory (Stevens, 1984, p. 20)." Levine's assumptions are implicitly related to commonplaces and include: (1) the person as a whole open system;

(2) the nurse as the provider of patient care; (3) health and disease as patterns of adaptive change; and (4) the nurse as an active participant in the patient's environment (Fitzpatrick & Whall, 1983).

EXTERNAL EVALUATION

Theory evaluation also necessitates an examination of external factors. These factors include reality convergence, utility, significance, capacity for discrimination, scope, and complexity (Stevens, 1984).

Reality Convergence

Principle
In viewing nursing as conservation, Levine stresses the idea that nursing supports the patient's level of adaptation that already exists. It provides an explanatory function by showing the need to maintain a balance between what the nurse does (interventions) and the patient's requirements for intervention (determined by the patient's level of participation). This also supports the holistic approach of Levine, because holism involves the concept of humans actively participating in their environment. What becomes impaired is the *level* of the patient's participation, not participation itself. Adaptation, inherent in Levine's theory, is a core explanatory principle of nursing in particular and life in general, for it involves the constant adjustment of the individual to changing circumstances or environment.

Interpretation
Although Levine's theory does not address nursing beyond the hospital setting, it does have a reality basis for the area it describes, the time period in which the theory was advanced, and the role of the nurse at that time. Many years after its original publication Levine's theory remains valid and has continued significance for nursing today. As such, it describes human experience and may be termed phenomenal. The phenomenal nature of the theory is especially evident in Levine's reappraisal of the conservation principals in the preceding chapter.

Method
The problematic method seemed helpful to Levine when she was creating an instructional text for beginning nursing students. This method is often effective in the instruction of first-year nursing students. Levine has been successful in using this method to accomplish another theory goal—dealing with the real world of nursing experience in the hospital-based setting. Here the nurse encounters the same patients as the physician but strives to meet nursing goals. As the agent of the physician in his or her absence, the nurse also directs his or her care toward the accomplishing of medical goals. These can be mutual because

they both address a central concern—the patient. This holistic focus is a satisfying way to approach nursing because the problem and the patient are not separated from each other.

Utility

Levine's theory facilitates the achievement of its socially prescribed nursing goals. Improved patient health and comfort result from nursing care and nursing interventions that evolve from this theory. The theory is constructed in the real world of nursing practice. It is extant in the respect that Levine's theory allows for the fact that what hospital-based nurses do changes with time but nursing in the hospital setting is a fact that persists with time. This real world basis is illustrated by the theory's strong reliance on the nine factors that Levine constructed. These factors are deeply rooted in scientific, psychological, and social principles. The utility is further illustrated in the use of the theory to teach beginning students the practice of clinical nursing. This theory could also serve as a useful basis for curriculum construction in a school of nursing. This would involve identifying vertical threads (form) using the conservation principles. It also would involve describing the horizontal threads (processes) of problem solving or problem elimination and nursing process or goal resolution. These processes would also include conservation (for the nurse) and adaptation (for the patient). Some may view Levine's theory as existing in the "ought to be" world due to its being designed for beginning students who are often taught the "ideal" versus the "real." However, the theory is useful to nursing activities in a variety of work world settings. It is reality based and far from esoteric. It is a theory designed to be used and its concepts are pragmatic.

Significance

This theory is salient because it concerns itself with the nurse-patient interaction and other core issues in nursing. It also contributes to nursing knowledge for nurses in general, not just the student for whom it was originally designed. Additionally, it has extensive research potential, because Levine places great emphasis on the scientific method. Although Levine does not explicitly address research, the nine factors have the potential to generate many research questions. Most of these questions would relate to the focus of her theory and the ill, hospitalized person.

Capacity for Discrimination

Levine's theory does not establish a boundary that adequately separates nursing from other disciplines and activities. In discussing differences between what nurses do versus what physicians do, she only briefly notes differences. These include the nurse acting as "the doctor's agent in his absence and directly responsible for the actual performance of the therapeutic measures he prescribes (Levine, 1973, p. 31)" She also identifies the physician's role as determining the medical diagnosis and planning medical care. Nurses, on the other hand, may construct an imprecise nursing diagnosis (initially introduced by Levine, 1973) as opposed to a medical diagnosis. The use of the term "nursing diagnosis" by Levine is in contrast to her use of the term "trophicognosis." Levine (1965) originally suggested trophicognosis—a scientific method for reaching a nursing care judgment—as an alternative to nursing diagnosis. Lack of specific boundaries is further demonstrated in the use of the conservation principles, which can apply to other professionals as well as nonprofessionals. This can be illustrated by considering the number of nursing skills identified by Levine that may be performed by others, such as nurse aides. The aide, like the nurse, is taught principles and also practices in the hospital setting, caring for patients at the illness end of the continuum.

Scope

Levine's theory is often criticized for having a limited scope. On the contrary, the scope of Levine's theory is good, because it covers a wide range of patient problems. These problems can be approached using the conservation principles, yet the use of these principles extends beyond Levine's nine factors. If a deficiency in scope exists, this concerns the limited setting for her theory—the hospital. This implies an illness-based concept of health. However, this is not really a deficiency, for her principles have universal application.

Complexity

This theory is not overly parsiminous. Although the theory elements are easily perceived the theory is not oversimplified. These elements could be readily developed in greater depth, but this would not be consistent with Levine's goal. If this were done it would not change the essence of the theory, a conservation schema, used with a health-illness continuum, and utilizing a problem-solving process. In addition, the theory is not excessive in its complexity, because the critical elements are clear. Also the interrelatedness of the principles is apparent. Levine's theory is well-balanced between the criterions of parsimony and complexity.

CONCLUSION

Overall, Levine's theory has made a positive contribution to theory development. It contains some valuable core ideas that have the potential for serving as a basis for additional efforts in theory construction. Essentially, these efforts would have to address today's changing health care settings, the focus on health promotion, and the transformed role of patient into client-consumer. This represents a challenging task to the potential theorist. Levine herself has made additional efforts toward further development and clarification of her theory. Among her more recent contributions have been the presentation of papers at the Second Annual Nurse Educator Conference (1978), Allentown College of St. Francis (1984), and the Nursing Theory Conference, Boyle, Letourneau Conference (1984). An especially valuable new contribution is contained in the preceding chapter of this text, which elaborates upon Levine's earlier writings and provides additional support for the continued use of the four conservation principles in nursing today.

REFERENCES

Bates, M. (1967, June-July). Naturalist at large. *Natural History, 76,* 10.

Bertalanffy, L. V. (1968). *General systems theory.* New York: Braziller.

Cannon, W. (1963). *The wisdom of the body.* New York: Norton.

Dubos, R. (1966). *Man adapting.* New Haven, CT: Yale University Press.

Dunn, H. (1961). *High-level wellness.* Arlington, Virginia: Beatty.

Erikson, E. (1963). *Childhood and society* (2nd ed.). New York: Norton.

Fitzpatrick, J., & Whall, A. (1983). *Conceptual models of nursing: Analysis and application.* Bowie, MD: Brady.

Hall, L. (1964, February). Nursing: What it is? *Canadian Nurse, 60,* 150–154.

Leonard, M. K. (1985). Myra Estrin Levine. In J. B. George (Ed.), *Nursing theories: The basis for professional nursing practice* (2nd ed., pp. 180–194). Englewood Cliffs, NJ: Prentice-Hall.

Levine, M. E. (1966). *Trophicognosis: An alternative to nursing diagnosis.* Presented at an ANA Regional Clinical Conference. Proceedings published in *Exploring progress in medical-surgical nursing* (vol. 2, pp. 55–70). New York: American Nurses Association.

Levine, M. E. (1967). The four conservation principles of nursing. *Nursing Forum, 6,* 45–59.

Levine, M. E. (1973). *Introduction to clinical nursing* (2nd ed.). Philadelphia: Davis.

Levine, M. E. (1978, December). Paper presented at the Second Annual Nurse Educator Conference, New York. Audiotape available from Teach 'em Inc., 160 E. Illinois Street, Chicago, IL 60611.

Levine, M. E. (1984, April). *A conceptual model for nursing: The four conservation principles.* In the proceedings from the Allentown (Pennsylvania) College of St. Francis Conference.

Levine, M. E. (1984, May). Paper presented at Nursing Theory Conference, Boyle, Letourneau Conference, Edmonton, Canada. Tapes available from Ed Kennedy, Kennedy Recording, R.R. 5, Edmonton, Alberta, Canada TSP4B7 (4030470-0013).

Maslow, A. (1970). *Motivation and personality* (2nd ed.). New York: Harper & Row.

Selye, H. (1956). *The stress of life.* New York: McGraw-Hill.

Stevens, B. J. (1979). *Nursing theory: Analysis, application, evaluation.* Boston: Little, Brown.

Stevens, B. J. (1984). *Nursing theory: Analysis, application, evaluation* (2nd ed.). Boston: Little, Brown.

Tillich, P. (1961, autumn). The meaning of health. *Perspectives in Biological Medicine, 4,* 92–100.

Levine's Conservation Principles

Using the Model for Nursing Diagnosis in a Neurological Setting

Joyce Waterman Taylor

In *Nursing: A Social Policy Statement* published by the American Nurses Association (1980), nursing is defined as the "diagnosis and treatment of human responses to actual or potential health problems (p. 9)." The phenomena of concern to nurses, according to the policy statement, include those responses resulting from the medical diagnosis and treatment as well as those that relate to the unique health-related needs and concerns of the individual and the family. A nursing diagnosis is the label given to a health problem or concern that relates to one or more of the "phenomena of concern (Gordon, 1982.)" The diagnostic statement includes the etiological or risk factors contributing to the diagnosis and the signs and symptoms, referred to as the "defining characteristics," that distinguish one diagnosis from another. The diagnostic statement, properly formulated, provides the rationale for nursing intervention (Gordon, 1982).

The process of diagnosis begins with the collection of data and the development of testable hypotheses about the patient and his or her need for nursing care (the first step in the nursing process). However, according to Levine, Gordon, and others (ANA, 1985; Gordon, 1982; Roy, 1975), one must first make decisions about the data to be collected and about the specific "provocative facts" (Levine, 1966) that are most relevant to nursing. This implies the availability of a conceptual framework or model that describes the phenomena of concern and provides a focus for assessment and a basis for decision making about the patient.

Gordon (1982) specifies that a nursing model, to be useful, must provide:

1. An abstract way of viewing the patient.
2. A statement of the ultimate goal or purpose of nursing care.
3. A focus for determining appropriate nursing interventions.

Such a framework allows the nurse to make *deductions* about the nursing problems (diagnoses) most likely to be found in a particular patient or patient population, and to prescribe nursing interventions most likely to achieve predetermined goals. It then becomes possible to validate the frequency of the diagnoses in that population, and to study, document, and compare the effects of various interventions so that nursing practice is scientific.

LEVINE'S CONCEPTUAL FRAMEWORK

Levine's model (1966, 1967, 1969, 1971), based on the four principles of conservation, views the patient *holistically,* postulating the unity and integrity of the individual as he or she interacts in complex ways with both the internal and external environments. The individual must be seen within the context of the environment, with both health and illness a product of a very personal pattern of adaptation. The individual "caught in the predicament of illness" (1967) responds "organismically" (1971)—that is, with the whole being. Levine describes four levels of response, physiologically determined, that enable the individual to make a viable adaptation to the constantly changing internal and external environments:

1. Response to fear (fight or flight).
2. Inflammatory response (energy directed toward removal or exclusion of an irritant or pathogen).
3. Response to stress (nonspecifically induced changes that allow adaptation to a variety of stressors over time).
4. Sensory response (recognizable interactions between the individual and the environment).

Nursing care, according to Levine, is focused on the individual and the complexity of his or her relationships with the environment. The goal of nursing care is to *conserve* or "keep together" the patient's biological, personal, and social integrity as he or she struggles (toward health and well-being) to achieve a positive adaptation. To keep together means to maintain a proper balance between active nursing intervention coupled with patient participation, on the one hand, and the safe limits of the patient's ability on the other. By entering the patients ecosystem, the nurse directs, activates, and sustains the organismic response as the patient strives for renewed well-being. When adaptation is no longer possible, the nurse supports the individual and family until care is no longer needed.

Nursing interventions are based on the four principles of conservation, which are discussed in the following sections.

Conservation of Energy

According to Levine (1967), all of life's processes are fundamentally dependent on the production and expenditure of energy. The ability of the individual to function is predicated upon his or her energy potential and the specific pattern of energy exchange available. A balance between energy production and energy expenditure is essential for all activity, but is particularly crucial for neurological functioning. Conservation of energy is a natural defense against the disease process. The lethargy and withdrawal observed in the acutely ill patient indicates a physiological response designed to prevent further damage and promote recovery. Therefore, for the patient with a neurological dysfunction the *commonly recurring nursing diagnoses* related to energy conservation are those that reflect a threat to a continuous supply of oxygen, glucose, and other nutrients and those that indicate an increase or decrease in energy utilization.

Nursing care of the neurological patient must be designed to conserve and mobilize the patient's energy resources to meet basic physiological needs, to promote healing, and to eventually allow an energy reserve sufficient to permit the regaining of physical, personal, and social integrity.

Conservation of Structural Integrity

The design or structure of the body determines the way in which it functions (Levine, 1967). Structural change, resulting from disease or injury (or even the normal developmental processes, including aging), leads to change in function. Conservation of structural integrity requires that the "wholeness" of the body be protected and that the normal physiological functions be maintained. For the neurological patient, the *commonly recurring nursing diagnoses* related to structural integrity are those that pose a threat of permanent damage to nerve tissue; those that relate to concurrent or complicating diseases; those that result from procedures or therapies that have both benefits and risks; and those relating to the immobility, impaired nutrition, and hydration that may result from the disease state.

Nursing intervention for such patients is based on the need to protect the patient from further damage or injury; to prevent iatrogenic or trophicogenic (Levine, 1966) complications; and for the presentation of basic physiological functions such as nutrition, hydration, mobility, rest, and sleep; and for the rehabilitative measures that will return the patient to a state of relative independence and well-being.

Conservation of Personal Integrity

Both survival and rehabilitation depend on the patient's energy resources and on some measure of structural integrity. But according to Levine (1967), the body cannot be separated from the mind, emotions, and the soul. The person who is the patient is dependent on the structural integrity of the brain itself and on the processes of the mind; the thoughts, emotions, sensations, experiences, and expressions that have accumulated over a lifetime. Each individual responds to illness on his or her own terms (Levine, 1967) and the nurse is responsible for interpreting the patient's behavior and responding to each need as it presents itself.

For neurological patients, the *commonly recurring nursing diagnoses* relate to the loss of critical functions such as language, memory, emotional control, and judgment; to abnormalities of perception and sensation; to changes in the level of responsiveness to internal and external stimuli; to sudden loss of body functions; to dependency in self-care; and to socially unacceptable problems such as incontinence.

All of these problems have a serious impact upon the patients self-concept and self-esteem and create feelings of isolation, guilt, and loneliness. The patient, helpless and vulnerable, depends on the nurse to cherish and protect his or her wholeness. The nurse communicates with the patient, often using what Levine refers to as the "silent language" (Kim & McFarlane, 1984), administering meticulous physical care with warmth and gentleness; preserving the patient's privacy and dignity; respecting his or her possessions, beliefs, and values; keeping the patient safe and secure in the environment; and in all of these ways helping to conserve and restore personal integrity.

Conservation of Social Integrity

The ultimate goal of all health care is to return the individual to the family and community in a state that will facilitate reentry into a productive and satisfying life (Levine, 1967). When this goal cannot be fully realized because of the patient's disease or prognosis (as is so often the case with neurologically damaged patients), an alternate goal is to help the patient and family cope adaptively to the inevitable outcome. For neurologic patients the commonly recurring nursing diagnoses related to the resocialization process result from the patient's communicative and cognitive dysfunction; social isolation and self-care deficits associated with changes in life style and role relationships. Nursing care will focus on helping the patient and family adapt to the new person the patient has become and on fostering a new realignment of roles and relationships. Teaching the patient to function outside the protected environment of the institution and to establish a modified version of the preferred life style is critical to the conservation of the patient's social integrity.

Thus, by incorporating the body of neuroscience nursing knowledge into the Levine model, the patient with neurological dysfunction will be approached with:

1. A view of the patient as an integrated individual, continuously interacting with the environment, and reacting and responding to every stimulous (including the "predicament of illness").

2. A defined purpose or goal: to conserve or keep together the patient's biological, personal, and social integrity when it is threatened by illness or injury.
3. A focus for nursing intervention: the four conservation principles, recognizing and supporting the four levels of organismic response as the patient struggles to maintain or regain integrity.

USING LEVINE'S MODEL TO ASSESS AND DIAGNOSE

As stated earlier, a fundamental purpose of a nursing model is to direct the collection of data, based on the *view of the patient*, the *purpose of nursing*, and the *focus of nursing concern*. By combining the concepts from Levine's model with knowledge of neuroanatomy and physiology, medical and nursing science, it becomes possible to select, from all of the possible facts one could collect about the patient, those that are most relevant to the purpose of nursing. Then, from the collected data, what Levine (1966) refers to as the "provocative facts" are isolated. In medical terminology, these might be referred to as the "positive findings." The provocative facts, analyzed and extrapolated, lead to a set of defining characteristics (Gordon, 1982; Kim & McFarlane, 1984) that differentiate the appropriate nursing diagnoses. By applying a knowledge of neuroscience one is enabled to arrive at the etiological (or risk) factors contributing to the diagnosis.

Thus, using the Levine model, the nursing assessment will focus on:

- Energy exchange
- Structure and function
- Self-identity (self-concept, self-respect).
- Social milieu (life style, relationships).

Table 30–1 is an assessment guide to help direct the data collection for a neurological patient. Not all data need to be collected on every patient. The experienced nurse can quickly focus on those items that would seem most relevant to the particular patient's situation. From the collected data the nurse can isolate the provocative facts that indicate the presence of a particular nursing diagnosis. These facts can then be summarized and used to develop the nursing care plan. Table 30–2 is an example of a plan developed in this way. The nursing outcomes described in the care plan reflect a knowledge of the medical diagnosis and prognosis for recovery and for return of function, while the nursing interventions listed are firmly rooted in a knowledge of both general and neuroscience nursing.

Since the early 1970s, the organization now known as the North American Nursing Diagnoses Association (Gordon, 1982; Kim & McFarlane, 1984) has been in the process of developing and updating standardized nomenclature for describing nursing diagnoses, including when possible a set of defining charac-

TABLE 30–1. NURSING DIAGNOSIS ASSESSMENT DATA*; IMPLICATIONS OF CONSERVATION PRINCIPLES IN A NEUROLOGICAL SETTING

I. Energy exchange (energy resources/energy expenditures)
   A. Oxygen supply
      1. Airway
      2. Respirations (rate, rhythm, volume)
      3. Arterial blood gases
   B. Nutrition
      1. Present nutritional status
      2. Nutritional intake
   C. Activity/rest/sleep
      1. Medically prescribed restrictions
      2. Physical restrictions/fatigue
      3. Effects of level of consciousness, mental status changes
      4. Effects of life style/patient goals
   D. Illness-related energy expenditures
      1. Fever/infection
      2. Seizures
      3. High stimuli environment (as ICU)
      4. High stress (physiological)
      5. Pain
      6. Metabolic abnormalities
II. Structure and function
   A. Integument
      1. Skin condition
      2. Mucus membranes, corneas
      3. Surgical wounds/injuries/tubes/catheters
      4. Skin turgor/tone/circulation
      5. Sensation (temperature, pain, touch, pressure)
   B. Musculoskeletal system
      1. Strength
      2. Tone
      3. Reflexes
      4. Abnormal movement
      5. Ability to initiate, sustain, control, and terminate movement
      6. Range of movement (all joints)
      7. Mobility/weight bearing
      8. Fractures/injuries
   C. Sensation/perception
      1. Vision
      2. Hearing
      3. Smell
      4. Touch
      5. Temperature
      6. Pain
      7. Proprioception
   D. Cerebral perfusion pressure
      1. Level of consciousness
      2. Blood pressure (lying, standing, sitting)
      3. Pupil size and reactivity
      4. Other cranial nerve function
      5. Posturing
      6. Intracranial pressure (when being measured)

(cont.)

TABLE 30-1. (*CONTINUED*)

   E. Elimination
     1. Bowel function
      (a) Bowel sounds
      (b) Stool (frequency, consistency)
      (c) Flatus
      (d) Control
     2. Urination
      (a) Amount/frequency/specific gravity
      (b) Bladder emptying
      (c) Evidence of infection
      (d) Control
   F. Fluids and electrolytes
     1. Fluid intake and output
     2. Weight
     3. Skin turgor
     4. Serum electrolytes/osmolality
   G. Treatment-related risks
     1. Steroid therapy
     2. Radiation/chemotherapy
     3. Invasive diagnostic/treatment procedures
III. Self-identity/self-respect/self-concept
   A. Mental status
     1. Orientation
     2. Memory
     3. Judgment
     4. Problem solving
     5. Emotional lability/catastrophic reactions
   B. Communication
     1. Language (verbal/written)
     2. Speech
     3. Gestures
     4. Facial expression
   C. Image of self
     1. Degree of independence
     2. Control of bodily functions
     3. Perceived relationships with family/others
     4. Congruence of previous and present life style/activity level/goals and aspirations
   D. Adaptation
     1. Evidence of grief reaction/resolution
     2. Coping strategies
IV. Social milieu/life style/relationships
   A. Family/significant others
     1. Availability of support systems
     2. Willingness/ability of family/significant others to provide care/ongoing support
     3. Coping strategies of family/significant others
   B. Social situation
     1. Financial status as effected by illness/disability
     2. Career status as effected by the illness/disability
     3. Living arrangements
     4. Role relationships/expectations

*In addition to routine nursing assessment.

TABLE 30-2. PLAN EXAMPLE

Trophicognoses (summary of "provocative facts")

Mrs. G. is a 73-year old widow, living alone, brought to the hospital by ambulance after being found unresponsive on the floor at home. Admitting medical diagnosis is probable left middle cerebral artery infarct. Recent cataract surgery. At time of admission is awake, but does not respond to verbal commands. Mutters unintelligibly and is very restless, attempting to get out of bed. The right arm and leg are flaccid with no spontaneous movement. There is a facial droop and absent gag reflex. Voided in bedpan which was placed under her, and was then noted to be less restless. Patient's daughter is the nearest relative. She became distraught (crying) upon seeing her mother. States that the family want "everything" done to make her mother well.

Nursing Care Plan—Nursing Diagnoses

I. Energy exchange
  A. High risk for secondary brain injury (recent CVA)
    1. Monitor vital signs, neuro status
    2. Maintain oxygenation (lung hygiene, avoid aspiration, avoid orthostatic hypotension)
    3. Minimize increased ICP (elevate head of bed, control agitation, avoid valsalva)
  B. Altered nutrition: potential for less than body requirements (anticipated difficulty chewing, swallowing)
    1. Mechanical soft diet
    2. Small frequent feedings
    3. Nutritional supplement anytime less than 50% of diet not eaten
    4. Feed patient from left side, placing food well back in mouth
II. Structural integrity
  C. Potential for injury: trauma (restlessness, visual impairment, right-sided weakness)
    1. Side rails at all times
    2. Posey vest
    3. Close observation
    4. Bedside table on left, within field of vision and within reach at all times
    5. Glasses on during waking hours
    6. Night light
    7. Offer bedpan; anticipate needs to reduce efforts to get out of bed
  D. Impaired physical mobility (flaccid paralysis of right extremities)
    1. Position in correct functional alignment
    2. Use pillows to support right arm/leg.
    3. Reposition Q 2 hours. Leave on right side no longer than 1 hour
    4. ROM all extremities Q 4 hours
    5. Refer to PT, OT as soon as condition stabilizes
  E. Potential for impaired skin integrity (restlessness, decreased muscle tone, immobility)
    1. Alternating pressure mattress
    2. Heel and elbow protectors
    3. Use turning sheet
    4. Reposition as above
    5. Examine all skin surfaces each time patient is turned
    6. Routine skin care, with gentle massage to bony prominances
III. Personal integrity
  F. Impaired communication (confusion, aphasia)
    1. Anticipate and meet needs for care
    2. Speak slowly, clearly, using one, two words (verbs, nouns). Use "yes," "no" questions.
    3. Use gestures and touch to communicate with patient
    4. Explain communication problem and management to daughter and other visitors
    5. Refer to speech pathologist as soon as condition has stabilized

(cont.).

TABLE 30–2. (*CONTINUED*)

    G. Dependency (self-care deficit: total)
       1. Provide needed care with gentleness
       2. Explain situation, procedures, etc in short, simple words
       3. As condition stabilizes, allow (do not force) patient to begin simple, nontiring self-care tasks
       4. Preserve patient's dignity (speak as to an adult, using proper title; offer choices; respect patient's preferences; provide privacy; maintain personal hygiene and appearance)
IV. Social integrity
    H. Altered family process (sudden illness of previously independent mother)
       1. Refer to social worker
       2. Begin exploring with daughter home/family resources for long-term care
    I. Anticipatory grieving: daughter (anticipated loss, permanent disability of mother)
       1. Provide opportunity for daughter to verbalize thoughts and feelings
       2. Discuss patient's condition, medical diagnosis, and prognosis with daughter and other family members
       3. Discuss options/alternatives including patient family wishes regarding resuscitation, use of life-support measures
       4. Respect/support family decisions. Assist family in arriving at realistic plan for ongoing care of mother

---

teristics and etiological factors. In 1985 the American Nurses Association and the American Association of Neuroscience Nurses cooperated in a joint project to publish a document to facilitate the implementation of the neuroscience standards of care (ANA-AANN, 1985). In analyzing the assessment data to formulate nursing diagnoses the nomenclature standardized in these published documents is used and is being tested in the clinical setting.

SUMMARY

Levine's nursing model provides a focus for collecting patient assessment data, for isolating the provocative facts that are of concern to nursing. The four levels of organismic response and the principles of conservation form the basis for decision making about the nursing care of patients. The Levine model facilitates and enhances the development of nursing diagnoses, and is an appropriate framework for organizing the standardized diagnosed nomenclature being developed by the North American Association for Nursing Diagnoses, the American Nurses Association, and the American Association of Neuroscience Nurses.

REFERENCES

American Nurses Association. (1980). *A social policy statement.* Kansas City, MO: Author.

American Nurses Association-American Association of Neuroscience Nurses. (1985). *Neuroscience nursing practice: Process and outcome criteria for selected diagnoses.* Kansas City, MO: Author.

Gordon, M. (1982). *Nursing diagnosis: Process and application.* New York: McGraw-Hill.

Kim, M. J., & McFarlane, A. (1984). *Pocket guide to nursing diagnosis.* St. Louis: Mosby.

Levine, M. E. (1966). *Trophicognosis: An alternative to nursing diagnosis.* Presented at an ANA Regional Clinical Conference. Proceedings published in *Exploring progress in medical-surgical nursing* (vol. 2, 55–70). New York: American Nurses Association.

Levine, M. E. (1967). The four conservation principles of nursing. *Nursing Forum, 6*(1), 45–59.

Levine, M. E. (1969). The pursuit of wholeness. *American Journal of Nursing, 69*(1), 93–98.

Levine, M. E. (1971). Holistic Nursing. *Nursing Clinics of North America, 6*(2), 253–264.

Roy, C. (1975). A diagnostic classification system for nursing. *Nursing Outlook, 23*(2), 90–94.

Orem's General Theory of Nursing
An Interpretation

Joan Riehl-Sisca

A synopsis of Orem's self-care theory is presented in this chapter. The purpose of including this is to assist those who are unfamiliar with the self-care framework to easily visualize and understand its structure and function. For others, it can be used as a reference in their own work and in teaching.

In her general theory of nursing, Orem (1971, 1980) describes three concepts: self-care, self-care deficit (dependent-care deficit), and nursing systems. These three concepts each have a central idea, propositions, and presuppositions. They constitute the structure of her model. Each concept has component parts. The process or function of the model indicates how the concepts are operationalized. Tables 31–1 through 31–6 contain a graphic representation of this framework. Much of the content in the tables is self-explanatory, but a supplemental discussion will be helpful. This is provided in the following narrative.

In Table 31–1 an overview of Orem's structure and process is shown. In it, the relationships between three theoretical constructs are evident. A health care focus is a part of people's lives and is of interest to nurses. It includes the first concept, that is, the self-care practices of individuals, and the second concept, when the self-care capabilities are greater than or equal to the therapeutic self-care demand. A nurse assisting focus emerges when the self-care capabilities are less than the therapeutic self-care demand. When the latter occurs between these two patient variables, it is referred to as the "self-care deficit theory." The resulting relationship between a patient's self-care deficit system and the nursing system is an interacting relationship.

Self-care systems and nursing systems are self-organizing action systems (Backscheider, 1974) that are influenced by the self-care requisites (SCRs) and the basic conditioning factors (BCFs). The BCFs modify the SCRs and are listed in Table 31–1. The SCRs are shown in Table 31–2 and are discussed here.

The process or operation utilized to implement the structure of Orem's

TABLE 31-1. OVERVIEW OF OREM'S STRUCTURE AND PROCESS

Structure *Self-Care Requisites* *(SCRs)*	*Basic Conditioning Factors* *(BCFs)*	*Theoretical Constructs*	

Universal	Modify the SCRs
	  Age
	  Sex
	  Developmental state
	  Health state
		Self-care system
		Deliberate action of individuals, family, community
			Health Care Focus

Developmental	Life experience
	  Sociocultural orientation
	  Resources
		Self-care capabilities (e.g., self-care agency [SCA]) $>$ Therapeutic self-care self-care demand (TSCD)	

Health deviation		SCA $<$ TSCD *Self-care deficit* Interacting relationship *Nursing systems* Nursing capabilities (Nursing agency) 1. Tridimensional 2. Types of systems	**Nurse Assist Focus**
Process/Operations Assessment/diagnosis	Design-prescribe/plan	Regulate-manage/intervene-evaluate	

TABLE 31-2. THE SELF-CARE REQUISITES

Universals	Developmentals	Health Deviations
Maintenance of air, water, and food Maintenance of a balance between rest and activity and between solitude and social interaction Provision of care associated with elimination Prevention of hazards Promotion of human functioning and development in accord with potential, limitations, and normalcy (Orem, 1980, p. 42)	A. Support and promote life processes including: Pregnancy, birth, neonates, infancy, childhood, adolescence, and adulthood B. Provide care in: Educational deprivation, social maladaptation, loss of family, friends, possessions and security, change of environment, status problems, poor health or living conditions, terminal illness (Orem, 1980, p. 47)	Secure medical assistance when exposed to pathology Attend to results of pathologic conditions Utilize medical therapy to prevent or treat pathology Attend to discomforting effects of medical care Modify self-image to accept care as needed Learn to live with pathology (Orem, 1980, p. 51)

TABLE 31-3. SELF-CARE DEFICIT ANALYSIS

Self-Care Capabilities		Therapeutic Self-Care Demand
(Self-care agency/dependent-care agency)	Abilities/limitations in 3 scales	
	Development, Operability, Adequacy	
Power Components		*Primary Prevention*
The ability to:		Therapeutic self-care demand is the action needed to meet the self-care requisites
1. Maintain attention		
2. Control body position		*Primary Prevention*
3. Be motivated		≥ is utilized when self-care is
4. Reason		> the TSCD
5. Make decisions		
6. Acquire and operationalize knowledge		
7. Order self-care actions to achieve goals		
8. Perform and integrate self-care operations into activities of daily living		
9. Regulate energy for self-care operation		
10. Utilize skills to perform self-care		
Self-Care Deficit Theory: Determine the deficit relatiionship between the self-care capabilities (self-care agency) and the therapeutic self-care demand	<	*Secondary and Tertiary Prevention* are utilized when an SCD exists

model is also identified in Table 31-1. It is reviewed in conjunction with the detailed presentation of the theoretical framework shown in Tables 31-4, 31-5, and 31-6.

THE SELF-CARE REQUISITES

Although Orem's model can be analyzed from several perspectives, the approach employed here is to first examine the self-care requisites, or requirements. The BCFs naturally follow because they modify the SCRs. The three concepts—self-care, self-care deficit, and nursing systems—are discussed last because they seem to build upon the foundation of the SCRs.

The SCRs with their component parts are given in Table 31-2. In one sense, they represent a continuum from the universals through the developmental to the health deviations. The requisites initiate the process or operation of the

TABLE 31–4. THE ASSESSMENT AND DIAGNOSTIC PROCESS

Nursing Capabilities
(Nursing agency)
	1. Tridimensional
	    Interpersonal
	    Social
	    Technical

	2. Types of systems
	    Wholly compensatory
	    Partly compensatory
	    Supportive-educative

Nursing Systems ***Process/Operations***	*Assess and diagnose* In addition to obtaining the self-care deficit data, the nursing situation by health care focus is assessed.

There are 3 dimensions	*and 7 groups that focus on:*
1. Presence/absence of disease	1. The life cycle
2. Quality of general health	2. Recovery from disease
3. Current changes and need for care	3. Illness of undetermined origin
	4. Genetic defects or developmental defects
	5. Regulation through treatment
	6. Restoration and stability
	7. Regulating processes that have disrupted human functioning to the degree that life cannot continue (Orem, 1980, p. 137)

health care focus for an individual, family, or community. Although the family and community are considered, Orem (1980) makes the point that: "The unit of a nurse's service may be an individual or a multiperson unit, but nursing ultimately is for human beings individually considered (p. 194)." This may pose a problem for nurses in community health who are assigned to care for families. From this quotation, however, it seems clear that when a nurse is involved in the care of a family, he or she is the dependent care agent for only one person at a time. For example, on a family visit, the nurse may give care directly to a youngster (a self-care agent) and to the parent (a dependent-care agent to the child). The care provided may vary. It could be wholly compensatory with the youngster and supportive-educative with the parent.

The SCRs can be viewed on a continuum, as mentioned earlier. The universals initiate the process, the developmentals assume a middle position, and the health deviations end the process. The universals and the elements listed under part A of the developmentals in Table 31–2 represent the behaviors that usually are considered within normal limits (WNL) for human beings. They are, therefore, essential to learn so that the professional nurse can readily identify limitations, deficits, or the abnormal. These begin to appear in part B of the

TABLE 31–5. DESIGN AND PRESCRIBE/PLAN THE NURSING CARE

Nursing Systems

Process/Operations   *Design and prescribe/plan*

A. 1. Calculate all the TSCDs
     Identify all the limitations in the self-care agency (SCA)
  2. Determine the best methods of helping to resolve the
     patient's self-care deficits

B. Set priorities

C. Determine the patient's role: the degree of development,
operation, and adequacy, and determine the nurse's
(or nonnurse's) role

D. This is the primary †, secondary ‡, and tertiary ∰ prevention
focus

A. 1. *To Calculate the TSCD*	A. 2. *Methods of Helping*	*Nursing System*
a. Identify the SCRs	1. Doing for	a. Wholly compensatory†
b. Identify the internal and external patient orientations that determine how each SCR is met	2. Assisting in meeting needs	b. Partly compensatory‡
c. Identify inter-relationships among the SCRs	3. Guide, teach, environmental support	c. Supportive-educative ∰
d. Determine if method used to meet a need affects other needs		
e. Determine action needed to meet SCR		
f. Formulate design for self-care action		

**TABLE 31–6. THE REGULATORY PHASE/INTERVENTION AND
EVALUATION OF NURSING CARE**

Nursing Systems	
Process/Operations	*Regulate or manage/intervene-evaluate*
	Regulate the patient's self-care agency and the therapeutic self-care demand and regulate the nurse and patient role relatiionships

developmental SCRs and are particularly obvious in the health deviation SCRs.

THE SELF-CARE SYSTEM

In the self-care system, the health focus of individuals is to maintain for themselves and their families a state of wellness. Orem's self-care construct is appropriately conceptualized as it applies to the individual because it refers to everyone's activities of daily living. In the theory of self-care, the key feature is the relationship between the deliberate action of a mature member of society and her or his development and functionability. This also applies to the care of the dependent family members in regard to promoting their development and functionability as well.

Self-care theory may be interpreted two ways from its key statement (Orem, 1980, p. 28). One is that the theory refers to healthy individuals and their families who are maturing and developing within normal limits. In the other, Orem infers that this concept refers to persons and their dependent family members whose health state is not, or at one time was not, within normal limits. Examples of the latter are individuals who have a chronic illness and women who are pregnant.

SELF-CARE DEFICIT THEORY

Table 31–3 affords a closer examination of the self-care deficit theory. Orem considers this to be her core concept because in it persons with health-derived limitations can benefit from nursing. In this concept, the therapeutic self-care demands (TSCDs), or actions needed to meet the SCRs, of a patient are examined and compared to his or her self-care agency or capabilities. When the TSCDs are sufficient to maintain a state of wellness, the evaluation is that the SCRs are being met. When limitations are noted in the self-care agency (SCA), a deficit relationship exists between the two. Different equations can further express this concept. For example, a TSCD − a limitation in the SCA can = a self-care deficit (SCD), or when the TSCD is < the SCA this can = a SCD. The former is illustrated thus: State the action needed (the TSCD) to meet an SCR, such as learning to live with a diagnosis − an unwillingness to change behavior to accommodate to the pathologic condition (SCA limitation) = a deficit or discrepancy between the two that must be resolved if life is to be sustained. Applying the latter equation would result in a statement like this: An individual needs to maintain himself on a diabetic diet (the TSCD); he is not motivated to do so (the SCA limitation), which = a deficit that needs attention.

To help identify the self-care agency and capabilities, the Nursing Development Conference Group (1979) identified ten power components, which are listed in Table 31–3. The abilites or limitations of a person's power components are classified into three scales and degrees of development, operability, and adequacy. The power components and scales are related to the therapeutic self-care demand. If there is a limitation in any of the power components in any of the three scales, there is a self-care deficit in the needed action.

One last consideration that can be injected at this point is the matter of the degrees of prevention utilized by nurses. Since primary prevention is employed when persons are generally in a state of wellness, it complements the situation that occurs when the self-care agency is about equal to the therapeutic self-care demand. For example, primary prevention is used in well-baby clinics. The secondary and tertiary preventions are mandatory when self-care deficits are present—that is, when the self-care agency is less than the therapeutic self-care demand.

NURSING SYSTEMS

The third concept of Orem's theory is nursing systems. It has two dimensions. One is tridimensional and consists of social, interpersonal, and technologic elements (Table 31–4). These three elements apply to the patient, the nurse, and their relationship. The social type of relationship is contractual for nursing. The interpersonal relationship is professional and helping in nature. In the technologic relationship, nursing is specified by the role sets of the nurse and the patient. To operationalize these elements, Orem (1980) consolidates the interpersonal with the social (contractual), places the technologic with professional, and then identifies a third category, which she entitles "types of operation." Examples of these are:

1. For the interpersonal-contractual, collaboration with the patient to assess what self-care the patient performs.
2. For technical-professional, identification of the patient's self-care limitations.
3. For types of operations: diagnosing the self-care agency.

The second dimension of the nursing systems concept is the types of systems, of which there are three: wholly compensatory, partly compensatory, and supportive-educative. These are reviewed in the next section.

The central theme of this concept is that nurses use their capabilities to implement the nursing process. In performing required actions, nurses regulate patients' self-care activities that are required to meet their SCRs.

THE NURSING PROCESS OR OPERATIONS

When the Nursing Development Conference Group (1979) discussed nursing systems, they defined it from the self-care agency perspective. They visualized this concept from two frames of reference. One analyzed the self-care agency from the individual's point of view. The other was the nursing system, which included the patient's therapeutic self-care demand and self-care agency. These interacted with the nursing agency. This interacting relationship (shown in Table 31–1) initiated the patient–nurse contact or nursing process. The word "patient" is used because this is the role assumed when a person moves from being a self-care agent to a receiver of care. The health care focus utilized by the self-care agent shifts to a nurse assisting focus at this point in time.

Orem identifies three steps in the nursing process. These are diagnostic and prescriptive, design and plan, and management, which includes evaluation. Orem classifies these terms as types of operations. However, because these terms can be equated with the steps commonly referred to as the nursing process—assess, diagnose, plan, intervene, and evaluate—they are so paired in Tables 31–4, 31–5, and 31–6 and in this discussion.

One of the first steps in the nursing process is an examination of the patient's health care focus in the nursing situation. In obtaining the patient's health history during assessment, the nurse reviews this focus, which contains three dimensions and seven groups. The three dimensions are (1) the presence or absence of disease; (2) the quality of the patient's general health; and (3) current changes and need for care. The seven groups that accompany these dimensions (listed in Table 31–4) serve as a guide for expanded inquiry and the plan of care.

An examination of the therapeutic self-care demand and the self-care agency initiates the diagnostic process per se, according to Orem. Because physicians are usually the first professionals seen by the patient, the nurse incorporates the physician's finding in deriving a nursing diagnosis. The physician's findings include the medical diagnosis, diagnostic tests, medications, and treatments. In the nursing diagnostic process, the nurse is aware that the patient's knowledge, skill, and attitude (KSA) determine the therapeutic self-care demand. The KSA is based on the power components. As mentioned earlier, each power component is viewed from these perspectives, namely, its degree of development, operation, and adequacy. The focal point of the diagnostic process is identification of the self-care deficit (dependent-care deficit), which is done by listing the limitations in the relationship between the therapeutic self-care demand and the self-care agency.

Before the diagnostic process is complete, a nurse seeks the answers to five questions:

1. What is the patient's therapeutic self-care demand?
2. Does he or she have a self-care deficit in meeting this demand?
3. What is the reason for and nature of the deficit?
4. Should the patient be helped to change the self-care practice, or should developed therapeutic capabilities be protected?
5. What is the patient's potential and willingness for performing self-care, increasing self-care knowledge, learning self-care techniques, and incorporating essential self-care measures into his or her activities of daily living? (Orem, 1980, p. 203)

Developing a design and plan of care follows this diagnostic process discussed above (Table 31–5). The nurse begins first by calculating all of the therapeutic self-care demands, identifying the limitations in the self-care agencies, and determining their deficit relationships. Secondly, the nurse determines the best method of helping. These two steps are necessary to design a therapeutic system of action to meet the self-care requisites.

In the design process, numerous factors are considered in calculating the therapeutic self-care demand before a plan of care is adopted. Among these factors are the internally and externally oriented behaviors required for self-care. An example of an internal orientation is "Learning activities related to the development of self-care knowledge, attitudes and skills," and an example of external orientation is "Activity to seek assistance to accomplish a self-care goal (Orem, 1980, p. 213)."

In classifying the methods of helping, secondary and tertiary prevention are used especially with self-care deficit theory. Primary prevention, on the other hand, is placed with self-care theory, because it is concerned with health maintenance before the onset of illness. This is not to say that there is no overlap among all three preventive methods used to promote self-care development of health.

The methods of helping consist of five categories and three divisions or types of nursing systems (Tables 31–4 and 31–5). The division is called "wholly compensatory." It requires the nurse to do everything, or nearly everything, for the patient. An example of this would be total care of a quadraplegic patient. The second division is known as "partly compensatory." In this situation, all five methods may be used, with the patient doing what he or she can and the nurse supplementing the activity. The knowledge, skill, and psychological set, or attitude, of the patient are determining factors. For example, a very young patient has to relearn to walk after a long hospitalization involving surgery. The primary method of helping in the nurse's role would be of physical and psychological support. The third and final division is called "supportive-educative." It involves guiding, teaching, and environmental support. The method of helping consists of assisting the patient in decision making, behavior control, and acquiring needed knowledge and skills—for example, teaching diabetic patients to give themselves insulin injections.

Setting priorities is another part of the design of care that is essential. In this realm, there is also the task of establishing completion dates for immediate goals and short-term and long-term goals. In setting priorities the nurse lists all the self-care deficits and rank orders them from most important to least important. Of course, those relating to life-threatening measures demand attention first, with immediate goals identified in regard to them. This is a judgment that becomes more precise as the nurse and patient increase their knowledge.

The prescriptive phase of the nursing process follows the design and plan of care. Although Orem considers the prescriptive phase with the diagnostic phase, in practice it follows or is a part of the design. This is true because to prescribe is to write down the rule of action (Webster's, 1983). A prescription consists of determining and writing out the patient's role in regard to his or her degree of development, operation, and adequacy. The nurse's or nonnurse's role is also determined and noted. Because this is the role of the dependent care agent, it may be assumed by a nonnurse, such as a parent. The role of the nurse and the other is prescribed in terms of meeting the methods of helping and the therapeutic self-care demands.

The tasks of managing and evaluating are the final steps in the nursing process (Table 31-6). In nursing systems theory, the product of nursing practice is a system in which a patient's capability to engage in self-care is regulated so that self-care is continuously developed in the patient. Managing consists of regulating (1) the nurse-patient roles to meet the self-care requisites; (2) the methods of helping; and (3) the therapeutic action systems.

In evaluating the outcomes of the nurse-patient interactions, changes are made when self-care deficits persist. The process is thus circular and may well include a closer look at all the self-care requisites as well as the self-care agency–therapeutic self-care demand relationship in redesigning a new plan of care.

REFERENCES

Backsheider, J. E. (1974). Self-care requirements, self-care capabilities, and nursing systems in the diabetic nurse management clinic. *American Journal of Public Health,* 64(12), 1138–1146.

Nursing Development Conference Group (1979). *Concept formalization in nursing* (2nd ed.). Boston: Little, Brown.

Orem, D. E. (1971). *Nursing: Concepts of practice.* New York: McGraw-Hill.

Orem, D. E. (1980). *Nursing: Concepts of practice* (2nd ed). New York: McGraw-Hill.

Webster's New Collegiate Dictionary. (1983, 9th ed.). Springfield, MA: Merriam-Webster.

Orem's Self-Care Nursing Theory

Rebecca Lynn Feathers

The purpose of this chapter is to evaluate Dorthea Orem's Self-Care Nursing theory according to criteria adapted from Stevens (1984). The internal evaluation examines the commonplaces, clarity, consistency, adequacy, logical development, and the level of theory development. The external evaluation analyzes the theory's reality convergence, utility, significance, capacity for discrimination, scope, and complexity.

After the evaluation, comparisons will be made, when applicable, to the work of Maslow, who has contributed to the development of Orem's theory through his efforts in the field of psychology.

INTERNAL EVALUATION

Commonplaces

The commonplaces in Orem's self-care theory are related to the concept of the nurse and nursing acts, the patient, health, the nurse-patient relationship, the nurse's relationship to health, and the patient's relationship to health.

The nurse acts in a deliberate and purposeful manner to provide assistance to those who are unable to meet their health-related self-care needs. Orem uses the term *nursing agency*, which Greenfield and Pace (1985) define as the "complex, acquired abilities of the nurse in designing, creating, providing, and managing systems of therapeutic care to individuals with self-care deficits (p. 188)." The nurse functions to evaluate any self-care deficits and to assess the patient's self-care abilities. According to Caley, et al. (1980), there are three levels of nursing care. Care is wholly compensatory when the nurse provides total care for the patient. Care is partly compensatory when performed by both the nurse and the patient. The educative or supportive approach is utilized when the nurse assists the patient in acquiring knowledge or skills related to self-care. The goal of the nursing agency is to provide the appropriate system of care until the self-care abilities of the patient are sufficient to meet his or her self-care demands.

The patient is viewed as a person or group of persons in need of assistance to perform self-care. Griffith and Christensen (1982) define self-care as those activities personally initiated to continually maintain life, health, and well-being. Orem (1971) relates self-care activities to self-care requisites, which are catagorized as universal, developmental, or health deviation. The self-care agency of an individual is the ability to perform the activities necessary to meet the self-care requisites. Self-care agency is affected by the individual's physiological state, intellectual capabilities, emotional and psychological states, and social and economic factors.

The concept of health is defined in terms of the ability to meet the universal, developmental, and health-related needs. Health exists on a continuum that is affected by the quality and quantity of self-care deficits and the ability to perform self-care activities. Levels of health are supported or altered through maintenance of normal functioning, compensation for disabilities, education, and psycho-social guidance.

According to Orem (1979), a valid relationship exists between the nurse and the patient when there is an "absence of the ability to maintain continuously that amount and quality of self-care which is therapeutic in sustaining life and health, in recovering from disease, or in coping with their effects (p. 70)." Nursing intervention only takes place when the individual's self-care demands exceed his or her abilities to meet those demands. A nurse-patient relationship is contractual in nature and is based on the ability to provide care and the acceptance of that care. The complexity of the relationship will vary with the nature and scope of the self-care deficits.

The nurse's relationship to health is based on achieving desired health results through the encouragement of self-care. Nurses contribute to the status of well-being by sustaining health, assisting with recovery, and by providing health education and support.

The relationship between the patient and health is continuous in nature, and self-care is viewed as the responsibility of each individual. An individual's ability to achieve or maintain their desired state of health may be limited or enhanced by factors such as age, developmental level, medical condition, cultural influences, or available resources. When health-related needs cannot be met it is the responsibility of the individual to seek appropriate assistance.

Clarity

The elements of the theory are clear in their meaning and can be easily understood. The content of the theory is limited to the foundations relevant to self-care. Self-care is defined as the activities that individuals perform to maintain their life, health, and state of well-being. The definitions given for key concepts allow for a clear reference point for establishing the relationships within the theory.

Consistency

The theory is consistent throughout its development. Key terms and concepts are defined and used in the same manner at all levels of the theory. An example is that "nursing agency" is consistently used only to refer to the abilities of the nurse.

The interpretation of reality falls within the scope of human experience. The fundamental principle of self-care, and the actions and thought processes involved in performing self-care activities, are experienced every day by most individuals.

The underlying principle of self-care maintenance is present throughout the theory. The actions of the nurse and the patient are directed toward meeting self-care demands.

The operational method of thought is used to develop the self-care theory. The capabilities of the self-care agent determine the subsequent actions to be taken. The concepts are differentiated on the basis of who provides care, what care is necessary, and how that care is given.

Adequacy

Orem's theory adequately relates to the real world of nursing and health. The basic concepts of self-care, self-care agency, therapeutic self-care demand, and nursing agency, form a realistic relationship between health care consumers and the nursing profession. These concepts are fully accounted for in the presentation of the theory.

Self-care is an acceptable premise on which to build a theoretical framework. A realistic function of nursing is to provide assistance in meeting self-care requisites. In any area of nursing practice the evaluation of self-care deficits can be utilized to provide the appropriate level of care to maintain or improve the self-care agency of the patient.

Logical Development

The theory is logically developed and its structure is based on the premise that self-care activities are performed to maintain a desired state of well-being. Self-care agency, self-care deficits, and nursing agency are logical concepts developed from the original premise of the application of self-care to nursing practice and are supported by the definition of self-care.

Level of Theory Development

Orem has developed a complete descriptive theory and also addressed several elements of explanatory theory. At the descriptive level the major elements are identified as the ability to perform self-care activities, what self-care activities are necessary to maintain life and health, how self-care may be limited, and what level of intervention is required to assist with self-care. These concepts are fully developed and are easily identified as the most significant constituents of the theory.

The descriptive theory is further developed to explain the relationships between the concepts and to interpret these relationships. An example is that the nurse agency assists the patient only when her or his self-care ability is less than the self-care demand. Cause and effect and predictions relative to future intervention could be established from the present level of theory development; however, these are not clearly established.

EXTERNAL EVALUATION

Reality Convergence

How well this particular theory reflects the real world of nursing and health will be evaluated according to principle, interpretation, and method.

The basic principle of self-care is an acceptable premise, because all capable adults perform certain activities to maintain their own or their dependent's well-being. Meeting self-care requisites is an integral part of our daily lives. Developmental and health-related needs are becoming increasingly important in our society. This is evidenced by the growing number of health education and support programs. The emphasis in providing health care has shifted toward increasing the self-care abilities of the patient, as seen by the growth of home health care agencies and visiting nurses associations. More individuals are now being educated to care for themselves in the areas of advanced nutritional support, dialysis therapy, and chemotherapy.

Orem's interpretation of the world of the nurse as it relates to the concept of self-care is appropriate. In view of the need to reduce hospital costs, patients must be encouraged to participate in their care. With more stringent regulations controlling hospital admissions, greater attention must be given to promoting the self-care abilities of the patient.

The method used to develop the self-care nursing theory easily lends itself to research and validation. Provision is made for the assessment of the self-care abilities and limitations of the patient, establishing levels of therapeutic intervention, achieving desired goals, and methods for the evaluation of care. Research designs can incorporate these concepts to study the level of care assessed by the client and the adequacy of care provided by the nurse.

Utility

The self-care theory meets all the criteria of utility. The theory is useful to the practitioner in all areas of nursing practice, and it provides a framework from which to view patients. The concepts related to self-care activities and nursing functions can be easily utilized to develop an individualized plan of care for a variety of clients. The selected concepts are both pragmatic and operationalized.

In clinical settings the self-care model can be utilized in the assessment of self-care deficits, in formulating a plan of care based on the level of nursing intervention necessary to assist with self-care activities, and in evaluating the effectiveness of the nursing process in meeting desired health goals. Orem's theory can also be utilized in the area of nursing administration to develop departmental philosophy, policies, and goals, and to establish staffing patterns for the delivery of nursing care. The concepts can be applied to both hospital and outpatient care settings. In the field of nursing education the self-care concept can be used to develop curricula and methods of teaching. The theory also provides a framework for research and investigation into various areas of nursing practice.

Patients are viewed from the perspective of their ability to meet their self-care requisites. Nursing intervention is not imposed, but is contractual. Because patients are viewed as being responsible for self-care activities they retain as much control as possible over their care.

The key theoretical concepts have meaning in the real world of nursing and are operationalized in a manner that facilities their practical application. To define nursing as assisting individuals with self-care activities is a pragmatic view of how nurses function in the real world. The concepts related to self-care—such as self-care agency, self-care deficits, and nursing agency—create an operationalized framework for the practical application of the theoretical concepts.

Significance

Orem's theory has significance for nursing because it deals with the essential issues concerning nursing practice. The nurse and nursing acts are clearly defined, and the method and levels of nursing care are also well-developed. These are central issues of any nursing theory because they establish what nursing is, what levels of nursing care are required, and how that care should be delivered. The relationship between nurses, patients, and the concept of health is a central issue to nursing theory because these relationships establish when nursing intervention is appropriate and how nursing care must be directed to reach desired health goals.

Capacity for Discrimination

Orem separates nursing from other health professions by characterizing nursing as a substitute for self-care. The level of substitution is dependent on the nurse's evaluation of the self-care deficits of the patient. It is the responsibility of the nurse to establish and deliver a system of care that will be therapeutic to the patient. This system may be wholly compensatory, partially compensatory, or supportive in nature. The various roles of the patient, family, and other health professionals are not viewed as conflicting with the role of the nurse. These other significant relationships help to define the pattern of nursing care. According to Greenfield and Pace (1985), the nurse is essentially viewed as the mediating system affecting the patient's self-care agency to ensure that the capabilities for self-care are equal to or greater than the self-care demands.

Scope

A nursing theory based on the concept of self-care may appear to be limited in scope. However, Orem's theory has been constructed to include a variety of concepts that provide an adequate framework for observing nursing as it relates to self-care. An example can be found in the levels of nursing care utilized to meet self-care requisites. These levels range from total care being provided by the nurse, to the nurse serving only as a resource for supportive or educational needs.

Complexity

Orem's theory contains the appropriate balance between complexity and parsimony. The number of key principles is limited to those that are essential to self-care nursing. Each concept is then further developed to explain many related variables. An example is found in the concept of self-care requisites. These requisites are used to determine the appropriate levels of nursing intervention. To fully account for the wide range of self-care activities, self-care requisites are related to the physiological, psychological, sociological, developmental, and health-related needs of the patient.

COMPARISON OF OREM AND MASLOW

The influence of psychology, particularly the work of Maslow, can be recognized in Orem's self-care nursing theory. This influence is seen primarily in the area of Orem's conceptualization of human beings and in the formulation of self-care requisites.

Maslow (1968) views people from the perspective of humanistic psychology. Using a philosophy based on human worth and dignity, this approach generates a new conception of people. Positive fulfillment is necessary to develop human potential for self-realization, and the uniqueness of each individual is not suppressed or denied. Self-actualization can be accomplished by promoting personal growth.

Orem utilizes the human need for positive fulfillment in the self-care nursing theory. Maintenance of self-care is viewed as the responsibility of each individual. Performance of self-care activities, or at least participation in self-care, allows patients to retain a sense of personal worth and dignity. Self-expression is encouraged and utilized in planning nursing care. Each patient is viewed individually in relation to his or her capacity for self-care.

The influence of Maslow is also evident in Orem's formulation of self-care requisites. Although Maslow (1970) uses different terminology, he identifies basic human needs as physiological needs, safety needs, belongingness and love needs, esteem needs, and the need for self-actualization. Orem's universal and developmental requisites correspond to these basic human needs. Universal requisites include physiological and safety needs. Developmental requisites include needs related to love, belongingness, esteem, and self-actualization. Orem uses the basic human needs identified by Maslow to develop self-care requisites and then relates them to nursing practice. Because Orem's focus is on self-care requisites as they relate to nursing, health deviation self-care requisites address the results of illness or injury.

Orem refers to the inability to meet self-care requisites as creating a self-care deficit. From the psychological perspective, Maslow (1971) developed the terms "deficiency needs" and "hierarchy of needs" to explain the motivation of behavior (p. 2). When a deficiency occurs at some level in the hierarchy of human needs, an individual must satisfy that deficiency before a higher level of needs will emerge. This concept has implications for the nursing assessment of self-care deficits. Priorities must be established to meet self-care requirements. A patient suffering from an acute asthma attack must receive adequate oxygen before any other self-care requisites can be addressed.

Orem's theory utilizes knowledge generated from various fields of study. Maslow's contribution from the field of psychology has been essential in the formulation of the self-care nursing theory.

REFERENCES

Caley, J. M., Dirksen, M., Engalla, M., & Hennrich, M. L. (1980). The Orem self-care nursing model. In J. P. Riehl & C. Roy, *Conceptual models for nursing practice* (2nd ed., pp. 302–313). East Norwalk, CT: Appleton-Century-Crofts.

Greenfield, E. & Pace, J. (1985). Orem's self-care theory of nursing: Practical application to the end stage renal disease (ESRD). *Journal of Nephrology Nursing, 2*(4), 187–193.

Griffith, J. W., & Christensen, P. J. (1982). *Nursing process: Application of theories, frameworks, and models* (pp. 13–14). St. Louis: Mosby.

Maslow, A. H. (1968). *Toward a psychology of being* (2nd ed.). New York: Van Nostrand Reinhold.

Maslow, A. H. (1970). *Motivation and personality.* New York: Harper & Row.

Maslow, A. H. (1971). *The further reaches of human nature* (pp. 1–49). New York: Viking.

Orem, D. E. (1971). *Nursing: Concepts of practice* (3rd ed., pp. 1–53). New York: McGraw-Hill.

Orem, D. E. (1979). *Concept formalization in nursing: Process and product* (2nd ed.). Boston: Little, Brown.

Stevens, B. J. (1984). *Nursing theory: Analysis, application, evaluation* (2nd ed., pp. 1–74). Boston: Little, Brown.

33

The Relationship Between Self-Care Theory and Empirical Research

Elizabeth Geden

A major concern expressed by graduate students and beginning researchers is the need for examples illustrating how self-care theory serves as a framework and stimulus for research. The purpose of this chapter is to provide these examples and to illustrate the relationship between self-care theory and empirical or data-based research.

No one research approach will be or should be touted as being superior. At this time in the development of nursing science, and in particular the development of self-care theory, all approaches are appropriate and necessary. Researchers should choose an approach consistent with their beliefs regarding the nature and existence of reality. For example, quantitative research is premised on the belief that reality exists independent of the research. Thus, the researcher must be objective, and the outcomes of the research are compared with this external referent—reality. Qualitative research—for example, the phenomenologic approach—on the other hand, is premised on the belief that reality is unknown and not independent of the human experience. Thus, the researcher must be unbiased, open to the full breadth of the experience of the phenomenon, and the outcomes of the research effort are validated through a process of consensual agreement, not by reference or comparison to an external criterion.

Readers interested in a more detailed discussion of qualitative approaches applicable to nursing research are referred to Omery (1983) and Davis (1978). Further, readers should be cognizant that my belief systems are more congruent with the quantitative perspective. This perspective will be reflected in the remainder of this chapter and become particularly apparent in the forthcoming discussion of the law of correspondence and its application within the research process.

GOALS OF THEORY

The goals of theory are to provide typologies, explanations, predictions, and a sense of understanding. Reynolds (1971) suggests that three attributes seem to facilitate the adoption of a theory, concept, or statement into the scientific body of knowledge: abstractness, intersubjectivity, and empirical relevance. Abstractness means that the concept or theory is independent of time and space. A theory would be of little use if it were bound to a particular time, nor could it possess the ability to predict future events if it were time-bound. Few would argue with the assertion that self-care theory possesses the attribute of abstractness.

Intersubjectivity, the second attribute, has two components: shared agreement and logical rigor. Shared agreement means that there is consensus and logical rigor. Shared agreement means that there is consensus regarding the meaning of the theory and of the terms or concepts within the theory. An example is the statement that a self-care deficit exists when a client's ability to care for self is not sufficient due to the magnitude of the therapeutic self-care demand or the quality of the client's self-care agency. Intersubjective agreement is most likely when the theory or concept is sufficiently explicit so that the scientific community may discuss the theory in detail using the terms to represent similar phenomena or events (for example, a self-care deficit). Logical rigor refers to another type of consensus—consensus within the theory or its internal consistency. Taylor and Taylor (1983) assessed the logical rigor of self-care deficit theory using symbolic logic and found the theory to be internally consistent. This process enabled them to remove the bias of language and use symbols to assess the relationships among and between concepts within the theory.

The third attribute, and the focus of this chapter, is empirical relevance. The essence of the evaluation of the correspondence between the theory and the results of empirical research constitutes the law of correspondence. The outcome of an assessment of empirical relevance influences one's degree of confidence in the theory. If correspondence or congruity between empirical research and the theory is found, one's confidence or belief in the usefulness and utility of the theory increases. Conversely, if little or no corresondence is found, one's confidence in the theory decreases. However, the finding of a lack of correspondence has the greatest potential for advancing the theory. This potential will be manifested only when the theory itself, or the concept within the theory, is questioned. All too often, researchers have such a high degree of confidence in the theory that they fail to examine the theory for its inability to account for the findings. More often, they fault themselves—small samples, weak instrumentation, and so on. This behavior is typical of researchers operating within the "normal science" period described by Kuhn (1970). Rather than being disappointed in having to reject one's research hypotheses, the reader should recognize that the researcher has the opportunity to make a substantive contribution by advancing the theory's development.

It is highly unlikely that any single research effort will test a theory in its entirety. The more prevalent approach is to derive a research question from the theory wherein an explicit link between the research question and the theory is present. Although no single approach is better or holds more promise than another, it is necessary and essential to be able to describe the present—what is (descriptive approach)—before one can ask the question—what could be (experimental approach). In the remainder of this chapter, I will present examples of different types of research derived from or related to self-care theory, and extend the discussion of the law of correspondence or congruity to elements (research question, assumption, and operational definition) within the research process.

CORRESPONDENCE OF RESEARCH ELEMENTS AND THEORY

To be able to assert correspondence of empirical outcomes and theory, all the elements within the research must be congruent with the theory. For example, one cannot examine the question of the effects of a nursing technology on patients without those patients or nurses being a part of a legitimate nursing situation. Nor may one be capricious in constructing operational definitions. A self-care deficit must be operationally defined so that this concrete concept (the operational definition) matches or corresponds to the abstract concept (theoretical concept).

One final example relates to the use of research assumptions. The law of correspondence or congruity must also be considered. It is probably obvious to most readers that research assumptions must also be congruent with the theoretical framework or theory. For example, it would be incorrect to make the assumption that all patients have self-care deficits or that all hospitalized individuals are assumed to be a part of a legitimate nursing situation. It may be appropriate to assume that when patients attribute a causal relationship between actions and self-care practices, the self-care practice represents deliberate action. It should be clear that the theoretical perspective and the specific components of the research plan must be in concert with one another in order for the researcher to be able to assert the correspondence or lack of correspondence of the outcomes of research with the theory.

EXAMPLES OF RESEARCH DERIVED FROM SELF-CARE THEORY

Not all research is a direct testing of theory. More frequently, research questions are derived from or related to a theoretical point of view. In these instances, the relationship of the research to the theory is frequently less evident. However, the link should be made explicit so congruity between the genesis of the question and the outcomes may be assessed. Hugo (1983) examined the effects of a moderate exercise program on the dietary intake of nursing home residents. A review of the literature indicated that malnutrition and lack of appetite were prevalent problems in this population. Hugo asserted that an imbalance between activity and rest may be a significant factor accounting for these problems. She was able to document through previous research that strenuous exercise depresses eating behavior, whereas the effects of moderate exercise were largely untested. Thus, Hugo argued for the need for this study within a nursing perspective and used self-care deficit theory to assert the study's potential to contribute to the development of a nursing technique.

Consider the following question: "What is the relationship between self-care practices and compliance with medical regimens?" This question has the potential of being incongruent with self-care theory if the researcher defines compliance as "the number of prescribed medications taken." Furthermore, the outcomes may be quite misleading if the researcher fails to consider whether the patient made a deliberate choice to engage in this therapy. It should be obvious that if patients decide not to accept a therapy, their compliance levels would be quite low, but their self-care agency may be quite high.

Basic research is frequently needed to provide a comparative base for more applied clinical research. My research is an example of basic research related to self-care theory. My students and I have conducted a number of studies examining the energy expenditure of common nursing techniques and comfort measures. These studies may be related to the universal self-care requisite of maintaining a balance between activity and rest or related to the power component of self-care agency, which states "ability to control the position of the body and its parts in the execution of the movements required for the initiation and completion of self-care operations (Orem, 1979, p. 195)." To date all our work has been conducted in the laboratory using healthy subjects. We determined the oxygen consumption necessary (1) to get out of bed using different lifting techniques (Geden, 1982); (2) to perform active and passive range-of-motion leg exercise (Hathaway & Geden, 1983); and (3) to bathe and be bathed in bed (Flanagan, 1983). Other questions that could now be asked are: What are the energy costs associated with lifting patients or bathing patients with a particular health problem? What is the effect on energy expenditure when patients who need to be moved or engaged in exercise have limited capacity to control the position of their bodies or parts of their bodies?

Descriptive research is also needed. Orem (1980, p. 28) presents an exercise to assist students in acquiring the concept of self-care. It consists of seven questions to be asked of patients, designed to elicit alterations and adjustments in patient's self-care practices. A sample question is, "Since the occurrence of (name the conditioning factor, disease, injury, etc), do you have to care for yourself differently than you did before its occurrence?" This exercise provides an excellent frame for the development of descriptive studies of the self-care practices of sets of patients. Data generated by these types of studies would be enormously helpful in understanding the changes patients make in response to their health state.

In the same vein, Orem (1980) asserts that: "Self-care and care of dependent family members are learned within the context of social groups by human interaction and communication (p. 28)." Comparative descriptive studies would be helpful to determine if differences in self-care practices among various social groups exist and the nature of those differences. If these data were available, nurses would be able to predict the impact of those self-care practices and perhaps the likelihood of other practices being adopted.

For readers interested in examining the nurse-patient relationship, Orem (1980) suggests that the constructs of intensity and extensity may be useful in explicating the relationship. *Intensity* refers to the meaning the nurse and patient ascribe to their role relation, and *extensity* refers to the extent or the number of aspects of the patient's daily life that are encompassed in the relationship. From the nurse's perspective, one could hypothesize that nursing situations with high intensity and high extensity, such as an ICU, would yield more frequent burnout, or that nursing situations with low intensity and low extensity would yield less job satisfaction. Geden and Begeman's findings (1981) on personal space preferences of hospitalized adults could be reinterpreted using these constructs. Intensity and extensity would explain the differences between preferences assigned to physicians and nurses. As few patients were able to cite the name of the nurse or attribute nursing care measures to a particular individual, it is likely that the patient's view of the nurse-patient relationship was both low intensity and low extensity. This discussion is not to suggest that intensity and extensity are the only constructs of interest in the nurse-patient relationship, but rather to illustrate the diversiy of the theory in its ability to generate research questions.

One final example of research completed using self-care theory is the work of Hanson (1981) and Bickel (1982). Their efforts, using a psychometric approach, offer a great deal of promise. The instrument they developed needs further work using discriminant and convergent validation approaches to ascertain its ability to classify patients according to their quality and level of self-care agency.

The examples presented illustrate both the breadth of research questions that may be generated from self-care theory and the multiplicity of research approaches that may be used. It must be emphasized that the prime requisite for scientific inquiry is knowledge of the subject matter. One must be knowledgeable both about self-care theory and the research approach chosen to explicate, examine, and test the theory and thereby make substantive contributions to its development.

REFERENCES

Bickel, L. S. (1982). *A study to assess the factorial structure of the perceptions of self-care aging questionnaire.* Unpublished thesis, University of Missouri-Columbia.

Davis, A. J. (1978). The phenomenological approach in nursing research. In N. Chaska (Ed.), *The nursing profession: Views through the mist.* New York: McGraw-Hill.

Flanagan, R. (1983). *Energy expenditure of normal females during three bathing techniques.* Unpublished thesis, University of Missouri-Columbia.

Geden, E. A. (1982). Effects of lifting techniques on energy expenditure: A preliminary investigation. *Nursing Research, 33,* 214–218.

Geden, E. A., & Begeman, A. (1981). Personal space preferences of hospitalized adults. *Research in Nursing and Health, 4,* 237–241.

Hanson, B. E. (1981). *Development of a questionnaire measuring perception of self-care agency.* Unpublished thesis, University of Missouri-Columbia.

Hathaway, D. K., & Geden, E. A. (1983). Energy expenditure during leg exercise programs. *Nursing Research, 3,* 147–150.

Hugo, N. (1983). *Physical activity and dietary intake in the aged.* Unpublished thesis, University of Missouri-Columbia.

Kuhn, T. S. (1970). *The structure of scientific revolutions* (2nd ed.). Chicago: University of Chicago Press.

Omery, A. (1983). Phenomenology: A method for nursing research. *Advances in Nursing Science, 5,* 49–63.

Orem, D. E. (Ed.). (1979). *Concept formalization in nursing: Process and product* (2nd ed.). Boston: Little, Brown.

Orem, D. E. (1980). *Nursing: Concepts of practice* (2nd ed.). New York: McGraw-Hill.

Reynolds, P. D. (1971). *A primer in theory construction.* Indianapolis: Bobbs-Merrill.

Taylor, S., & Taylor, T. (1983). *Orem's theory and structure.* Unpublished manuscript.

The Riehl Interaction Model
An Update

Joan Riehl-Sisca

> To take what there is, and use it, without
> waiting forever in vain for the
> preconceived—to dig deep into the actual
> and get something out of that—this
> doubtless is the right way to live.
>
> *Henry James*

Any number of approaches may be used, singly or in concert, in organizing material to describe and analyze nursing models. Stevens (1984), Crane (1985), Meleis (1985), and Fawcett and Downs (1986) are among those who have presented guidelines for analysis. It is not surprising to find some overlap in their recommended methodologies. The Riehl Interaction Model (RIM) presented here is couched in an analytical framework that utilizes two of the perspectives cited, those of Crane and Stevens. Crane's precept, covered in the first part of the chapter, was developed primarily for nursing but has broad application to many areas of human endeavor. Stevens' contributions, discussed in the second part, are directed exclusively to nursing theory.

PART ONE: CRANE'S PERSPECTIVE

The traditional lag between the results of research and the actual application of findings has been evidenced in nursing as elsewhere. Crane's (1985a) efforts to increase research utilization resulted in a report on four nursing demonstration projects. In each project, she employed a different research utilization model based on general knowledge. The four models used by Crane (1985b) were: (1) research, development, and diffusion; (2) social interaction and diffusion; (3) problem solving; and (4) linkage.

The first model promoted research utilization in a rational sequence in which basic and then applied research were utilized over a period of time. These were followed by conversion and design, development, and finally diffusion of new knowledge. This entire process was directed toward the target population.

The second model was developed to highlight the way new research knowledge was diffused throughout a social system. Herein Crane identified the processes involved, the roles of opinion leaders, and the factors that influenced the success of the change agents who promoted the diffusion.

Crane's utilization of the third and fourth models was of particular interest because it applied to the framework of this chapter. Crane's third model was the problem-solving model. The benchmark of this paradigm is found in planned change, which begins with an identified need espoused by a member of the target population. It is then translated into a diagnostically oriented statement of the problem, which leads to a solution (innovation) to satisfy the identified need. The solution is shaped to meet the person's need in such a way as to assure the most facile implementation of the innovative measures and to allow for a thorough evaluation of its effectiveness (Havelock & Havelock, 1973). Thus, the stated needs determine the problem-solving processes. Internal resources are utilized in conjuction with applicable external resources including consultation with others. A key factor in this model is that the person-initiated and self-applied solution results in the greatest commitment and long-term survival of the problem resolution (Havelock, 1969).

The fourth model, linkage, was developed by Havelock and incorporates the strongest points of the other three models in that it links the user with the basic resources from which the new knowledge was generated. Four primary components form the core of this model and link the user (the client, patient, or family) to the resource (the nurse). These components demonstrate that a reciprocal relationship exists between the user and the resource person. This permits a cooperative arrangement in which each component can simulate or take on the role of the other in the problem-solving process.

The essential components of the linkage model are:

1. The user has identified needs, internal problem-solving abilities, and the willingness to seek external assistance.
2. The resource locates solutions relevant to the problems identified by the user.
3. A process of communication is established between the resource and the user wherein knowledge is transmitted regarding problem identification, a proposed solution is introduced, implementation of the solution is initiated, and the effectiveness of the solution is assessed.
4. A process is confirmed that disseminates new knowledge, skill, attitudes, and products from the resource to the user in an immediate and assistive fashion (Havelock, 1969; Havelock & Havelock, 1973).

One obvious value of this model lies in the reality that the user-resource relationship is greater than that which is obtained from models in which the patient is nothing more than the receiver of nursing orders. It is one that calls on and improves the problem-solving skills of all involved persons and results in far more lasting changes. Further, it requires that each member of the arrangement continues to learn from every other member. Thus, the effectiveness of the resource knowledge communicated reciprocally, allows for adjustments as needed in the concepts and strategies of the changes introduced as resolutions to identified problems.

PART TWO: STEVENS' PERSPECTIVE

Jacobson's (1987) recent research project, which involved a national survey of users of models in nursing, provides an excellent introductory foundation to a discussion of the Riehl Interaction Model. The 691 respondents to Jacobson's survey revealed that those who were users of nursing models were enthusiastic about their value. Eighty-seven percent of these respondents regarded the development of conceptual models in nursing as being of great importance to the advancement of nursing. Although Jacobson's study may represent but one small sample of the total population of professional nurses, it does provide sound rationale to pursue this endeavor and serves to motivate those who expend time and energy serving as resource persons in nursing theory.

Nursing models as we know them today have been on the scene for over 15 years, so it is not surprising that analytic criteria for assessing them are available. As stated in the introduction, the measures recommended by Stevens are presented in this section.

Stevens (1984) identifies and discusses several analytical mechanisms that can be employed in examining nursing theories. The first two are structural schemes and the second two are analytical devices that provide criteria to describe and evaluate theories. In one structural scheme, form, process, and context are addressed, and in the other scheme theories are viewed in terms of agency. *Agency* is the state or action of the patient and the nurse. The approach to the relationship between the two parties may be labeled as the nursing domain. When theories are described analytically, principles, interpretation, and methods are applied. When theories are evaluated, two guidelines are provided: internal and external criticisms. Both of the structural schemes and the analytical devices are discussed in this chapter as they apply to the Riehl Interaction Model.

Form, Process, and Context

As defined by Stevens, these three terms can easily be related to by curriculum developers. Stevens equates form to vertical/progressive threads, process to horizontal/pervasive threads, and context to the environment or background as interpreted by this author.

Form
Form includes a discussion of the organizing structure of the RIM based upon the social psychological theory of symbolic interaction. Essential components

of this structure are the assumptions and commonplaces or terms with their key concepts and definitions. Proponents of symbolic interaction theory include Mead (1934), Coutu (1951), Rose (1962), Manis and Meltzer (1967), Blumer (1969), and Wells and Marwell (1976), to name a few. This theory is defined as the interaction that occurs between human beings who interpret each other's actions instead of just reacting to them. Thus, their responses are based on the meanings they attach to such actions. This indicates that a process of interpretation occurs in each and every interaction. According to Rose (1980), symbolic interaction emerged as an alternative to psychological theory grounded on assumptions about vertebrate behavior and research on animals other than humans. In their research, the behaviorists usually study small animals and the Gestaltist study large animals such as apes. When investigating human behavior, they examine that which people share with animals and they use middle-range rather than large-scale theories. Although some principles may apply to people in their research and theory analysis, no reference is made to distinctive human characteristics. The latter underlie the assumptions of social psychological frameworks as seen in psychoanalysis and symbolic interaction theory.

Assumptions. Rose (1980) has identified analytic and genetic assumptions of symbolic interaction (SI). They represent the basic assumptions in the RIM. They are listed in Table 34–1; for a discussion, see Rose (1980) and Riehl (1980).

Commonplaces. The commonplaces or terms for the RIM are defined below.

PERSON: A human being, a genetically and socially emergent self.

ENVIRONMENT: The conditions influencing the emergent self that continuously interact with the internal and external factors and parameters.

NURSING: Therapeutic action that guides the nurse-patient interaction toward the highest quality of a patient's health potential. The nursing act (domain) is classified as enhancement.

HEALTH: A wellness-illness process on a continuum monitored by a person's view of self and formulated in communication with others. There are three influencing concepts: communication, self, and role.

The definitions are naturally congruent with symbolic interaction theory and the assumptions stated earlier. In the definition of *environment*, there is reference to factors and parameters that are the variables addressed in the assessment tool. Examples of this tool are given in the following chapters. The definition of *nursing* includes a comment about the nursing domain. This is one of the structural schemes referred to earlier and will be discussed momentarily. The definition of *health* contains three terms: communication, self, and role. These are key concepts in symbolic interaction and in the RIM. Communica-

TABLE 34-1. ASSUMPTIONS USED IN THE RIEHL INTERACTION MODEL

Analytic Assumptions:

1. Humans live in a symbolic environment as well as a physical environment and can be stimulated to act by symbols as well as by physical stimuli

2. Through symbols, people have the capacity to stimulate others in ways other than those in which they are themselves stimulated

3. Through communication of symbols, people can learn huge numbers of meanings and values—and hence ways of acting—from other people

4. The symbols—and the meanings and values to which they refer—do not occur in isolated bits, but often in clusters, sometimes large and complex

5. Thinking is the process by which possible symbolic solutions and other future courses of action are examined, assessed for their relative advantages and disadvantages in terms of the values of the individual, and one of them chosen for action

Genetic Assumptions:

1. Society—a network of interacting individuals—with its cultures—the related meanings and values by means of which individuals interact—precedes any existing individual

2. The process by which socialization takes place can be thought of as occurring in three stages . . . in the development of the infant

3. Socialization is not only into the general culture but also into various subcultures

4. Although old groups, cultural expectations, and personal meanings and values may be dropped, in the sense that they become markedly lower on the reference relationship scale, they are not lost or forgotten

tion is the ability to convey verbal and nonverbal meaning to the self and others. It is essential in the health field where, for example, doctor-nurse synergy impacts on the patient's progress (Pennsylvania Nurse, 1987). The self and role concepts warrant further commentary to illustrate their significance.

Self-concept is a mirrored image of the self conveyed by others, which results in a negative to positive self-concept that can lead from an external to an internal locus of control and from being dependent to being independent. In the RIM, the symbolic interaction position is taken—that is, the definition of the self is from the social-psychological versus the psychological-phenomenological perspective. In self-growth, self-behavior is thinking behavior, not habitual. A person therefore acts rather than reacts. The self-concept is the key between action and the social group the individual is in—that is, what one does in any interaction is based upon the self-concept in that situation. In acting, a person interprets or defines actions of others rather than just reacting to them. A response is based on the meaning an action has and the response is the result of an interpretation process. The interpretive thinking process includes analysis of a situation, the self-concept in a situation, decision making, and responsive behavior.

Role is an assigned or assumed part taken by an individual that displays socially acceptable behavior, which is determined by status in a society. For every role there is an opposite role—that is, one does not exist without the other.

Examples are parent-child, teacher-learner, nurse-patient, decision maker-decision taker, and coper-copee. The latter refers to a strong to weak ability to cope with stress; the coper focuses away from the cause of stress to strengthen the coping resources in the copee. Roles assumed vary from one to many. In illness, roles assumed decrease in quantity and quality. The goal is to return the person to previous roles assumed when possible. In SI, social action is studied in terms of how it is formed—that is, it is necessary to trace the way an action is actually developed. To do this, one must see the situation as it is seen by the actor. This means that role-taking, or taking the role of the other, is involved. This may be an overt or covert action. Studying action in terms of how it is formed is a different approach to that taken by some social scientists and psychologists. They focus on the formation of social action as the product or the antecedent factors to explain the causes of behavior.

There is a relationship between the three concepts of communication, self, and role. When fewer roles are assumed, in general, there is a lowered self-concept and a decrease in communication. Table 34–2 elaborates on the component parts of the three key concepts and illustrates their relationship. Although the concepts appear uni-dimensional in Table 34–2, in reality they are multi-dimensional and fluid or dynamic. For example, the appropriate role emerges or dominates as the need arises. The communication steps accelerate or vary depending on the situation or problem complexity, with some steps being omitted if not appropriate. Comminication determines the self-concept, which in turn guides the role assumed in every encounter.

Inherent in each role are several steps. In decision making, some of the steps in the bioethical process as described by Thompson and Thompson (1985) are appropriate. These steps include review of the situation; gathering needed additional information; identifying values of the nurse, patient, and family; determining value conflicts; diagnosing pertinent problems; recognizing the need for change; identifying the possible actions, anticipated outcomes, and who should determine the problem-resolution approach; deciding on a course of action; implementing it; and evaluating the results. It is obvious that this is similar to problem solving, which is the initial approach used in the RIM. The decision making steps are more explicit but are appropriate because they exemplify the potentially important differences in persons (patient, family, and nurse) whose values and problem solving may vary. These differences must be identified and resolved in order to proceed effectively. When they are not resolved, evaluation results are often poor. For good results in symbolic interaction, the nurse must "get inside the skin" of the other to understand that position and how the other sees the world.

Decision making was selected advisedly as an example. The decision making process falls within the purview of professional nursing and is a concern and interest of those who promote nursing's professional autonomy. In a recent study conducted on the clinical decision making of staff nurses, Prescott, Dennis, and Jacox (1987) discussed staff nurse satisfaction with the decision-making process of nurses employed in different hospital units. Those in intensive care were more satisfied with their decision-making involvement than

TABLE 34–2. THE NURSE-PATIENT-FAMILY RECIPROCAL RELATIONSHIP

Emerging Roles		Communication Stages/
Patient/Family	*Nurse*	Level of Interaction
1. Aware health problem exists; Problem resolution seeker	1. Problem solver	1. Individual/family tries to solve health problem by self and with input from others
2. Care receiver	2. Care provider	2. Nurse encounters problem when patient and family seek professional help
3. Learner	3. Teacher	3. Situation assessed, problem identified and diagnosed, care plan developed and implemented, care evaluated for acceptance or rejection of problem resolution. If rejected, reassess, etc. Use FANCAP
4. Copee	4. Coper	4. Low or negative self-concept. External locus of control range (may be temporary)
5. Decision taker	5. Decision maker	5. Change in self-concept from negative to positive (lower to higher)—e.g., closed family to open family relationships
6. Change agent novice	6. Change agent	6. Change in roles from few to more assumed
7. Seekers of guidance to maintain health	7. Consultant to patient & family	7. Change in roles to match change in self-concept
8. Observers to doers	8. Role model for patient & family	8. Change in external to internal locus of control
9. Support advocacy, friend/ acquaintance	9. Patient & family advocate, professional friend	9. Continue to set short- and long-range goals and accomplish them

The number assignments are somewhat arbitrary. The primary goal throughout is an improved level of health. This is achieved by means of communication, which is inherent in this model.

were nurses in the medical-surgical units. An interesting point made in the study was that "physicians generally resisted the decision making discretion of nurses (p. 56)." Trust, control, knowledge, skill, and authority needed for decision making in patient care were also discussed. Physician-nurse synergy was not addressed, but in the study reported in the Pennsylvania Nurse (1987) study the synergistic variable was the only component that explained the differences in patient deaths in intensive care units. Good doctor-nurse interaction, coordination, and communication—the human element—resulted in a lowered patient death rate. This study indicates that it behooves these two professional groups to resolve any differences they may have and pool their resources for the good of their patients.

Process

Process refers to the acts or behaviors of the agent (patient, family, or nurse) and the method utilized in a given theory. Stevens (1984) makes the point that the problem-solving approach and the nursing process approach are the two methods most commonly employed in nursing today. However, there are some structural differences between the two, which she identifies and discusses. She notes, among other things, that the nursing process is a logistic method. In the RIM, the process utilized is that of problem solving, a form of the problematic method.

Context

Context represents the background or environment in a model. For the RIM, a comprehensive view of health is taken. Smith (1981) has identified four models of health from the narrowest to the broadest view: the clinical, role-performance, adaptive, and eudaimonistic models. The latter, the most comprehensive, is well illustrated by the comment "health transcends biological fitness. It is primarily a measure of each person's ability to do what he wants to do and become what he wants to become (Pepper, quoting Dubos, 1986, p. 15)." Although role is an important concept in the RIM, it is subsumed under health. From Smith's perspective, the RIM is classified as a eudaimonistic model of health. Viewed from another perspective, context encompasses the nursing domain.

Nursing Domain

This classification represents the second structural scheme identified by Stevens (1984). It addresses agency or the state or action of the patient, family, and the nurse. Stevens identifies patient-nurse relationships. These are enumerated and briefly defined below. In addition, some suggestions of nurse theorists in each domain are provided.

1. Intervention, in which action and decision rest with the nurse. Nursing model examples are found in Johnson (1980) and in Chapter 9 of this text.
2. Conservation, in which preservation of beneficial aspects of a patient's situation occurs. Chapter 28 of the present text provides a nursing model example.
3. Substitution, in which the nurse does for patients that which the patients cannot do for themselves. A nursing model example is found in Orem (1971).
4. Sustenance, in which the focus is on support-building and coping mechanisms, and the goal is to assist the patient in coping with stressful situations. Rubin (1968) offers a nursing model example.
5. Enhancement, in which nursing is a means of improving the quality of a patient's life. The primary aim is to make a change for the better, which

is internal to the person, under the person's control. A nursing model example is given in Chapter 16.

The definition of nursing given earlier reveals that the RIM focuses on actional principles. As in Hall's (1966) model, these principles are a part of the agent and a patient's self-mastery is expected. Actional principles are characterized by human drives, motives, needs, and will power. On the other hand, in models where homeostatsis, equilibrium, or exchange are evident, reflexive principles apply (Stevens, 1984).

With self-mastery and actional principles in mind, an examination of Stevens' classifications given earlier indicate that the RIM is readily placed in category five, enhancement. However, the lines become a bit blurred at times and other approaches appear to be in evidence, such as sustenance, as when an interim involves assisting a patient to cope in stressful situations. It should be remembered, however, that as the stress subsides, the goal of ultimately improving the quality of life again predominates the approach.

Principles, Interpretation, and Method

Principles, interpretation, and method represent the first set of two analytical descriptors of models. Principles may be equated with the assumptions in a model. Interpretation refers to the philosophical perspective of the theorist. Method reveals the way theorists reason. Identifiable thought patterns emerge from their assumptions to application of their frameworks (Stevens, 1984).

Principles
There are two sets of assumptions, or principles, that are an inherent part of symbolic interaction and are, therefore, an inherent part of the RIM. When only one set of assumptions is considered by others in the application of this theory, a part of the foundation on which this model is built is violated. It is possible to focus on one set in a research project, for example; but one must nevertheless be cognizant of all of the assumptions. For this reason, the analytic and genetic assumptions were restated in Table 34–1.

Figure 34–1 illustrates how the nurse-patient-family interaction functions. The assumptions in this model indicate that every person is a member of a family or group, and therefore no one is viewed in isolation. As emphasized in Figure 34–1, the patient and the patient's family are considered a unit. The interaction between the nurse, patient, and family, which is often used in resolving problems, is role-taking. Roles are taken by the patient, members of the family, and by the nurse to achieve a goal. The ultimate goal is an improved state of health. As indicated in Figure 34–1, a part of the definition of self is evident: one moves from being dependent to being independent as the self-concept becomes more positive and an internal locus of control emerges.

Interpretation
Interpretation may be viewed as the philosophical perspective of the theorist. There are two main types of philosophy addressed: (1) phenomenal, which is

392

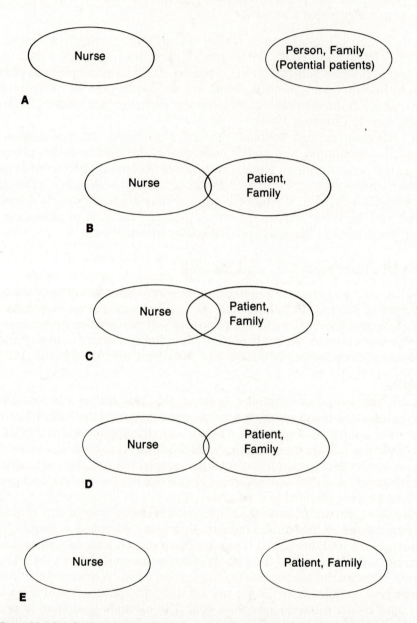

Figure 34–1A to E. Nurse-patient-family interaction relationship. **A.** Initial contact: Patient, family, and nurse have independent roles. **B.** Assessment and beginning involvement as person, family assumes patient(s) role in interacting with the nurse. **C.** Almost total interaction and dependency role assumed by patient, family in nurse-patient-family relationship. **D.** Patient, family again assuming independent role in nurse-patient-family interaction on way to discharge and recovery. **E.** Patient, family is once again independent from the nurse, and the nurse is independent from the patient, family.

within human experience and (2) transcendental, which is beyond human experience (Stevens, 1984).

In the phenomenal philosophy, the theory is classified as either existential or essential. In existentialism, the subject matter is considered to be in the human agents acts. In the essential position, nursing is explained by reference to the situation in which it occurs. Examples are changes in body temperature due to internal and external factors, and locus of control that can also be attributed to internal and external components.

In transcendental philosophy, there are also two classifications: ontic and entitative. In the ontic interpretation, nursing reality is larger than life—behavior is described in terms of life phases. In the entitative interpretation, reduction occurs. It consists of many units in which behavior is described by multicomponents. Nursing models that fit this category are usually complex and detailed in description.

Method

According to Stevens (1984), based on work by McKeon, there are four main methods of thought that can be used to categorize nursing models. These methods are the dialectic, logistic, problematic, and operational. In the dialectic method, the whole is greater than the sum of its parts. Using this method, the study of life phases is selected to blend and synthesize knowledge in theory and practice into a unifying whole. In a curriculum, the subject matter may be taught on a continuum of wellness to illness or birth to death. The aim is to teach the student nurse to interact effectively with the total patient and family.

In the logistic method, the parts organize the whole. This is the opposite of the dialectic method. Both differ from the problematic and operational methods, in that the structure of the former two are independent of the agent whereas in the latter two the agent is a part of the method. In the problematic method, problems are solved through interaction of the problem solver with concerned others in the environment. Solutions to one set of problems may well be applied to other similar situations. In this way, working toward a whole may emerge. The problematic and operational methods differ in that with the problematic approach, interaction occurs between the agent and the environmental situation, whereas in the operational method the agent determines how a process will proceed based on an either-or perspective.

Summary

The underlying philosophical perspective in the RIM is more transcendental than phenomenal. The rationale for this is that human behavior is described by life phases, which are influenced by the culture and environment. The essential versus the existential component of the phenomenal philosophy is evident, however, in that the concept of internal-external locus of control is a factor in the RIM's decision-making process. The ontic versus the entitative component of the transcendental philosophy predominates because behavior is described in life phases as is evident in the stated assumptions. In utilizing the life phase and wellness-illness continuum, by definition the dialectic method is applicable. In this method, the art or practice of logically examining opinions or ideas is based on principles. In questioning an idea or event, the opposite view emerges, which results in a reconciliation of differences. This underlies the principle of taking the role of the other expressed in symbolic interaction. In the Riehl Interaction Model, the dialectic method encompasses the problem-solving approach, which is the initial point of departure in nurse-patient-family interactions.

Application of Theory into Practice

There are three stages in the problem-solving process (Stevens, 1984). The process is initiated when a problem is encountered. Secondly, there is as much discussion as necessary among the patient, family, and nurse to identify the problem and possible solutions. Finally, and most importantly, the correct diagnosis of the problem must be determined. This is more vital than the solution, because diverse paths may be taken to attain the goal. Utilizing familiar words to apply this knowledge would result in the following. Assessment would begin when an obstacle arises among the patient, family, and nurse. Identifying the problem is an informal process. Deciding on what the problem is naturally results in the label of diagnosis. A plan for the solution also fits into this group. Implementation and evaluation follow until another obstacle is encountered. A tool is utilized to guide the nurse through the assessment process. This, plus a problem diagnosis, a plan for a solution to the problem, implementation, and evaluation, are addressed in more detail in the following sections.

Assessment Tool

The tool used to assess the patient and family captures the essence of the principles, interpretation, and method. The RIM assessment tool is composed of factors and parameters that form a matrix (*see* Table 34–3). The factors consist of the mnemonic FANCAP, which stands for fluids, aeration, nutrition, com-

TABLE 34–3. THE ASSESSMENT MATRIX IN THE RIEHL INTERACTION MODEL

Factors	Parameters				
	Physiological	*Psychological*	*Sociological*	*Cultural*	*Environmental*
Fluids					
Aeration					
Nutrition					
Communication					
Activity					
Pain					

munication, activity, and pain. The parameters are the physiological, psychological, sociocultural, and environmental items that are addressed. For further elaboration and discussion, see Abbey (1980), Riehl (1980), and subsequent chapters in this text that illustrate the use of the tool in clinical and research situations.

One example that may be given here, however, refers to the pain factor. Melzack and Wall's 1965 gate-control theory of pain can be utilized when a patient is experiencing this physiologically based phenomenon. Their concept of pain involves "the interaction of many different neural systems—not only the parts of the brain involved in pain's sensory component but also the parts involved in attention, memories, emotions and even ideas indoctrinated by cultural training (Warga, 1987, p. 55)."

Nursing Diagnosis, Plan, and Care

Nursing diagnoses readily emerge when an anlaysis of the data from the assessment tool is completed. These are prioritized and a plan of care is made. At this point, all of the available knowledge in the participants' repertoire is brought to bear for a solution to the problem(s). In the RIM, knowledge is classified by the matrix mix—that is, from the cross tabulation of the factors with the parameters. For example, knowledge is needed regarding the physiology of fluids as in electrolyte imbalance. In the psychological category, information about alcoholic fluid intake may be required. For further illustration, see Chapter 37. The diagnosis and plan of care are the most important elements in this problematic process. When the care is implemented according to a knowledgeable plan, the evaluation of results should prove to be successful. Guidelines for the plan of care are presented later in the chapter.

Internal and External Analysis

Stevens' (1984) internal and external criteria for evaluating nursing models represent the second and final set of analytic descriptors discussed. Her internal evaluation terms are clarity, adequacy, logical development, level of theory development, and consistency. These terms are briefly defined as follows. *Clarity* indicates that the theory is understood. *Adequacy* is deemed to be present if the theory accounts for all the aspects of the subject matter that the model introduces. *Logical development* illustrates that a systematic design is evident—that is, do the conclusions follow the premises? *Theory development* determines if the model is at the descriptive or explanatory level. And *consistency* addresses a myriad of facets seeking an appropriate level of symbiosis between and among terms, definitions, approaches, principles, interpretations, and methodologies. The presence of consistency certifies that these terms are used the same way throughout the presentation and discussion of the model. Its importance suggests that this criterion especially be identified in an analysis of all the nursing frameworks.

In the RIM, effort has been made to convey meaning in terms and definitions in a way that is clearly understood. The RIM is broad in scope due to the fluidity of the changing interaction process, and it remains adequate as long as it has applicability to all clinical nursing situations. The model has been logically developed from symbolic interaction theory. The philosophy, assumptions, and all other essential entities flow from this theory. The RIM is in the second or explanatory level of development, in that in addition to providing a description of the model, research suggestions and implementation in various clinical settings are available, as in the following chapters. To assure that the consistency criterion is met throughout the model, the assumptions and common terms are reviewed before any additions or changes are created.

Stevens' (1984) external evaluation terms are: reality convergence, utility, significance, scope, complexity, and capacity for discrimination. *Reality convergence* refers to principles, interpretation, and method and the question is asked: Are all three of these components apparent in the real world? Because these three topics have been discussed and will be illustrated from the external perspective in the subsequent chapters, no further comment is included here. The *utility* criterion seeks to determine if the theoretical model can be operationalized in the practice setting. The model is *significant* if it contributes to nursing knowledge through research. *Scope* addresses the broadness of the range of concepts, and *complexity* ranks the model on a bipolar scale ranging from parsimonious to complex. Of these criteria, utility and significance, as applied to RIM, are demonstrated in the chapters that follow. Brief but pertinent comments on the scope, complexity, and capacity for discrimination criteria are included below.

Scope

The scope of this model midline between limited and broad. Jacox (1974) has recommended that nursing utilize middle-range theories that focus on limited scope such as pain alleviation, teaching health measures, or socialization of patients into the health care delivery system. These are utilized in this model. On the otherhand, Ellis, (1968) has suggested that nursing remain broad in scope and focus on explaining the relationship between biological and behavioral observations. As the parameters in the assessment tool of this model indicate, data are collected in both the biological and behavioral areas. As a result, the potential for examining relationships between these two exists, although the research done to date addresses behavioral observation, which tends to weight the model slightly toward the limited side in scope. This rank is appropriate because this model is in the middle-range theory area at this time.

Complexity

In addressing complexity versus parsimony, the concepts in the RIM are sufficiently complex to provide for subcomponents without changing the basic outline of the model, which is essential. However, an effort has been made to keep the concepts parsimonious for purposes of describing and explaining the theory components. According to Stevens (1984), "parsimony has the advantage of clearly separating figure and background, of setting the critical elements of nursing in relief so that they are more easily perceived and understood (p. 71)." This statement leads to the final and perhaps the most important of the external evaluation criteria.

Capacity for Discrimination

The particulars discussed here were selected because of their application to the RIM. In the capacity for discrimination, one must determine if the proposed theory differentiates nursing from other health professions and from other care-tending acts. A discriminating theory explains role differences and sets boundaries for nursing practice. For example, when nurses are compared to physicians, the term *care* is applied to the former and cure of pathological conditions is assigned to the latter. By keeping this in mind, nurses can clearly differentiate the nursing role from the physician's role.

A second point of departure that is evident in the RIM is that the nurse-patient-family relationship is reciprocal. This infers that all parties share in and contribute to the relationship and the decision-making process. A third point is that there are short-, medium-, and long-range goals established together. These goals enable nurses to work with patients and families in acute and long-term care situations. Acute care may be provided in a hospital or in the community—when patients are assisted in a crisis situation, for example. Long-term care commonly falls into the purview of community nursing. Communication between nurses in acute care and community settings becomes increasingly important for continuity of care. This communication task is difficult but essential if nurses are to accomplish the goals set with patients for follow-up care.

Although there are three categories of care goals, the nurse-patient-family situation always remains fluid and ever-changing in the interaction process. This indicates that the nurse must be alert for potential problems and reorder current ones on a continuing basis as needed. With a focus on care and prevention of health problems, establishing acute community care teams would improve the nursing care provided. With this goal in mind, nurses can focus on salutogenesis rather than pathogenesis. The opportunity for new insights into health care will thus be enhanced. Remembering that not all stress is harmful, nurse educators and practitioners may be well advised to shift away from the causes of stress and concentrate on strengthening the coping mechanisms already developed in the patient and family. When new ones are needed, they can be learned. In general, this positive approach may very well accelerate the nursing discrimination process. Although what is suggested is not necessarily new, without continuous management and evidence of caring such problems as lack of compliance persist.

A final item that discriminates nursing practice is the development of a nursing taxonomy. Like nursing models, these too are being critiqued. In a discussion on this topic, Rasch (1987) reviewed the differences between natural versus artificial, hierarchic versus nonhierarchic, and deductive versus inductive criteria. Natural characteristics are fundamental while artifical are arbitrary. In a hierarchic taxonomy, the characteristics of the group are increasingly more inclusive and general, such as occurs in classifying plants and animals. In non-hierarchic taxonomies, sets of external attributes apply, such as placing nursing diagnoses in alphabetical order. The latter and a deductive method was utilized at the First National Conference on Classifying Nursing Diagnoses (Gebbie & Lavin, 1975). On the other hand, when natural criteria are used essential characteristics of entities and inductive approaches apply. An advantage of the latter is that additional types may be added to existing groups and new groups may be formulated. In this way, the taxonomy continues to develop and change and the goal of the taxonomy—which is improved communication—can continue to be clarified. In a critique of the North American Nursing Diagnosis Association (NANDA) taxonomy, Rasch (1987) states that it "is not a taxonomy of nursing diagnoses. It is a taxonomy of Human Response Patterns that was deductively created (p. 148)." Porter (1986) indicates that "what nurses diagnose is specific human-environment interactions (p. 138)." This position may not apply in all nursing situations but it is certainly worthy of consideration. The critiques by Rasch and Porter alert us to premature closure on the matter of taxonomies. Sometimes, in an eagerness to crystalize our nursing science, we may mistakenly rush to this end.

With the above comments and critiques in mind, a taxonomy for the RIM was initiated. An attempt has been made to keep it natural, hierarchic, and inductive, as defined by Rasch. The results of this taxonomy are shown in Table 34–4. The categories listed roughly correspond to the roles and communication stages given in Table 34–2. An example of the statement that additional types may be added to existing groups is supplied by Bruner, Olver, and Greenfield (1966) in their book entitled *Studies in Cognitive Growth*. In it, they discuss a multistage theory of cognitive growth in children. According to this theory, a child successively employs three models: (1) the enactive (thinking through action, such as riding a bicycle); (2) the iconic (thinking through images); and (3) the symbolic (thinking through language). This may be considered as an expansion of item seven in Table 34–4, which addresses age and development of family members. This example is important in that it reinforces the genetic assumptions and serves as a reminder that youngsters as well as adults are considered in the taxonomic structure of the RIM.

Although at the first reading of Table 34–4 it may appear as though some interactions are nurse determined, it must be remembered that the decisions made at each phase are shared by the patient, family, and nurse. For example, when the nurse assumes the teacher role, it is with the consent or request of the other.

A final comment about Table 34–4 is in regard to the classification of knowledge referred to in the section on plan and implementation of care. At the outset, it should be remembered that there is overlap in utilization of information, but for purposes of discussion content is placed into "little boxes" according to the

TABLE 34-4. PROPOSED TAXONOMIES/MANAGEMENT STRATEGIES FOR USE IN PLANNING NURSING INTERVENTIONS IN THE RIEHL INTERACTION MODEL

1. Listen to the patient, family, accept, believe, and trust them. Use communication theory throughout

2. Support problem identification and plan for resolution. Promote early problem or potential problem awareness in the patient, family and willingness to seek help for preventive health deviation problems

3. Support acceptance of care from others when indicated to accelerate problem resolution and to conserve energy in illness. Perform skilled nursing care as indicated

4. Identify coping mechanisms in the assessment. The planned strategy for intervention is to strengthen the past or present coping mechanisms already established in the patient, family repertoire. If new ones must be learned, these are taught and utilized in current and future situations. Crisis theory may be used

5. Encourage decision-making ability in the patient, family. Employ a decision-making process

6. Support change in self-concept from negative to positive. The theory of change is used. Once the change occurs it is practiced until it is a well-established part of the patient, family repertoire

7. Consider increasing or varying the roles assumed to ensure the quality and quantity of life of the patient, family. The quality or quantity of life is one variable in the life style, health practices, age, etc, of the patient, family

8. Match the roles and self-concept of the patient, family to reinforce self-confidence

9. Promote external to internal locus of control by encouraging choice determination in the patient, family

10. Encourage compliance to the treatment plan by education and involvement of the patient, family in the plan of care

11. Discuss and consider alternatives to the plan of care offered by the patient, family or nurse

12. Patient, family and nurse should prioritize and implement each plan of care as it is formulated

13. Patient, family and nurse should evaluate the implemented plan. If not successful, reinitiate the process

14. Listen to the patient, family, accept, believe, and trust them to know what is best for them after all recent knowledge and alternatives have been discussed. It is their choice. It is their life

Several theories have been identified. Others may apply. These may serve as guidelines in working with patients and families. When the persons involved—the patient, family, and nurse—are mentioned in the above statements it is done as a reminder and does not mean that some or all of these persons are excluded from the other categories.

parameters in the assessment tool. The result is that item 3 (skilled nursing care) is placed in the physiological group. From the communication theory perspective, item 3 and items 1 (listening to the patient and family), 2 (support patient and family identification of problem and plan), and 14 (listen to and accept their decisions) are placed in the sociological group. Item 4 (identify and support coping mechanisms) is in the psychological category. Items 5 (encourage decision making), 9 (promote an internal locus of control), 10 (encourage compliance), 11 (consider alternatives), 12 (prioritize), and 13 (evaluate) involve decision making that is influenced by the sociocultural component. Finally, item 6 (encompassing self-concept and change theories) and items 7 and 8 (addressing role theory) are placed in the sociocultural-

environmental group. Hopefully, the rationale for these placements is sufficiently obvious to negate further discussion.

PART THREE: NURSING THEORY AND RESEARCH

Walker and Avant (1983) have identified four levels of theory in nursing.
These are:

1. Meta theory—a theory about theories.
2. Grand theory—conceptualizes general prescriptions for nursing practice.
3. Middle-range theory—an intermediate theory comprising a conceptual
   scheme derived from a large cluster of empirically observed social
   behavior (Merton, 1957).
4. Practice theory—the process of developing and testing hypotheses in nursing practice settings, called the clinical experimental
   method (Wooldridge, Leonard, & Skipper, 1978). As hypotheses cluster, they may become middle-range theory (Bullough & Bullough,
   1984).

The Riehl Interaction Model can be considered as a combination of a grand
theory and a middle-range theory. This statement supports the comments made
earlier by Jacox (1974) and Ellis (1968) in the section on external analysis.
Grand theory applies as concepts are utilized to prescribe general nursing actions. Middle-range theory is dominant, however, in that clusters of empirically
observed social behavior comprise the conceptual schema housed in symbolic
interaction. This middle-range theory classification is the result of the hypotheses being developed and tested in nursing practice settings. With a symbolic
interaction foundation guiding the research, and new knowledge being utilized
as it fits the framework of the RIM, a variety of nursing research projects have
been completed and others are in progress.

Another view for research in this model is evident in a perusal of the science-
into-art elements. However, prior to application, research needs to be done in
the known knowldege areas for validity and reliability of the diagnoses and
plans of care. After the nursing assessment is done, an eclectic array of knowledge is utilized in the diagnosis and planning process. One example of current
research applicable to item 8 (locus of control) in Table 34–2 is the hardiness
personality studies. Fischman (1987) summarized the research by Maddi of the
University of Chicago and Kobasa of the City University of New York in an article entitled "Getting Tough: A personality that Resists Sickness." Another example of hardiness research was reported by Rich and Rich (1987). Their article
was entitled "Personality Hardiness and Burnout in Female Staff Nurses." And
finally, Lambert and Lambert (1987) wrote a paper entitled "Hardiness: Its
Development and Relevance to Nursing."

It is suggested that all the items in Tables 34-2 and 34-4 are on the artist's palette and have research potential in the Riehl Interaction Model. Selecting choices from this palette immediately infers that research may be practice or theory based, inductive (from observations in practice) or deductive (from rational or ethical principles), originating from "what is" (what nurses do) or "what ought to be" (what nurses do right), or any combination of these (Stevens, 1984).

Most theories originate in the classroom and from "what ought to be." With a commitment from nurse administrators, the nursing profession may well advance more rapidly and judiciously from "what is," with nursing care, education, administration, and research proceeding from observations of our extant practice. Informed changes would be directed from that point of departure. A step in the direction of theory based-practice is demonstrated in the clinical research reported in the chapters that follow.

REFERENCES

Abbey, J. (1980). FANCAP: What is it? In J. P. Riehl & C. Roy (Eds.), *Conceptual models for nursing practice* (2nd ed.). New York: Appleton-Century-Crofts.

Bruner, J. S., Olver, R. R., & Greenfield, P. M. (1966). *Studies in cognitive growth.* New York: Wiley.

Blumer, H. (1969). *Symbolic interactionism: Perspective and method.* Englewood Cliffs, NJ: Prentice-Hall.

Bullough, V. L., & Bullough, B. (1984). *History, trends, and politics of nursing.* East Norwalk, CT: Appleton-Century-Crofts.

Coutu, W. (1951). Role-playing versus role-taking. An appeal for clarification. *American Sociological Review, 16,* 180-187.

Crane, J. (1985a). Using research in practice: Research utilization-nursing models. *Western Journal of Nursing Research, 7*(4), 494-497.

Crane, J. (1985b). Using research in practice: Research utilization: Theoretical perspectives. *Western Journal of Nursing Research, 7*(2), 261-268.

Ellis, R. (1968). Characteristics of significant theories. *Nursing Research, 17*(3), 221.

Fawcett, J., & Downs, F. S. (1986). *The relationship of theory and research.* East Norwalk, CT: Appleton-Century-Crofts.

Fischman, J. (1987, December). Getting tough: A personality that resists sickness. *Psychology Today,* 26-28.

Gebbie, K. M., & Lavin, M. A. (1975). *Classification of nursing diagnosis: Proceedings of the first national conference.* St. Louis: Mosby.

Hall, L. E. (1966). Another view of nursing care and quality. In K. M. Straub & K. S. Parker (Eds.), *Continuity of patient care: The role of nursing* (pp. 47-66). Washington, DC: Catholic University Press.

Havelock, R. G. (1969). *Planning for innovation through dissemination and utilization of knowledge.* Ann Arbor, MI: Center for Research on Utilization of Scientific Knowledge, Institute for Social Research, University of Michigan.

Havelock, R. G., & Havelock, M. (1973). *Training for change agents.* Ann Arbor, MI: Center for Research on Utilization of Scientific Knowledge, Institute for Social Research, University of Michigan.

Jacobson, S. F. (1987). Studying and using conceptual models of nursing. *Image, 19*(2), 78–82.

Jacox, A. (1974). Theory construction in nursing: An overview. *Nursing Research, 23* (1), 12.

Johnson, D. (1980). The behavioral system model for nursing. In J. P. Riehl & C. Roy (Eds.), *Conceptual models for nursing practice*, (2nd ed.). New York: Appleton-Century-Crofts.

Lambert, C. E., & Lambert, V. A. (1987). Hardiness: Its development and relevance to nursing. *Image, 19*(2), 92–95.

Manis, J. G., & Meltzer, B. N. (1967). *Symbolic interaction.* Boston: Allyn & Bacon.

Mead, G. H. (1934). *Mind, self & society.* Chicago: University of Chicago Press.

Meleis, A. I. (1985). *Theoretical nursing: Development & progress.* Philadelphia: Lippincott.

Merton, R. K. (1957). *Social theory and social structure.* Glencoe, IL: Free Press.

Orem, D. E. (1971). *Nursing: Concepts of practice.* New York: McGraw-Hill.

Pennsylvania Nurse. (1987, October). Doctor/nurse synergy reduces hospital patient deaths, *42*(10), 12. Harrisburg, PA: Pennsylvania Nurses Association.

Pepper, J. M. (1986). The essential ingredient in curriculum design: The organizing framework. In E. A. Pennington (Ed.), *Curriculum revisited: An update of curriculum design.* New York: National League for Nursing.

Porter, E. J. (1986). Critical analysis of NANDA nursing diagnosis taxonomy I. *Image, 18* (4), 136–139.

Prescott, P. A., Dennis, K. E., & Jacox, A. K. (1987). Clinical decision making of staff nurses. *Image, 19*(2), 56–62.

Rasch, R. F. (1987). The nature of taxonomy. *Image 19*(3), 147–149.

Rich, V. L., & Rich, A. R. (1987). Personality hardiness and burnout in female staff nurses. *Image, 19*(2), 63–66.

Riehl, J. P. (1980). The Riehl Interaction Interaction Model. In J. P. Riehl & C. Roy (Eds.), *Conceptual models for nursing practice* (2nd ed.). New York: Appleton-Century-Crofts.

Rose, A. M. (1962). *Human behavior and social processes.* Boston: Houghton Mifflin.

Rose, A. M. (1980). A systematic summary of symbolic interaction theory. In J. P. Riehl & C. Roy (Eds.), *Conceptual models for nursing practice* (2nd ed.). New York: Appleton-Century-Crofts.

Rubin, R. (1968). A theory of clinical nursing. *Nursing Research, 17*(3), 210–212.

Smith, J. A. (1981, April). The idea of health: A philosophical inquiry. *Advances in Nursing Science, 3,* 43–50.

Stevens, B. J. (1984). *Nursing theory: Analysis, application, evaluation* (2nd ed.). Boston: Little, Brown.

Thompson, J. E., & Thompson, H. O. (1985). *Bioethical decision making for nurses.* East Norwalk, CT: Appleton-Century-Crofts.

Walker, L. O., & Avant, K. C. (1983). *Strategies for theory construction in nursing.* East Norwalk, CT: Appleton-Century-Crofts.

Warga, C. (1987, August). Pain gatekeeper. *Psychology Today,* 50–56.

Wells, L. E., & Marwell, G. (1976). *Self-esteem.* Beverly Hills: Sage.

Wooldridge, P. J., Leonard, R. C., & Skipper, J. K. (1978). *Methods of clinical experimentation to improve patient care.* St. Louis: Mosby.

Working with the Riehl Model of Nursing[1]

Peter Aggleton
Helen Chalmers

Models of nursing differ from one another in terms of the emphasis that they give to systems within the person, processes of development, and the human ability to communicate and interact. A number of nurse theorists therefore differentiate in their work between systems, developmental, and interactionist nursing models (Aggleton & Chalmers, 1986; Fawcett, 1984; Thibodeau, 1983). In reaching decisions about which model of nursing to work with in particular care setting, nurses should be guided not by past precedent or intuition but by whichever of these emphases they feel is most appropriate in meeting the needs of their patients.

Recent developments in nursing practice in both Britain and America (Ceccio & Ceccio, 1982; Faulkner, 1984; Smith & Bass, 1982) have highlighted the role that good interpersonal relations and effective communication between patient and nurse can play in facilitating recovery from ill health. Increasingly, it is also being recognized that patients' perceptions of themselves, those around them, and the situations they are in, are significant factors in influencing recovery from illness and adjustment to new health-related demands (Bergsma & Thomasma, 1984). Such insights call for the critical evaluation of nursing models that take seriously these aspects of human functioning. In this article, therefore, we hope to contribute to such a process by examining in detail one of the better known interactionist models of nursing—that was developed by Riehl (1980)—in order to explore its usefulness in offering guidelines for planning and delivering high-quality nursing care.

Key Concepts Within Interactionist Theory

According to those who have developed and worked with interactionist models of nursing, people behave as they do not because of the operation of systems within them (be these biological, psychological, or social), but because it is *meaningful* for them to do so. According to interactionist social scientists such as Mead (1934), an important human quality is the capacity to understand the world in terms of *symbols*—words, images, and actions that stand for something else. Humans communicate with one another using symbols and they come to understand themselves and other people through the symbols that they give off.

Because symbols such as words, signs and actions do not have any intrinsic meaning, they must be *interpreted* by those who encounter them. The meanings associated with, for example, particular words, facial expressions, and gestures are not fixed but vary widely across cultures and throughout history. How a particular symbol is interpreted, therefore, depends on whether or not it is familiar and what the past experience of similar symbols has been (Blumer, 1969). Within health-care settings, there is ample opportunity for people to encounter symbols that are unfamiliar to them. The signs and notices identifying wards, specialized care areas, and clinical departments in a general hospital often appear bewildering even to those who work within them. Imagine, therefore, how they can appear to patients and visitors. If qualified nurses working in routine ward environments sometimes find the technical equipment of the intensive care unit unfamiliar and frightening, how might this same area appear to others?

When confronted with unfamiliar symbols, people try to make sense of them as best they can by drawing on their past experience. Hence, patients and nurses unfamiliar with high-technology care environments may liken these to the sets we see in science fiction films. Similarly, regimented and restricted care regimens may be perceived as "prison-like" by those nursed within them.

According to another early interactionist social scientist, Cooley (1909), people actively build up understandings of themselves by imagining how others might see and judge them. We therefore develop *looking-glass* selves built up out of the various reflections we see in other people's reactions towards us. Within health-care settings, the behavior of nurses and other health care workers towards patients can therefore have important consequences for the type of self-image the latter develop.

Our anticipation of how others see us contributes at least in part to how situations come to be *defined*. If we believe that others are behaving negatively towards us, we may adopt quite different forms of behavior (perhaps hostility, aggression, or withdrawal) from those that might otherwise be exhibited. If we believe that others think we will not recover from a particular illness or medical procedure, then it is all the more likely that with time we too will subscribe to that particular interpretation of events. According to Thomas (1923), situations defined as real therefore become real in their consequences.

By putting these various ideas together, we can begin to see how important the reactions of health care workers can be for the development of patients'

self-understanding. Through interaction with those around them and by interpreting the behavior given off in their presence, patients not only learn particular self-understandings but to adopt *roles* congruent with these.

Within the context of a chapter such as this, it is not possible to do more than
sketch out some of the key ideas with which interactionist models of nursing
are likely to operate. Nevertheless, in Riehl's model of nursing it is possible to
make commitments such as those described to work within an innovative and
sensitive approach to nursing care.

Riehl's Model of Nursing

In order to identify a number of significant dimensions within Riehl's model of
nursing, we will consider what it has to say about seven key components of
nursing care (Aggleton & Chalmers, 1986). The first two of these components
focus on the nature of people and the causes of problems likely to require
nursing intervention. The next four identify what the model has to offer
nurses interested in working with a problem-solving approach to care. The
final dimension points to the implications of this model for the role of the
nurse.

The Nature of People

Riehl's model of nursing argues that those receiving nursing care are individuals constantly striving to "make sense" of the world around them. People
are, above all, "givers of meaning" to the situations they find themselves in.
They differ from one another, however, in terms of how they make sense of
events affecting them. Within a health care context, people are particularly
likely to try to understand the cause and nature of their state of ill health as well
as its likely duration.

Part of the nurse's task must therefore be to try to enter into the subjective
world of the patient in order to see things as they do. Only by doing this can
the nurse make an accurate assessment of an individual's needs. Without such
an assessment, an appropriate series of nursing interventions cannot be
planned.

The Causes of Problems Likely to Require Nursing Intervention

According to Riehl's model, nursing problems arise when there are disturbances within one or more of three aspects of a person's behavior—the physiological, the psychological, and the sociological. These aspects, or *parameters* as
they are called, are closely related to one another in their functioning. Disturbance within one of them can have consequences for how the others operate.
Of these three parameters, the psychological and sociological are critical determinants of human behavior. Many health-related needs create disturbance
within either or both of these aspects of human functioning. These disturbances can, in turn, give rise to new health-related demands.

The Nature of Assessment

For nurses working with Riehl's model of nursing, assessment is likely to be a two-stage process. At the first stage, nurses are likely to ascertain whether a need exists for nursing intervention. At the second, nurses will try to gain insight into a patient's subjective perceptions of problems affecting them.

The Riehl model advocates a systematic approach to nursing assessment, and the FANCAP system of assessment (Abbey, 1980) has been cited with some approval in early descriptions of this model (Riehl, 1980). This encourages patient assessment under each of six headings—fluids, aeration, nutrition, communication, activity, and pain (FANCAP). The use of this mnemonic device as a guide to assessment encourages nurses to pay attention not only to physiological aspects of those in their care but to psychological and sociological dimensions as well (Fig. 35-1). Thus, an assessment of fluids requires the nurse not only to assess drinking needs but also the changeability (fluidity) of the patient's behavior. Likewise, in assessing respiration, the nurse should focus not only on breathing needs but also on those associated with the ventilation of feelings and emotions. Other assessment systems may be used with this model providing they remain sufficiently sensitive to the subjective experiences of those receiving nursing care.

Having identified problems affecting the patient, nurses working with this model will next be interested in exploring the *roles* the patient has previously adopted in coping with problems similar to these. Throughout assessment, therefore, nurses will be interested in gaining both an *intersubjective understanding* of how patients see the situation they are in, and an appreciation of the *role performances* that are available as coping responses to these perceptions. By carrying out an effective second-stage assessment, the nurse should be able to determine the degree of role flexibility open to the patient. This should allow for the anticipation of problems that may later arise when patients are encouraged to develop new roles.

The Nature of Care Planning

Because Riehl's model of nursing emphasizes the importance of a developing relationship between patient and nurse, the use of jointly negotiated short-term

Liquids, drinking	**Fluids**	Changeability, lability
Respiration	**Aeration**	Ventilation of feelings
Food, calorie intake	**Nutrition**	Cared for, not deprived
Sense organs, nervous system	**Communication**	Perception, interpretation
Physical exertion	**Activity**	Conversing, learning
Accompanying injury, lack of oxygen	**Pain**	Distress, grief, fear

Figure 35-1. FANCAP, a system for the assessment of patient needs. Nurses assess each of the six aspects of patients specified by the mnemonic FANCAP, paying particular attention to the range of functions covered by each element in the mnemonic.

goals is likely to be of considerable value. Their use allows care planning to remain sensitive to patient's changing needs. The Riehl model advocates that goals should be written in patient-centered terms for each problem identified during nursing assessment.

The Focus of Nursing Intervention

For nurses working with this model, most nursing interventions will aim to help patients develop role-flexibility to cope with health-related demands. Some of the new roles that a person may need will be associated with the individual's medical condition. Others may relate to the effects of hospitalization or the special demands that nursing care imposes on an individual.

Many nursing interventions will involve *role-taking*. This requires the patient and nurse to think about a situation from another's point of view. By involving the patient in role-taking, the nurse encourages patients to perceive their present situation in alternative ways and to explore alternative roles they could adopt within this particular situation. Additionally, role-taking will allow nurses themselves to gain greater insight into patients' perceptions and needs.

Evaluating the Quality and Effects of Care

Nursing evaluation customarily involves an examination of the extent to which nursing interventions have been successful in meeting goals set earlier during care planning. For nurses working with Riehl's model of nursing, evaluation is likely to involve a consideration of the extent to which patients have developed role performances or acquired role flexibility to cope more adequately with health-related demands. In the light of findings arising from evaluation, there may be a need to reassess patient needs and plan future care. It may be useful to draw a distinction between ongoing *formative* evaluation and *summative* evaluation. The former is likely to take place as nurses monitor the effectiveness of their interventions in meeting individual patient needs. The latter is more likely to involve a consideration of the appropriateness of a particular nursing model for the planning and delivery of care within a particular area or nursing speciality.

The Role of the Nurse

Riehl's model emphasizes the need for nurses to involve themselves fully in the subjective worlds of their patients. Only by doing this will they be able to accurately assess patients' needs. Such an emphasis is quite different from that suggested by some other health-care models, many of which argue for the cultivation of *distance* between health-care professionals and their clients. Furthermore, because this particular nursing model argues that patients *and* nurses should involve themselves in role-taking, it highlights a complementary role for nurses in their negotiations with those in receipt of nursing care. Nurses working with Riehl's model should therefore aim to be empathetic and supportive in their relations with patients within an overall framework of trust and equality.

USING RIEHL'S MODEL OF NURSING IN PRACTICE

Riehl's model of nursing advocates a nursing role in which nurses try to enter the subjective world of patients. To demonstrate how this model might be applied in clinical practice, a nursing process approach to care will be used, because this offers nurses a systematic way of planning and delivering nursing care.

In order to illustrate the use of Riehl's Interaction model of nursing with the nursing process, two examples will be cited that take their origins from care plans that were developed and used by two practicing nurses with whom we have worked in the United Kingdom. Both care plans used the FANCAP system of patient assessment. The first example describes the nursing care planned and delivered to a married woman in her late 30s who was admitted to a surgical ward for a segmental mastectomy following the discovery of a lump in her left breast. In the second example, care was offered in a coronary care unit to a man of 54 years who was admitted with severe chest pain. He was later medically diagnosed as having a myocardial infarction.

Assessment

Nurses working with Riehl's model of nursing are more likely to engage in continuous assessment rather than a staged collection of data because an ongoing assessment process is more at one with the notion of a developing relationship between patient and nurse. Initial assessment, however, will be required to determine whether there is a need for nursing intervention. Subsequent assessment may be organized around a systematic tool such as FANCAP to identify key areas of concern.

Those working with Riehl's model of nursing, however, are not encouraged to be prescriptive in their actions. Rather, the nurse and patient together will reach decisions about the appropriateness, or otherwise, of the roles that the patient will be encouraged to adopt in particular situations. The nature of the physiological, psychological, and sociological parameters having an effect on the patient will be crucial in suggesting the appropriateness of particular forms of nursing intervention.

Following nursing assessment, the 36-year-old woman was identified as experiencing role conflict between her usual role as a mother and her present need for support and care from her immediate family. Further discussion led to greater understanding by the nurse of the patient's perception of her mothering role. Assessment indicated a lack of role flexibility with, in this patient's eyes, the role of mother equating closely with that of protector. Thus it became clear that the nature of the woman's medical problem and its possible implication for her immediate future had not been communicated either to her husband and children or to her father and brother. Assessment therefore led to the identification of problems within both psychological and sociological parameters.

These affected the patient's ability to ventilate her feelings (the aeration component of FANCAP).

For our second example of Riehl's model of nursing in practice, we shall turn our attention towards a nurse working in a coronary care unit who was involved in assessing a man who had recently been admitted to hospital. Because it appeared initially that he was not fulfilling his usual role as a verbal communicator, subsequent assessment initially proved difficult. Nevertheless, using observational skills, the nurse was able to determine that the man's chest pain was inadequately controlled. This was thought to be standing in the way of his usual ability to communicate verbally. A communication problem was thereby identified, largely based within the psychological parameter but exacerbated by the presence of physical pain. Subsequent assessment, once the man in the coronary care unit was able to fulfill his normal role as a verbal communicator, revealed that the pain had indeed proved a barrier to communication, not only because of its physical severity but also, and perhaps more importantly, because it induced in him a considerable fear of death.

The value of gathering information to aid intersubjective understanding between patient and nurse cannot be overstressed. A nurse working with Riehl's model of nursing aims to use assessment to gain a better understanding of the patient's actions from the *patient's* own point of view. As a result, within this model both verbal and nonverbal communication between nurses and their patients take on a special importance.

Setting Goals and Planning Care

Once a degree of intersubjective understanding has been achieved between patient and nurse, and problems have been identified, it is possible to set goals and plan care. In doing this, the nurse should negotiate with the patient a series of short-term goals as well as some long-term ones.

The use of short-term goals allows for flexibility within care planning because they can be quickly modified as intersubjective understanding between nurse and patient develops. Because Riehl's model of nursing underplays a traditional nursing emphasis on restoring balance within and between physiological systems, goals should be patient-centered and behavioral in their emphasis.

The initial short-term goal negotiated with the woman approaching surgery in connection with a lump in her breast was that she should consider the effect that withholding information from her family might have on her present relationship with them. Then, in the light of this consideration, a further goal was set—that she would choose whether or not to discuss her medical condition and proposed care with her family.

The nurse working in the coronary unit negotiated as a short-term goal with her patient that he would feel able to communicate verbally if and when he wished. Additionally, care planning enabled the identification of other short-term goals relating more specifically to the prompt relief of his chest pain.

Nursing Intervention

By gaining a better understanding of how people see the situation they are in, nurses put themselves in a position to offer care to extend the range of role behaviors open to their patients. For those working with Riehl's model, nursing intervention therefore aims to help the patient achieve the goals negotiated and set at the planning stage. Such goals will usually be concerned with patients' acquiring new role performances or extending existing ones. Riehl's model of nursing advocates the use of role-taking as an effective way by which nurses can alert a person to the possibilities associated with developing new role performances. Role-play may also be used as a means of intervention.

In keeping with interventional commitments such as these, the woman awaiting surgery for the removal of a breast lump was encouraged to put herself in the place of her relatives so that she could imagine the situation as they might see it. She was also encouraged to think about the nurse's view that the sharing of information might be beneficial because it might result in greater support and nurturance for her from her family. It was further suggested that the patient might try to look forward to the role performances that she would need to adopt in the light of her decision about whether to confide in her relatives or not. She was thus provided with opportunities in which to rehearse the kind of behaviors that might suit each situation, and to evaluate their relative strengths and weaknesses for her own sense of well-being.

To meet the short-term goal set initially for the man being nursed in the coronary care unit, nursing intervention involved administering prescribed analgesia, making the man more comfortable in bed, and remaining in the area of his bed to offer comfort and support. In the longer term, it was important that a closer relationship should develop between the patient and the nurse so that each could come to understand the situation from the other's point of view. Once the nurse was cognizant of the close relationship that the patient perceived between severe pain and impending death, it was possible to offer kinds of support more in tune with the patient's needs. Following discussion between patient and nurse about the nature of the mechanisms by which chest pain occurs and the range of methods available to relieve it, the patient being nursed in the coronary unit was also able to better understand the situation from the nurse's point of view. Nursing intervention in this case also involved the sharing of views about the value of communication between nurse and patient. Similarly, role-taking by the nurse helped her to better understand the barriers to communication perceived by the patient.

Evaluation

Formative evaluation with Riehl's model of nursing is likely to focus on whether, following nursing intervention, short- and long-term goals have been achieved. Decisions about this will usually be made after observing the patient's behavior to see whether there is any evidence of new or extended role performances.

Self-evaluation also has a role to play in Riehl's model because it emphasizes the importance of the patient's perception and understanding of the situation. It is likely, however, that both nurse and patient will only consider care to have been successful when the role performances adopted enable the patient to cope more effectively with his or her health-related needs.

Following nursing intervention, the woman in the surgical ward thought carefully about the possibility of telling her relatives more about her medical problem, but in the event chose not to do so prior to surgery. She was, however, able to appreciate the effects that this particular decision might subsequently have on her relationship with them. In the light of this, she planned to give more thought to her decision during the postoperative period when she felt she would have more definite information to share.

The short-term goal set for the man in the coronary care unit was rapidly met in that his physical pain was markedly reduced following nursing intervention. However, his psychological pain and distress was initially much harder to ease, because his fear of death was more deep seated. In the longer term, however, a relationship developed between the nurse and patient that facilitated an increase in understanding by both parties. Verbal communication became easier and more productive for both of them.

Summative evaluation is also esssential with any nursing model in order to identify its strengths and weaknesses in offering effective guidelines for the planning and delivery of nursing care. In both of the examples given, the nurses working with the model found themselves excited by the possibilities offered by an interactionist model of nursing. For the nurse working in the surgical ward, it proved a most challenging model with which to work, demanding from her levels of social skill that are not always perceived as necessary in acute care settings. Her conclusion was that her successful use of the model had reinforced her belief that nursing is best considered as a series of meaningful interactions between two people.

Similarly, the nurse working in the coronary care unit felt that the use of Riehl's model had helped her remain alert to the importance of psycho-social processes in caring for patients in this particular setting. In an environment where the focus of care is often of a physical nature, she too found that Riehl's model highlighted important areas of concern that might otherwise have been overlooked.

ENDNOTE

[1]We owe a debt to Jenny Phillips of Bristol and Weston Health Authority and Margaret Wicks of Bath District Health Authority whose work provided us with illustrations of Riehl's model of nursing in practice.

REFERENCES

Abbey, J. (1980). FANCAP: What is it? In J. P. Riehl & C. Roy (Eds.), *Conceptual models for nursing practice* (2nd ed.). East Norwalk, CT: Appleton-Century-Crofts.

Aggleton, P. J., & Chalmers, H. A. (1986). *Nursing models and the nursing process.* Basingstoke, England: Macmillan.

Bergsma, J., & Thomasma, D. (1984). *Health care: Its psychosocial dimensions.* Pittsburgh: Duquesne University Press.

Blumer, H. (1969). *Symbolic interactionism: Perspective and method.* Englewood Cliffs, NJ: Prentice-Hall.

Ceccio, J., & Ceccio, C. (1982). *Effective communication in nursing.* New York: Wiley.

Cooley, C. (1909). *Social organization: A study of the larger mind.* New York: Scribners.

Faulkner, A. (1984). *Communication.* London: Churchill Livingstone.

Fawcett, J. (1984). *Analysis and evaluation of conceptual models of nursing.* Philadelphia: Davis.

Mead, G. (1934). *Mind, self and society.* Chicago: University of Chicago Press.

Riehl, J. P. (1980). The Riehl interaction model. In J. P. Riehl & C. Roy (Eds.), *Conceptual models for nursing practice* (2nd ed.). East Norwalk, CT: Appleton-Century-Crofts.

Smith, V., & Bass, T. (1982). *Communication for the health care team.* London: Harper & Row.

Thibodeau, J. A. (1983). *Nursing models: Analysis and evaluation.* Monterey: Wadsworth.

Thomas, W. I. (1923). *The unadjusted girl.* Boston: Little, Brown.

The Riehl Model in Practice
With Families and With Staff

Utharas Arumugam

My first experience with the use of the Riehl model was in mid-1984, when I used it to deliver nursing care for a small group of patients in a medium- and long-stay rehabilitation ward (Arumugam, 1985). The experience with the use of this model helped make my nursing actions more meaningful. It shifted my personal perspective from a behavioral to symbolic interactionism approach. I began to appreciate the model's potential usefulness in an acute psychiatric environment. I decided to work with the Riehl (1980) model in the mother and baby unit for several reasons. The bulk of problems we dealt with were interactional in nature. The staff was not familiar with any nursing models. It appeared as though when the patient was acutely ill the medical model emerged as a dominant model (tranquilizers, antidepressants, and electroconvulsive therapy may be used). When the crisis was over and the patient was more manageable, a broader psycho-social model was more apparently needed (conjoint sessions, family therapy, social skills, and so forth). One other major reason for the choice of the Riehl model was that it encouraged the staff to not only consider the patient's viewpoint seriously but also to empathize with the patient.

The Riehl model is a dynamic interations model, constructed around the theory of symbolic interactionism. Blumer (1969) defined *symbolic interactionism* as the interaction that occurs between human beings who interpret or define each others actions instead of just reacting to them. Apart from reflecting its theoretical origins, all nursing models include assumptions, values, goals, assessment process, intervention focus, and evaluation. It is not within the scope of this chapter to elaborate on the various aspects of the Riehl model, but I will attempt to highlight the usefulness of the model in facilitating the delivery of a much more meaningful nursing care for a patient in the mother and baby unit.

The following is a brief outline of what I intend to cover in this chapter. After the assessment of the patient, I will endeavor to bring to the fore and discuss some of the experiences the patient perceived to be significant. In this instance, the patient's experience was of childbirth in the maternity ward. Assessment in the Riehl model also involved exploring the patient's medical status, psychosocial problems, assertaining the roles she had adopted in the past and those she was currently displaying, problem-solving abilities, adaptability, role flexibility, and the defining processes by which a person comes to understand his or her present status. From these assessments short-term nursing diagnoses were formed.

The following is some general information, all obtained from the patient herself, followed by an assessment using FANCAP (Abbey, 1980). Jane was the eldest of four children. She worked as a secretary to a bank manager and supervised a staff of about ten. Jane married Clive about 2 years ago, her second marriage. Her first marriage to Dave lasted about 6 years (no children). He "left her for another woman." Jane described her present marriage as "fine" and her pregnancy was a planned one. She had never experienced any "psychiatric" problem in the past. The consultant psychiatrist suggested this admission after a home visit.

Assessment of the patient was a process largely organized around FANCAP as described by Abbey (1980). This is a mnemonic arrangement to aid the memory of staff involved in giving direct patient care. Briefly, FANCAP is divided into parameters and factors. Parameters cover the physiological, psychological, and social aspects of care. They may be central, proximal, or distal in the influence on the actor concerned. Factors in FANCAP are fluids, aeration, nutrition, communication, activity, and pain. These factors of care are the "do not miss" requirements for nursing. Factors can refer to normal definitive terms or broad associative terms. For example, "fluids" may be used to mean the intake of liquids or the constantly changing (fluid) nature of the patient's perceived problems.

Assessment Using FANCAP

Fluids
There were no apparent problems in the literal meaning of the word. However, the patient experienced her environment as constantly changing—fluidlike. The patient reacted to this changing nature of her perception of her environment; hence in the same morning she might experience her environment as hostile and at another moment herself as "unwell" and the environment as supportive.

Aeration
The patient experienced difficulty in ventilating her feelings. She attempted to release emotion by tensing her muscles, especially in her arms, and shook herself and sometimes banged the table (but well-controlled) while talking. At

times she cried aloud but without tears. She talked constantly as another mode of releasing tension.

Nutrition

Under normal circumstances the patient was well aware of the need for a balanced diet. This became less of a priority when she was preoccupied with personal problems. In terms of "psychological nutrition" she felt had had a very happy childhood. Her relationship with parents was very good—"can rely on their support." She was well accepted by friends and colleagues at work. Concerning "spiritual nutrition," she was a Methodist by religion and sometimes said her prayers by her bed. She perceived her parents as offering similar sustenance.

Communication

She was verbally very articulate. She appeared to talk to herself—constantly reassured herself of her identity and of her whereabouts, wanting others "to know" these were not "made up." She communicated a pressing need to sort out her "problems" and constantly asked herself "what have I done?" Sometimes she stated that she was distressed because she was "very confused." It appeared as though the patient's denial of her baby and her husband may have indicated a refusal on her part to acknowledge her new role and all the activities and responsibilities that went with it. There was another level of anlysis of the same actions, discussed later under "Psychosocial Problems."

Activity

Work, under normal circumstances, took up most of the patient's time. Jane's role as a secretary was a demanding one. Her responsibilities included supervising other staff. She was very happy at work, and had been at the same branch for 12 years. She enjoyed amateur dramatics. Since the birth of her baby, she maintained only minimal social contact and activities. She lost her self-confidence and generally became unable to cope. Jane called in her mother to help a week prior to her admisssion. Her baby was about 6 weeks old at this time.

Pain

Jane expressed two kinds of pain. First, her breast was engorged and it hurt (she had recently started bottle feeding). The second type of pain was psychological in nature, and sometimes so unbearable that she requested on several occasions to be given drugs "to put me to sleep" (she was not actively suicidal).

Further Assessment

Medical Status

Although Jane initially refused to come into the hospital, she relented after persuasion by her general practitioner and psychiatrist. Jane's understanding of

herself as being "mentally ill" appeared to have been either confirmed or initiated during this visit. Subsequently, it was reiterated by significant others.
She was told that she was "mentally unwell" and was prescribed Chlor-
promazine 100 mg three times daily and Temazepam 20 mg at night. Her medical status was only important insofar as it may have contributed to her ongoing
evaluation of her "present status"—that is the extent to which she viewed her
plight as a medical problem.

Psycho-Social Problems

Jane wanted a baby from her previous marriage to Dave, which she did not
have. "Dave wasn't keen on the idea." She felt she had yet to "work him out of
my system." In her highly aroused state she becomes confused, saying "Dave
did not want this baby" and being unsure who Clive was. Sometimes she
thought he was Dave and refused to acknowledge him. While in crisis she perceived her present situation in the context of her previous (perhaps more
meaningful) relationship.

Jane was admitted late in the evening. She had not heard of the hospital
where she was admitted. On the way there she was a signboard reading "Long
Ashton Research Station" (an agricultural research station). While on the unit,
she saw a notice that read "Agfa Minerva (EMI) Ltd" and "instruction for
operation" (a fire notice). Jane interpreted all these symbols to mean she had
been brought to a place where research was carried out, and she would be
operated on when she was asleep; hence her refusal to go to sleep. Jane initially
interpreted the staff as research assistants and showed a marked degree of anxiety when in contact with them. Her perceptions were sustained by the "fact"
that she did not "feel real"—her "parts" (breasts) did not feel as though they
belonged to her.

Jane perceived her parents as "staff." They were "treating me like a child."
She constantly wanted to know from them if she had done anything wrong and
if that was the reason they had brought her here. Under normal circumstances,
her relationship with her family and Clive was described as very good. However, Jane felt Clive was reluctant to get help (she actually meant help from
her parents; Clive had involved the general practitioner and the psychiatrist).
Jane perceived this act as one designed deliberately by Clive to "put me away."
Clive felt the family was "elbowing" him out of the way, and he was not in
control.

Role

Jane perceived herself as a competant working woman. She felt able to interact
with others on an adult-to-adult basis. She acknowledged that the "mothering"
role would be different and difficult to take on but wanted it all the same.

Role Flexibility

Under normal circumstance she felt able to move from one role to another with ease. She experienced no conflict between her role as daughter (she loved her parents very much) and her role as a wife. She cited her involvement in amateur dramatics as having improved her ability to assume different roles.

Problem Solving

Jane was a "well-adjusted" and self-confident person. She was able to assert herself appropriately without causing undue anxiety in others. She perceived herself as being able to look after her own interests and resolved problems to her satisfaction. She stated she usually resolved any problems in interpersonal relationships fairly quickly, and did not leave "any unfinished business" if she could help it.

Defining Processes

This is a method by which a person comes to understand his or her present status. Jane was generally puzzled about what was happening to her. She felt her husband was getting exasperated with her. She was feeling strange bodily sensations—things did not seem real and people significant to her started to treat her differently. She was not in control. Jane began to distrust her husband; she wanted her parents. She wanted someone to tell her what was going on. Two authoritative figures appeared—her general practitioner and the consultant psychiatrist, who explained the situation to her and assumed control. Jane felt relieved that someone had taken control of her situation. She understood that she was not well. She was suffering from a mental illness, puerperal psychosis.

In this admission, two lengthy (40-minute) sessions were utilized to explore Jane's subjective experience while she had been in the maternity ward. One session occurred on the fourth day and the other on the seventh day. In the first session, Jane recalled her experience "as a whole" as a pleasant one. She explained that "boredom" was her only "major problem." However, she proceeded to explain that she had been admitted for high blood pressure rather unexpectedly 2 weeks prior to delivery after a routine outpatient consultation. This she understood now to be preeclampsia. Jane stressed that she had not understood the seriousness of her condition and the threat to her baby. However, she had wondered about other mothers admitted for high blood pressure being allowed to go home. Jane construed from this that she was a lot worse than she imagined.

During the second session, Jane explained that she could not "take in" what the nurses and other staff members were saying and that everything appeared confusing. She felt that contradictary advice was given by different people and that her confidence was undermined. This was a very contrasting experience to what she was accustomed to in her role as a secretary.The sudden realization of a sense of no control or helplessness in an environment that was not only alien but also surrounded by "bizarre rituals" and unfamiliar symbols appeared to have evoked in Jane a sense of not belonging, of "being in a strange place." Although Jane could not remember how anxious she was, it would be reason-

418

TABLE 36–1. CARE PLAN FOR JANE AND FAMILY

Date	Nursing Diagnosis	Goal	Nursing Intervention	Date	Evaluation
Feb. 15, 1987	(Fluid problem) 1a. Patient (Jane) perceives her environment as working against her interest	1a. Patient will appreciate the unit environment as generally therapeutic	1a. Staff to explain the function of the unit, and why other patients are here. Explain the role of staff. Enlist other patients to reassure Jane	Feb. 22, 1987	1a. Understands the unit as part of a larger psychiatric hospital. Able to discuss her initial feelings about the place
	(Communication problem) b. Misinterprets signs on the unit, and any other incidental cues	b. Patient will understand the signs and the reason for being up	b. Staff to work through with Jane all the signs she misinterprets and explain why they are put up (e.g., "fire instructions ")		b. Jane says she is less anxious because she knows what these signs are about and they are up for "good reasons"
		c. Patient will interpret symbols (incidental cues) in her environment appropriately	c. Staff to deal immediately with Jane when she misinterprets cues (e.g., brown-colored water from hot water tap is not blood but a little rust and will clear)		c. No further misinterpretation of symbols or incidental cues observed

(cont.)

TABLE 36–1. *(CONTINUED)*

Date	Nursing Diagnosis	Goal	Nursing Intervention	Date	Evaluation
Feb. 15, 1987	(Communication problem) 2a. Perceives the unit as a research center	2a. Patient will understand her environment as the mother and baby unit. Will appreciate that the research station she saw on her way in is an agricultural research station, about half a mile down the road	2a. Staff to take Jane down for a walk to the agricultural research station. Explain that it is a separate establishment and show Jane the signboard she saw on the night she was admitted	Feb. 27, 1985	2a. Jane is able to laugh about thinking about the unit as she did. Acknowledges that the unit has nothing to do with the research station
	b. Not sleeping because she feels she will be operated on when she goes to sleep. Suspicious about her breast not feeling part of her	b. Patient will go to sleep without feeling of fear that something will happen to her	b. Staff to discuss with Jane about the way she feels about her body. Staff to explain to Jane why her breast feels the way it does—it is engorged with milk		b. Jane's breast is hurting less—can understand why she thought her breast did not belong to her. Remembered one night at home when she woke up in the middle of the night frightened, because her breast hurt—she had just stopped breast feeding

(cont.)

TABLE 36–1. (*CONTINUED*)

Date	Nursing Diagnosis	Goal	Nursing Intervention	Date	Evaluation
Feb. 18, 1987	(Communication and nutrition problems)				
	3. Requires constant re-assurance/input regarding:				
	a. Her belief that her baby is dead	3a. Patient will understand her baby is alive and well	3a. Staff to re-assure and encourage Jane to talk about her baby, Richard. Encourage Jane to handle her baby. Jane to under-take as much baby care as able to	Feb. 27, 1987	3a. Expressed relief that Richard was alive. Appears very fond of him. Willing to care for him—requires supervision
	b. Husband "don't exist"	b. Patient will acknowl-edge and relate with her husband	b. Staff to encourage Jane and husband to spend time together on their own—talk about their ordinary domestic situation		b. Appears to be relating to her husband reasonably comfortably. States she knows he has been good to her
	c. "What have I done, why am I here?"	c. Patient will appreciate that she has done nothing wrong, and that she is in the unit because she needed help and support from the unit	c. Reassure Jane that she is not here to be punished and that she has done nothing wrong		c. Does not appear to be a problem. Not express-ing any wrong doing

(*cont.*)

TABLE 36–1. *(CONTINUED)*

Date	Nursing Diagnosis	Goal	Nursing Intervention	Date	Evaluation
	d. Wants people to believe her	d. Patient will feel that the staff does listen to her and accept what she is saying	d. Staff to listen and encourage in Jane the feeling that she is important, and staff should accept what she is saying		d. Communicates well with staff and other patients
Feb. 18, 1987	(Aeration and activity problems)				
	4. "Pressure" to talk to release emotion	4. Jane will use talk as a useful tool to explore and express feelings	4. Staff will encourage Jane (20 minutes each shift) to talk about her feelings	Mar. 5, 1987	4. Jane uses her opportunities well to talk about her feelings and why she acted and felt the way she did
	5. Conjoint sessions needed	5. The couple will explore how they feel about their recent experiences	5. Staff will undertake at least 3 conjoint sessions with Jane and her husband before Jane's discharge		5. Jane appears happy with the way things have turned out. Feels has learned a lot about self and relationship with husband. Clive feels it a profound experience for him. Surprised at Jane's resourcefulness. Both will return to unit for two more weekly sessions

able to assume that she may have experienced a high level of anxiety—hence her inability to grasp what was said to her.

Jane politely smiled at everyone around her and gave the impression that she fine. Perhaps more significantly, especially in the light of Jane's subsequent experience, was the sensation that she did not "really feel" herself. There was no "emotion" and she felt that her physical body somehow was not part of her—it "felt as though they were quite separate." Seemingly this was a meaningful way for her to deal with her distress. I refrained from probing about how she felt when physically examined (all the poking and prodding)—she may have "sunk" even further away from her body. However, during the hospitalization before delivery, Jane was able to "hold her own." She then appeared together and composed and acted as expected.

At this juncture a brief mention about the care plan is in order. Table 36-1 partially illustrates this. In the Riehl model the objectives are not just patient objectives. Objectives may also be negotiated for the staff with specific patient problems. In a similar vein, nursing intervention may also be directed at changing staff attitudes and actions. The process of discovering problem areas and setting goals was negotiated actively between actors (staff, patients, and significant others). Setting priorities is perhaps a feature in most models. In the Riehl model, priority will largely depend on the actors' perceived need. Thus, the process of prioritization was a constantly changing activity.

Intervention in the Riehl model generally took the form of staff members attempting to "experience" the defining processes as experienced by the patient. This process may involve all concerned (staff, patients, and significant others) in role-playing each other's position to aid mutual (intersubjective) understanding.

To evaluate the patient's progress, I compared her feelings, attitude and actions with the nursing diagnosis and goals that had been established. In a formatative evaluation, two questions may be asked: have the goals that were originally set been achieved and is the patient now adopting a role appropriate to the situation (Aggleton & Chalmers, 1986). In practice, the changeable nature of perceptual problems did not readily lend themselves to the process of evaluation in objective terms. To a large extent, a reassessment was involved. From past experience in the use of the model, I accepted the patient's own subjective evaluation of progress. Perceived problems were often redefined and goals renegotiated. Hence, the theoretical perspective of symbolic interactionism was maintained throughout.

REFERENCES

Abbey, J. (1980). FANCAP: What is it? In J. P. Riehl & C. Roy (Eds.), *Conceptual models for nursing practice* (2nd ed.), (pp. 107–118). New York: Appleton-Century-Crofts.

Aggleton, P. J., & Chalmers, H. A. (1986). *Nursing models and the nursing process.* Basingstoke, England: Macmillan.

Arumugam, U. (1985, May 22). Helping Harry to relate. *Nursing Times,* 43–45.

Blumer, H. (1969). *Symbolic interactionism—Perspectives and methods.* Englewood Cliffs, NJ: Prentice-Hall.

Riehl, J. P. (1980). The Riehl Interaction model. In J. P. Riehl & C. Roy (Eds.), *Conceptual models for nursing practice* (2nd ed.), (pp. 350–356). New York: Appleton-Century-Crofts.

The Riehl Interaction Model Prenatal Family Assessment Tool for the Childbirth Educator

Donna G. Knauth
Ella B. Gross

The childbirth health educator needs to utilize a comprehensive assessment tool that can identify the health education needs of the pregnant woman and her family. Assessment tools that are currently used by childbirth educators mainly seek demographic information and focus primarily on the expectant mother and not on the total family as a unit of interacting individuals. A need exists to develop a theoretically based family health assessment tool. Such a tool could assist the educator to meet three goals: (1) to guide the educator's nursing practice toward a family-centered approach; (2) to encourage the development of family diagnoses; and (3) to plan interventions that contribute to positive pregnancy outcomes.

This chapter examines how the basic assumptions of the Riehl Interaction Model (RIM) can be operationalized within the context of an assessment tool and how it can be utilized in a clinical setting by the childbirth educator (Riehl, 1980). The tool was piloted with 35 families in the outpatient department of a university medical center in Pennsylvania. A case study of one of the families clarifying its application is presented later in the chapter.

RIM, which is based on symbolic interaction theory, is an appropriate conceptual framework for this assessment tool, because it focuses on the social processes between individuals. By analyzing roles and relationships, RIM enhances an active interaction between the childbirth educator and the family. To accurately assess educational needs, it is not sufficient for the childbirth educator to only observe and assess the behavior of the individuals within the family. The educator needs to also identify the meaning and value placed on that behavior within the context that it occurs. The childbirth educator must "get inside" the defining process of the expectant mother and her family in order to understand the symbols and meanings that comprise their world (Blumer, 1969). Through the act of role-taking, the nurse can attempt to understand the family's perspective. The nurse must realize that assessment is incomplete until this understanding is validated with the family members.

RIM directs the educator to alter problems by effecting intervention strategies that add resources to the family. This increases role-taking and interpersonal competence skills through deliberately planned socialization experiences, and by changing the family members' definition of the situation.

Review of the Literature

Evidence of a recent trend encouraging childbirth educators to base their practice on theoretical frameworks can be found in the literature. For example, Nichols (1984) implicitly states that childbirth educators need to base their research and practice on certain integrated components. The most important is a sound theoretical base that when implemented in practice will contribute to the professional growth of the childbirth educator. The American Society for Psychoprophylaxis in Obstetrics (ASPO), the International Childbirth Education Association (ICEA), and the Council of Childbirth Education Specialists (C/CES), are three of the leading organizations that represent the majority of childbirth educators in the United States. A review of their literature reveals that assessment tools currently available are demographic in scope. Kitzinger (1979), a noted British anthropologist and childbirth educator, highly endorses an interview assessment with expectant parents. Kitzinger gives suggestions to guide the assessment; however, it is not theoretically based.

Nursing literature is replete with assessment tools and strategies for the inpatient and outpatient clinical setting. Most of these assessments focus on the individual and are not specific for educational needs that the childbirth educator must address. Community health nursing assessments are more family focused and interventions are directed toward helping the family grow in its abilities to meet its health responsibilities. Friedman (1981) introduces an assessment guideline that encompasses the family unit in a composite setting. The assessment process includes the environmental, structural, functional, and cultural diversity of the family as a group. Friedman discusses the significance for the family health nurse to utilize the nursing process on two levels: the individual family member and the family as a group. This dual focus will be complex, but a necessary direction for nursing to take if it wants to consider its approach "family centered" and not just a worn out cliché.

The Institute of Medicine's (1985) report on preventing low birth weight identifies weaknesses in the health system to meeting the needs of the childbearing family. The lack of early and individualized efforts on the part of health care providers to provide health education is repeatedly identified as the greatest problem in planning effective interventions to prevent low birth weight. Ooms (1981) states that the health professions' myopic view of pregnancy, particularly for the adolescent, is restrictive and has bypassed the family concept. Using a family perspective is the most beneficial approach because it permits the health care provider to assess the way family members interact with each other.

There have been many theoretical approaches for viewing the family. As has been stated, symbolic interactionism was chosen because of its focus on the family as a set of interacting personalities within a psycho-social setting. Clements and Roberts (1983) describe symbolic interactionism as a conceptual framework that lends itself very well to assessing influencing factors on the family. It also provides the nurse with two possible levels of analysis: (1) the individual and his or her perception of an event; and (2) the pattern of interaction between two or more individuals. The second level of analysis helps the nurse to understand the behavior between family members. Jones and Dimond (1982) describe the significance of the interactional approach and its emphasis on role. Interactional theorists assess the family in relation to communication processes, problem solving, and decision making. Gilliss (1983) states it is important to find a perspective that allows the nurse to view the family in a framework that is more than just the sum of its parts. The interaction approach is the framework that incorporates the dynamic individual, the dynamic unit (family), and their interrelatedness.

Basic Assumptions of Symbolic Interaction Theory

RIM, with symbolic interaction theory as its underlying perspective, was chosen as the conceptual framework for the prenatal family assessment tool for two reasons. It emphasizes social processes and the methodological principle, which seeks to understand interactions that occur between individuals in the family unit. It also focuses on the individual's interactions with his or her environment. The following basic assumptions of symbolic interactionism were operationalized within the context of the prenatal family assessment tool.

1. The individual enters the world as an asocial being and must be socialized into the general culture and into various subcultures within the environment.
2. The individual lives in a symbolic as well as in a physical environment and can be stimulated to act by symbols as well as by physical stimuli. Having the capacity to think and use a complex language is unique to human beings. This enables people to learn symbols, their meanings, and values from other people with whom they interact. This set of meanings and values is part of the group's culture (Clements & Robert, 1983).
3. The individual is reflexive and capable of introspection. This enables the individual to distinguish between her or his own personal self and others. This leads to a dynamic definition of self. Self-concept is the key

link between behavior and the social organization to which the individual belongs. Self is designated in terms of observable behavior. Self behavior is viewed as conscious, thinking behavior.
4. Through symbols, individuals have the capacity to stimulate others in ways other than those in which they themselves are stimulated.
5. Through communication of symbols, individuals can learn many meanings and values and new ways of acting from other individuals.
6. The meanings and values of these symbols do not occur in isolation but rather in complex clusters.

The expectant mother defines herself, others, and the action of others. She comes to her pregnancy with her own self-concept, which defines her as a unique person. She sees herself in the role of a pregnant woman through the eyes and actions of those around her. The roles of pregnant woman, laboring woman, mother-to-be, and partner to father or significant other, all have socially prescribed behaviors that she has learned from her cultural patterns and nuclear family interactions. The pregnant woman reacts not only to the physical sensations of pregnancy (such as fetal movement, decreased muscle tone, and increased pelvic pressure) but also to the meanings and values she has learned for the many symbols of childbearing and parenting (for example, being pregnant, giving birth, becoming a parent, and growing larger).

For the pregnant woman, the childbearing year brings a language of its own that represents symbols that have unique meanings and values for each family. In order to understand the family's symbolic environment, the childbirth educator needs to try to learn and see the world from the family's point of view. The educator needs to "take on" the role of pregnant woman to fully understand the pregnant woman's behavior. Childbirth educators need to put themselves in the pregnant woman's place.

The childbearing family may be entering the subculture of the health care system for the first time. The family needs to learn what is expected of it and how to most effectively function in this system. The family needs to learn what to expect during pregnancy, birth, and parenthood. Through assessing the family's perceptions and expectations early in pregnancy and evaluating the educational needs, the childbirth educator can plan interventions for learning and care with the family to ensure more positive pregnancy outcomes. The childbirth educator can make it possible for the childbearing family to discuss these roles, expectations, and educational needs, and encourage participation through role playing.

The Riehl prenatal assessment tool focuses on the expectant mother within the context of her family and seeks to address her individual needs. Without this type of tool, too often the health care provider facilitates the system instead of the family seeking care within the system.

OPERATIONALIZATION OF THE RIM IN THE PRENATAL FAMILY ASSESSMENT TOOL

The three parameters of the RIM framework were used in operationalizing the model in the prenatal family assessment tool: the physiological, sociocultural-environmental, and psychological parameters. Within each of these parameters are six factors, which are represented by the mnemonic FANCAP: *f*luids, *a*eration, *n*utrition, *c*ommunication, *a*ctivity, and *p*ain. The assessment tool incorporates each factor of FANCAP into the broader concepts of the RIM parameters. For example, a question developed to assess the nutrition factor in the physiological parameter was "What do you eat?" The question developed to assess the nutritional factor in the sociocultural-environmental parameter was "When and with whom do you eat?" The psychological nutrition parameter concerned "How do you feel about weight gain?"

These questions developed for each of the factors in the RIM parameters are designed to identify the meanings and values placed on pregnancy and childbirth by the pregnant woman and the members of her family. They seek to provide insight into the pregnant woman's behavior and how she interprets and interacts with the family. They are designed to assess family behavior and the cultural significance of their interactions. With this information, the childbirth educator is able to formulate nursing diagnoses that focus on the family. Educational interventions to meet the childbearing family's needs can then be planned.

IMPLEMENTATION OF THE RIM ASSESSMENT TOOL

The RIM assessment tool (Fig. 37–1) is designed to be used in an interview format with an individual family. The pregnant women in the 35 families to whom the assessment tool was administered ranged in age from 14 to 40 years. This sample included primiparas, multiparas, and married and single women from different socioeconomic groups. All families who came to the outpatient department were invited to attend this interview and class with the childbirth educator. Participation was voluntary.

The responses to the questions on the assessment tool should be scored on completion of the interview and class, in order to promote an informal, relaxed atmosphere conducive to learning. Each of the three RIM parameters is tabulated using a Likert scale, which is designated in the tool as A (always), O (often), S (sometimes), and N (never). A point score from 4 to 1 is tallied for each item. Total scores can also be subgrouped in each of the three RIM parameters. The score reflects whether the factor is positive or negative. The range of scores is from a high of 336 to a low of 84. A high score overall (greater than 252) would indicate few or no educational deficits or interventions necessary. A lower score would indicate increased areas of edu-

```
┌─────────────────────────────────────────────────────────────────────┐
│       RIEHL INTERACTION MODEL PRENATAL FAMILY ASSESSMENT TOOL          │
│                        Foundation Data                                 │
│                                                                        │
│  Family Name: _____         │
│                                                                        │
│  Mother's Name: _____   Father's Name: _____      │
│                                                                        │
│  Support Person: _____         │
│                                                                        │
│  Address: _____   Phone:  (H) _____      │
│                                                                        │
│           _____          (W) _____       │
│                                                                        │
│           _____                                          │
│                                                                        │
│  Employment: _____          │
│                                                                        │
│  # Hours/Week: _____   Best Time to Contact: _____      │
│                                                                        │
│  EDC: _____  Gravida: _____   Para: _____      │
│                                                                        │
│  Date of First Prenatal Visit: _____          │
│                                                                        │
│  ═══════════════════════════════════════════════════════════════      │
│                                                                        │
│  FAMILY COMPOSITION:                                                    │
│                                                                        │
│        NAME         DOB    RELATIONSHIP   OCCUPATION   EDUCATION        │
│  1.                                                                     │
│  2.                                                                     │
│  3.                                                                     │
│  4.                                                                     │
│  5.                                                                     │
│  6.                                                                     │
│                                                                        │
│  _____       _____       │
│  R.N.                                    Date                           │
│  Nursing Care Plan:                                                     │
└─────────────────────────────────────────────────────────────────────┘
```

Figure 37-1A-D. A. Riehl Interaction Model prenatal family assessment tool. **B-D.** Case study using RIM.

PHYSIOLOGICAL FANCAP

Concerns about:				A O S N	DIAGNOSIS/SCORE

F. 1. Changes Digestion: a. nausea `1 2 3 4`
  Or b. appetite `1 2 3 4`
  c. vomiting `1 2 3 4`
P   Swelling: d. hands `1 2 3 4`
R e. feet `1 2 3 4`
O f. face `1 2 3 4`
B g. tingling `1 2 3 4`
L   Vaginal: h. discharge `1 2 3 4`
E i. bleeding `1 2 3 4`
M   Bowel: j. constipation `1 2 3 4`
S k. diarrhea `1 2 3 4`
  Bladder: l. infection `1 2 3 4`
  m. burning `1 2 3 4`
  n. stress incontinence `1 2 3 4`
  TOTAL: _____

A. 2. Changes Chest: a. breathing `1 2 3 4`
  TOTAL: _____

N. 3. Eat balanced diet: a. `4 3 2 1`
  * Weight distribution: b. `4 3 2 1`
  ** Medications: c. `1 2 3 4`
  Daily diet include: d. calories `4 3 2 1`
  e. protein `4 3 2 1`
  f. calcium `4 3 2 1`
  g. vitamins `4 3 2 1`
  TOTAL: _____

+**C.** 4. Speech: (difficulty) a. `1 2 3 4`
  TOTAL: _____

A. 5. Changes due to a. physical/activity `1 2 3 4`
P b. regular/exercise `4 3 2 1`
R c. energy/tiredness `1 2 3 4`
E d. practice/relaxation `4 3 2 1`
G e. changes/sexual `1 2 3 4`
  (difficulties)
  TOTAL: _____

P. 6. Pregnancy has a. discomfort `1 2 3 4`
  caused: b. pain `1 2 3 4`
  c. backache `1 2 3 4`
  Uterus: (signs of d. contraction `1 2 3 4`
  preterm labor)
  TOTAL: _____

PHYSIOLOGICAL TOTAL: _____

*Refers to knowledge of distribution of maternal weight gain in pregnancy.
**Refers to ingestion of over the counter drugs not those medically prescribed.
+Refers to presence of speech problem which physically interferes with ability to communicate.

Figure 37–1B. *(CONTINUED).*

SOCIOCULTURAL/SITUATIONAL-ENVIRONMENTAL FANCAP

Concerns about:			A O S N	DIAGNOSIS/SCORE
F. 7. Adequate fresh water:	a. drinking		4 3 2 1	
	b. bathing		4 3 2 1	
		TOTAL:	_____	
A. 8. Adequate living				
Space:	a.		4 3 2 1	
Quality:	b. air		4 3 2 1	
Presence of:	c. passive smoke		1 2 3 4	
		TOTAL:	_____	
N. 9. Shared meals:	a.		4 3 2 1	
Access food stores:	b.		4 3 2 1	
Resources	c. adequate		4 3 2 1	
Meals eaten away from home	d.		4 3 2 1	
		TOTAL:	_____	
C. 10. Accessible				
* support: available	a.		4 3 2 1	
** Comfort in this	b.		4 3 2 1	
		TOTAL:	_____	
+A. 11. Daily				
Employment	a.		1 2 3 4	
Adequate rest	b.		4 3 2 1	
Adequate sleep	c.		4 3 2 1	
Leisure time self	d.		4 3 2 1	
Shared time with family	e.		4 3 2 1	
Time with partner	f.		4 3 2 1	
		TOTAL:	_____	
P. 12. Family concerns:	a. divorce		1 2 3 4	
	b. death		1 2 3 4	
	c. problem pregnancy		1 2 3 4	
		TOTAL:	_____	
		SUM TOTAL:	_____	

*Asks who comprises support system.
**Asks whether woman finds comfort in these relationships.
+See type of work and hours employed from face sheet of RIM assessment tool (strenuous or full time employment can be added risk factor).

Figure 37–1 C. (*CONTINUED*).

PSYCHOLOGICAL FANCAP

Concerns about:				A O S N	DIAGNOSIS/SCORE
F. 13. Alcohol:	use	a. individual		1 2 3 4	
		b. partner		1 2 3 4	
		c. family		1 2 3 4	
Drugs:	use	d. individual		1 2 3 4	
		e. partner		1 2 3 4	
		f. family		1 2 3 4	
			TOTAL:	_____	
A. 14. Smoking:	use	a. individual		1 2 3 4	
		b. partner		1 2 3 4	
Drugs:	use	d. individual		1 2 3 4	
		e. partner		1 2 3 4	
		f. family		1 2 3 4	
			TOTAL:	_____	
N. 15. Positive feelings:		a. individual		4 3 2 1	
(weight gain)		b. partner		4 3 2 1	
		c. body image		4 3 2 1	
			TOTAL:	_____	
C. 16. Ease of shared		a. health care			
communication		providers		4 3 2 1	
		b. partner		4 3 2 1	
		c. family		4 3 2 1	
			TOTAL:	_____	
A. 17. Positive feelings:		* a. Work/home			
		or school		4 3 2 1	
		b. sexual		4 3 2 1	
Sleep:		c. quality		4 3 2 1	
Problem with		d. nightmares		1 2 3 4	
**relaxation:		e. awareness		4 3 2 1	
+Participate		f. individual		4 3 2 1	
		g. partner		4 3 2 1	
		h. family		4 3 2 1	
			TOTAL:	_____	
P. 18. Recognize stress		a. awareness		4 3 2 1	
in life:		individual		4 3 2 1	
		b. partner		4 3 2 1	
		c. family		4 3 2 1	
Available coping		d. individual		4 3 2 1	
skills		e. partner		4 3 2 1	
		f. family		4 3 2 1	
			TOTAL:	_____	
			SUM TOTAL:	_____	

*May only score one.
**Refers to how well stress is handled in daily life.
+Refers to use of relaxation technique by individual, partner, family.

Figure 37-1 D. *(CONTINUED).*

cational needs and the need for more interventions by the health care provider.

The families in the sample that scored less than 252 met with the childbirth educator or other appropriate health care providers on a weekly basis in the outpatient department in order to address their individual needs. The childbirth educator met with all the families after delivery to evaluate their childbirth experience and assess early parent-infant attachment and parenting skills.

The interviewers acknowledge the subjective nature of the responses to the assessment tool questions. They recognize the importance of addressing needs in a systematic, theoretically based format. This approach facilitates the formulation of nursing diagnoses and effective individualized plans of care. A copy of the assessment tool is given in Figure 37–1 with footnotes explaining how to implement and score the assessment. An example of a completed assessment from the case study is given in Appendix A.

CASE STUDY USING THE RIM PRENATIAL FAMILY ASSESSMENT TOOL

ZL was a 14-year-old, gravida 1, 26 weeks gestation, who attended the outpatient early pregnancy interview and class with her mother. They expressed an initial interest in attending a series of childbirth classes but transportation difficulties made attendance impossible. The mother was grateful for the outpatient class because her daughter "didn't know anything about pregnancy or birth." The RIM assessment tool was used as the initial guide for the childbirth educator who was able to identify numerous educational needs for this family and the pregnant teen.

ZL was living at home with her divorced mother, a teenaged "retarded" brother, and an unmarried sister who had three children under the age of 6. None of the family members had completed high school and ZL was attempting to complete the seventh grade for the third time. She became pregnant because of failing to take birth control pills on a regular basis. The father of the baby, who was in his late teens, was at the time of the interview not involved with the family.

ZL was treated for frequent urinary tract infections during the pregnancy. ZL's knowledge regarding nutrition was very inadequate and weight gain was well below the norm. The pregnancy had caused a marked change in her activity level and also had caused her to drop out of school. Fatigue and inertia were identified as frequent problems, and there had been one hospitalization for preterm labor, which had been attributed to a back injury caused by the brother.

The family had moved frequently in the past months and were hoping for a more permanent situation where ZL could have her own room for herself and the baby. Passive smoke was a constant problem as all the adults in the home situation were smokers. Resources for meals were scanty and access was limited by transportation difficulties. ZL's statement regarding her intake of vegetables and fruit was, "Sure I like'm, but you can't eat'm if you ain't got'm." The mother explained that Women, Infants and Children (W.I.C.) food supplements were often consumed by others in the family and there was no way to reserve them for ZL. The mother was supportive of ZL and gave her the opportunity to talk in the class, but the mother described her situation as being very compromised by her older daughter and "slow" son. ZL led a very solitary existence that resulted in few interactions with peers. She spent most of her day watching TV and eating "junk foods."

Alcohol and drugs did not appear to be a problem within the family. Weight gain was immediately identified by ZL as "getting fat" and "not being able to wear my jeans." ZL was a reluctant communicator. The mother stated that ZL was very shy and usually quiet around people who were new to her. ZL had no concept of relaxation skills or stress-reducing activities. She did express than when she gets angry she just yells and screams and cries. "That's what everyone does around the house!"

The following nursing diagnoses were developed after the use of the RIM assessment tool (*see* appendix A for the completed assessment):

1. Noncompliance in health management related to a lack of information and the perception that health care providers would not be helpful and accepting. This was evidenced by ZL not seeking care until late in her pregnancy and also by many missed appointments.
2. Potential for injury related to environmental hazards. Passive smoke was seen as a potential hazzard and the abusive relationship with her brother.
3. Nutrition, alteration in, less than body requirements related to inability to procure foods because of lack of money, and the lack of knowledge regarding adequate nutrition during pregnancy as evidenced by poor weight gain.
4. Potential for infection related to past history of urinary tract infection and renal disease.
5. Potential alteration in parenting related to age, single parent, level of completed education, sense of powerlessness, lack of knowledge regarding parenting, and economic problems.
6. Knowledge deficit of the physical and psychological changes of pregnancy related to being a poor reader, having dyslexia, and being only 14 years old.
7. Disturbance in self-concept related to stress, pregnancy, and having to repeat a grade level in school.
8. Social isolation related to loss of contact with peers and frequent moves.
9. Ineffective individual and family coping related to inadequate resources, being a single parent, poor economic status, and history of abusive relationship with sibling.

Evaluation of the RIM Assessment Tool. The use of the Rim assessment tool guided the childbirth educator to plan successful interventions with ZL and her family. The tool also facilitated interactions with other members of the health care team who were involved with the care of ZL.

1. *Successful outcome.* ZL delivered a healthy infant, at term, 7 pounds 2 ounces, with apgars of 7 and 9.
2. *Change in behavior.* Repeated contacts with ZL at scheduled appointments indicated an improved level of communication, more questioning, positive responses, and fewer missed clinic appointments.
3. No additional hospitalizations for preterm labor.
4. No additional urinary tract infections.
5. *Improved weight gain.* Prepregnancy weight was 88 pounds. From the time of assessment, an additional 12 pounds were gained during the pregnancy.

6. ZL was able to verbalize an increased understanding of changes in pregnancy and the birth process.
7. ZL was able to demonstrate use of relaxation and breathing patterns during labor.
8. ZL verbalized to the childbirth educator that the birth had been a positive experience. This contributed to ZL's feeling of increased self-esteem, confidence, and acceptance.
9. Positive interactions between ZL and her mother were enhanced. The mother was a very supportive labor partner, and the mother's self-esteem was also improved from positive feedback by the staff.
10. Adjustment to the parenting role was facilitated. The childbirth educator worked with the whole family to give positive support and encouragement.
11. The family's awareness of hospital and community resources was enhanced through a multidisciplinary approach with social workers, public health nurses, and the church.

CONCLUSION

Based on the positive responses from families with whom the Riehl Interaction Model Prenatal Family Assessment Tool was used, strong support can be shown for the use of the tool in identifying and implementing effective educational interventions for the childbearing family. The tool allows for individualization of care, and can be successfully implemented by other health care providers who desire a comprehensive tool based on a theoretical model of nursing. It also provides a framework for a more complete utilization of the childbirth educator's knowledge and skill in the complex and dynamic area of prenatal education for the client and her family.

Familiarity with the tool allows for tremendous flexibility in the assessment process and contributes not only to enhanced nursing diagnostic skill but makes a meaningful contribution to more positive health outcomes for the childbearing family.

REFERENCES

Blumer, H. (1969). *Interactionism: Perspective and method.* Englewood Cliffs, NJ: Prentice Hall.

Clements, I., & Roberts, F. (Eds.). (1983). *Family Health: A theoretical approach to nurssing care.* New York: Wiley.

Friedman, M. (1981). *Family nursing: Theory and assessment.* East Norwalk, CT: Appleton-Century-Crofts.

Gilliss, C. (1983). The family as a unit of analysis: Strategies for the nurse reearcher. *Advances in Nursing Science, 5*(3), 50–59.

Institute of Medicine. (1985). *Preventing low birthweight.* Washington, DC: National Academy Press.

Jones, S., & Dimond, M. (1982). Family theory and family therapy models: Comparative review with implications for nursing practice. *Journal of Psychological Nursing and Mental Health Services, 20*(10), 12–19.

Kitzinger, S. (1979). *Education and counseling for childbirth.* New York: Schocken.

Nichols, F. (1984). Translating research findings into practice. In D. Ewy (Ed.), *Expanding horizons in childbirth education.* Alexandria, VA: American Society for Psychoprophylaxis in Childbirth/Lamaze.

Ooms, T. (1981). *Teenage pregnancy in a family context.* Philadelphia: Temple University Press.

Riehl, J. (1980). The Riehl Interaction Model. In J. P. Riehl & C. Roy (Eds.), *Conceptual models for nursing practice.* New York: Appleton-Century-Crofts.

Appendix 37–A

Example of Case Study Assessment

<u>RIEHL INTERACTION MODEL PRENATAL FAMILY ASSESSMENT TOOL</u>

<u>Demographic Data Cover Sheet</u>

Family Name: Leiders

Mother's Name: Zellie   Father's Name: Craig

Support Person: Mother - Helen

Address: Small town in Pennsylvania   Phone: (H) No phone

(W) Contact neighbor: Joe
Barley 672-4113, p 7 pm

Employment: No

Hours/Week: _____   Best Time to Contact: _____

EDC: March 1986   Gravida: 1   Para: 0000

Date of First Prenatal Visit: December 1985

FAMILY COMPOSITION:

NAME	DOB/AGE	RELATIONSHIP	OCCUPATION	EDUCATION
1. Zellie	14	daughter	student	7th grade
2. Helen	42	mother	housewife	10th grade
3. Bob	19	brother	home	9th grade
4. Ann	18	sister	home	11th grade
5. Sue	5	niece	home	
6. Peter	3	nephew	home	
7. John	1	nephew	home	

E. B. Gross
_____
R.N.

December 1985
_____
Date

Nursing Care Plan (see Case Study) is
based on total assessment scores:
ZL had 206 of a possible 336.
A 252 minimum is desired.

TOTAL SCORE: 87
                    47
                    <u>72</u>
                    206 out of 336

Physiological FANCAP

Concerns about:

A O S N   **DIAGNOSIS**

F. 1. Changes   Digestion:

- a. nausea   1 2 ③ 4
- b. appetite   1 2 ③ 4
- c. vomiting   1 2 ③ 4

Swelling:
- d. hands   1 2 3 ④
- e. feet   1 2 3 ④
- f. face   1 2 3 ④
- g. tingling   1 2 3 ④

Vaginal:
- h. discharge   1 2 ③ 4   #4
- i. bleeding   1 2 3 ④

Bowel:
- j. constipation   1 2 3 ④
- k. diarrhea   1 2 3 ④

Bladder:
- l. infection   1 ② 3 4
- m. burning   1 ② 3 4
- n. stress incontinence   1 2 3 ④

TOTAL: **48**

(P R O B L E M S)

A. 2. Changes Chest:
- a. breathing   1 2 3 ④

TOTAL: **4**

N. 3. Eat balanced diet: a.   4 3 ② 1
Weight distribution: b.   4 3 2 ①
Medications: c.   1 2 3 ④   # 3
Daily diet includes:
- d. calories   4 3 ② 1
- e. protein   4 3 ② 1
- f. calcium   4 3 ② 1
- g. vitamins   4 3 2 ①

TOTAL: **14**   #6,7

C. 4. Speech: (difficulty) a.   1 ② 3 4   Reading difficulty

TOTAL: **2**

A. 5. Changes physical   a. activity   1 ② 3 4
regular   b. exercise   4 3 ② 1
energy   c. tiredness   ① 2 3 4
practice   d. relaxation   4 3 2 ①
changes   e. sexual   1 2 3 ④
(difficulties)

TOTAL: **10**

P. 6. Pregnancy caused:
- a. discomfort   1 2 ③ 4
- b. pain   1 2 ③ 4
- c. backache   1 ② 3 4

Uterus:
- d. contraction   ① 2 3 4   #2,9

TOTAL: **9**

PHYSIOLOGICAL TOTAL: **87** (out of 128)

Sociocultural/Situational Environmental FANCAP

Concerns about:			A O S N	DIAGNOSIS

F. 7. Access fresh water:
    a. drinking   ④ 3 2 1
    b. bathing   ④ 3 2 1
    TOTAL: 8

A. 8. Adequate living
    space: a.   4 3 2 ①
    Quality: b. air   4 3 ② 1
    Presence of: c. passive smoke   ① 2 3 4   **# 2**
    TOTAL: 4

N. 9. Shared meals: a.   4 3 ② 1
    Access food stores: b.   4 3 ② 1
    Resources: c. adequate   4 3 ② 1
    Meals eaten away   d.   4 3 ② 1   **#3,5**
      from home   *TOTAL:*   8

C. 10. Accessible
    support: available   a.   4 ③ 2 1
    Comfort in this   b.   4 ③ 2 1
    TOTAL: 6

A. 11. Daily employment*   a.   1 2 3 ④
    Adequate rest   b.   4 ③ 2 1
    Adequate sleep   c.   4 ③ 2 1   **#5,8**
    Leisure time self   d.   ④ 3 2 1
    Shared family   e.   4 3 ② 1
    Partner   f.   4 3 2 ①
    TOTAL: 17

P. 12. Family concerns: a. divorce   ① 2 3 4
    b. death   ① 2 3 4
    c. problem   **# 9**
      pregnancy   1 ② 3 4
    TOTAL: 4

    SUM TOTAL: 47   (out of 80)

*See type of work and hours employed from face sheet of RIM assessment tool (strenuous or full time employment can be added risk factor).

Psychological FANCAP

Concerns about:				A O S N	DIAGNOSIS

F. 13. Alcohol: use
- a. individual — 1 2 3 ④
- b. partner — 1 2 3 ④
- c. family — 1 2 ③ 4

Drugs: use
- d. individual — 1 2 3 ④
- e. partner — 1 2 3 ④
- f. family — 1 2 3 ④

TOTAL: *23*

A. 14. Smoking: use
- a. individual — 1 2 3 ④
- b. partner — ① 2 3 4
- c. family — ① 2 3 4

Drugs: use
- d. individual — 1 2 3 ④
- e. partner — 1 2 3 ④
- f. family — 1 2 3 ④

TOTAL: 14   #2

N. 15. Positive feelings: (weight gain)
- a. individual — 4 3 ② 1
- b. partner — 4 3 2 ①
- c. body image — 4 3 ② 1

TOTAL: *5*   #3

C. 16. Ease of shared communication
- a. health care providers — 4 3 ② 1
- b. partner — 4 3 2 ①
- c. family — 4 3 ② 1

TOTAL: *5*   #8

A. 17. Positive feelings:
- a. work/home* — 4 3 2 1
- a. school* — 4 3 2 ①
- b. sexual — 4 3 ② 1

Sleep:
- c. quality — 4 ③ 2 1

Problem with
- d. nightmares — 1 2 ③ 4

Relaxation:
- e. awareness — 4 3 2 ①

Participate
- f. individual — 4 3 2 ①
- g. partner — 4 3 2 ①
- h. family — 4 3 2 ①

TOTAL: 13   #7

P. 18. Recognize stress in life:
- a. awareness individual — 4 3 ② 1
- b. partner — 4 3 2 ①
- c. family — 4 3 ② 1

Available coping skills:
- d. individual — 4 3 ② 1
- e. partner — 4 3 2 ①
- f. family — 4 3 ② 1

TOTAL: 10   #5, 7, 9

SUM TOTAL: 72 (out of 128)

*May only score one.

Problem-Solving Style and Nursing Theory Choice

Doris J. Wiegand

"Nursing theory determines what goals are selected and what ways they are approached (Stevens, 1980, p. 3)." Every area of nursing practice, therefore, should contain an element of theory as the basis of nursing actions. Many nursing theories have been developed. The challenge now is to apply those theories to the practical realm. To do so some nurses may ask, "Where do you start?" "How do you begin?"

One approach may consist of finding out if a nursing theory does, in fact, exist prior to the formal introduction of the concept of nursing theory. To determine if such was the case, an investigation was undertaken to see if any threads of a nursing theory were present and operating in practice. The study had two parts. The first part was directed toward identifying nursing theory choice, and the second part related the nursing theory choice to problem-solving styles.

THE PROBLEM

Development of nursing theory in the nursing profession is in the beginning stages. Theories have been developed and are continuing to be developed. Some of these theories have been implemented into practice, education, and research. Nursing practice, however, has not implemented theory to the extent that education and research have. More awareness of nursing theory is needed in nursing practice before nursing theories will ever be able to be implemented.

Knowledge of the existence of nursing theories is present in the educational realm more than in the clinical practice realm. Education often bases a nursing curriculum on a nursing theory. As more nurses become educated through these systems that are based on nursing theory, knowledge of nursing theory will increase. There are many nurses in practice who never have been exposed to nursing theories in their education. This population includes nurses of all levels, from staff to top management. It is this group of nurses who have to be addressed in the efforts to increase the awareness of, and need for, theory-based nursing practice.

As the concepts of theory-based nursing practice become more of a reality, the profession of nursing will evolve into its own identity with clearer boundaries. Nursing as a profession, and nurses individually, must identify the basis of their existence. Clarity must be given to questions such as "What is nursing?" and "What prompts nursing actions?" The consequences of focusing on these questions will lead nursing in a more self-directed and independent path.

AN INVESTIGATION

Research Question

Despite the fact that nursing theories have not always been articulated, nursing has always been an integral aspect of life and of society. Commonalities, both conceptual and practical, have always existed in the delivery of care. The research question, therefore, is "Are there any threads of a nursing theory present and operating in the nursing department of a 300-bed general hospital in Western Pennsylvania?"

If any threads are identified, the results could be the basis for initiating the process of implementing a nursing theory in the nursing department of the hospital. Investigating this question could also increase the awareness among nurses that there are nursing theories, and emphasize the importance of theory-based practice.

At the end of the study a correlation would be made using the data of the study and using information about the problem-solving styles of the management group of that hospital. The purpose of this investigation was to see if there was any relationship between problem-solving style and choice of nursing theory.

Summary

Greater awareness and increased application of nursing theory in nursing departments is needed. Awareness is beginning, but only to a small extent. Threads of nursing theories may exist among nurses because nursing has always been an essential component of society. This study attempted to see if there were any threads present in the nursing department of a hospital, and if there was any relationship between problem-solving style and nursing theory choice. This activity may help to begin the process of implementing a nursing theory. It may increase the awareness of nursing theory and the importance of theory-based practice.

Some limitations of the study were that because nursing theory is a complex topic, it is difficult to summarize statements about the components of theory into brief statements and yet capture the essence of the content of the theory. Time is also a factor, and consideration has to be given to the population being studied. Statements about the topic have to be brief enough and clear enough that an unrealistic amount of time is not required for the collection of data. Theoretical topics are usually lengthy and complex, and they do not lend themselves to brevity.

Literature Review

In searching the literature, information was found about nursing theories in general. When the theories were critiqued efforts were given to the application of the theory to practice. Riehl and Roy (1980) and Riehl-Sisca (1985) have a considerable amount of information on how the various nursing theories relate to practice and how they could be implemented in community nursing, education, and in health care settings. There are also a few articles written in which a hospital nursing department actually applied a nursing theory in their hospital setting. Mastal, Hammond, and Roberts (1982) used a pilot study to apply the Roy model in one unit of a small community hospital. Capers et al (1985) implemented the Neuman Systems Model in the nursing department of a general hospital. Schmieding (1984) also implemented a nursing theory in a practice setting. The theory in this case was Orlando's theory. Finally, Orem's theory was initiated at Toronto General Hospital (Campbell, 1985). These four examples represent implementation of theory into a part of the structure of a nursing division. There were no studies found that addressed the relationship of problem-solving styles to the choice of nursing theory. The literature review is far from complete due to time restraints. There may be more information in the literature on this topic.

Research Design

Instrumentation

For this study, a questionnaire on nursing theories was developed. The purpose of the questionnaire was to identify if there were any threads of a nursing theory presently operating in a selected nursing department. The developed tool addressed four questions:

1. What is your definition of nursing?
2. What situations or events determine your nursing interventions?
3. What is your view or definition of person?
4. What does health mean to you?

There were seven responses to each of these four questions. Each forced-choice response represented an actual theorist as stated in Fitzpatrick and Whall's book *Conceptual Models of Nursing: Analysis and Application* (1983). An example of the questionnaire can be found in Appendix 38-A.

The names of the theorists were not included on the questionnaire, only statements of their answers to the four questions as given in Fitzpatrick and Whall. In choosing the specific responses to the questions, an emphasis was placed on statements that were relatively brief so that the questionnaire would not be too lengthy. The investigator and two other nurse researchers made the final choice of statements to use in the questionnaire. The result was that the seven nurse theorists selected were King, Levine, Neuman, Nightingale, Orem, Orlando, and Roy.

Directions on the questionnaire indicated that for each of the four questions, the participants were to order by rank their choices from 1 to 7, with 1 being the most favored response and 7 the least favored. If none of the responses were chosen, the participants were directed to mark "other" with an X and give an explanation in the space provided for comments. This approach was taken because only seven theorists were chosen and because there are many more than seven, the participants' added viewpoints might reflect the thinking of other theorists and could be tracked if sufficient in number.

Responses of specific theorists were not always assigned the same letter in each question. This was done intentionally so that participants would not choose answers by letter if they saw a pattern. Emphasis was placed on the fact that the choices reflected personal opinion, and that there were no right or wrong answers. The participants were requested to identify themselves by name and by nursing area so that commonalities could be made.

The responses to the questions were rated from 1 to 7. Because there were 7 choices, the first choice was given 7 points and the last choice was given 1 point. See Tables 38–1 and 38–2 for examples.

Method

A 300-bed general hospital in western Pennsylvania was selected for data-collection purposes. Prior to distribution, the questionnaire was given to two nurses from staff development. They were asked to give feedback on clarity of information and directions, and on the length of time needed to complete it. Their critique was that it was clear and that it took approximately 20 to 30 minutes to finish.

TABLE 38–1. NUMERICAL VALUE OF RATED RESPONSE

Choice Number	Weighted Value
1	7 points
2	6 points
3	5 points
4	4 points
5	3 points
6	2 points
7	1 point

TABLE 38-2. COMPLETED RESPONSES AND THEIR NUMERICAL VALUES

Response	Weighted Value
A. 5	3 points
B. 2	6 points
C. 4	4 points
D. 1	7 points
E. 6	2 points
F. 3	5 points
G. 7	1 point

Following this, the questionnaire was given first to each member of the nursing management group individually by the investigator. The purpose of this was to emphasize the importance of the study and to respond to any question that any of them might have. It was felt that if the management people understood the purpose and significance of the study, they would support the research efforts and communicate that support to the staff.

After the nursing management group completed the questionnaire the head nurses were given enough questionnaires for each part-time and full-time registered nurse on their area. They were responsible for distributing them to the staff and having them returned within 2 weeks. At the end of 2 weeks, the questionnaires were obtained from the nursing areas. A total of 225 questionnaires were distributed, and 131 (58 percent) were returned.

As the questionnaires were received they were given a number and kept in the category of their nursing area. Files were established for each nursing unit. In each file a data-collection sheet was used. The seven nurse theorists were identified on the data-collection sheet. Each question was tallied separately. The numerical values were then tallied for the four questions for each nurse theorist. Finally, each of the nursing area results were combined for the total population responses (*see* Table 38–3).

Data Analysis

The data obtained from the questionnaire showed that the Neuman model had the greatest number of points. This pattern was true of the whole research population except for pediatrics and the recovery room. Pediatrics choose Roy first, with 57 points, and Neuman second, with 56 points. The recovery room chose Orlando first with 83 points, Roy next with 79 points, and then Neuman with 77 points.

The Neuman theory totaled 2735 points. This represents 19.4 percent of the total responses. The choice that followed Neuman was Roy, with 2315 points or 16.4 percent. Table 38–4 indicates the total points of each of the nursing theorists and the corresponding percentage.

TABLE 38-3. TOTAL RESPONSES OF ALL NURSING AREAS: NURSING THEORY QUESTIONNAIRE

Area	All RN's						
	Nightingale	*Orlando*	*Levine*	*Orem*	*Roy*	*Neuman*	*King*
Management							
Total	268	366	407	328	482	520	394
Return	96.15%						
Med-Surg							
Area #1	126	162	157	124	176	183	136
Area #2	42	52	63	55	79	115	70
Area #3	67	105	102	89	113	161	108
Area #4	118	132	152	123	164	188	133
Area #5	74	98	92	74	98	132	86
Area #6	33	35	25	28	32	47	24
Area #7	140	219	182	180	257	290	189
Area #8	28	46	44	46	56	65	51
Total	628	849	817	719	975	1181	797
Return	62.50%						
Critcal Care							
ICU/CCU	83	104	127	96	166	175	141
Emer.	62	82	70	59	75	106	50
Telem.	96	104	133	103	125	160	122
Total	241	290	330	258	366	441	313
Return	31.43%						
Maternal/Child							
OB	103	154	127	133	157	200	131
PEDS	31	49	51	38	57	56	50
Total	134	203	178	171	214	256	181
Return	54.55%						
Surgery							
OR	120	150	145	122	142	197	118
Recovery	62	83	56	49	79	77	42
Amb.	39	43	53	40	57	63	43
Total	221	276	254	211	278	337	203
Return	89.47%						
Total % Return	58.22%						
Total Responses	1492	1984	1986	1687	2315	2735	1888

TABLE 38-4. NURSING THEORISTS' TOTAL POINTS AND PERCENTAGE

Theorist	Type	Points	Percent
Neuman	Systems	2735	19.4
Roy	Systems	2315	16.4
Orlando	Interactional	1984	14.1
Levine	Interactional	1986	14.1
King	Systems	1888	13.4
Orem	Interactional	1687	12
Nightingale	Developmental	1492	10.6

The data were than converted into three broad categories as recommended by Riehl and Roy (1980). The categories were developmental, interactional and systems theories. Developmental theory included Nightingale. Interactional theories included Orlando, Levine, and Orem. Systems theories included Roy, Neuman, and King. The results showed that the responses favored the systems theories with 49 percent, the interaction theories with 40 percent, and the developmental theories, 11 percent. The developmental theory category, however, contained only one theorist, whereas the systems category and the interactional category each had three theorists represented in the group.

Comments were also given. Many of the comments revolved around the statement by Nightingale that nursing is a profession for women. Eight of the respondants disagreed with the statment because men are also a part of the profession. A summary of other comments can be seen in Table 38-5.

Finally, one more topic that deserves comment is the percent of return. In Table 38-3, the total responses were divided into the categories of management, medical-surgical, critical care, maternal-child, and surgery. Specific units under each category can be seen there. Management had a 96 percent return rate, surgery a 90 percent return, medical-surgical a 63 percent return, and maternal-child a 56 percent return. However, critical care had only a 31 percent return. Critical care consists of ICU/CCU, telemetry, and the emergency room. Telemetry is half medical-surgical. Telemetry's return was 56 percent. ICU/CCU's response was 23 percent, and emergency room response was 26 percent. Telemetry falls closer to medical-surgical responses. ICU/CCU and emergency room were the low responders.

Critical care nurses, especially ICU/CCU and emergency room nurses, can relate strongly to the medical model. Often times their concern and priority is the medical problem and the technical aspects of a patient's care. Sometimes this cannot be avoided. However, when nursing concerns revolve around the medical model, nursing theories become confusing and nursing boundaries are difficult to define. Possibly the critical care nurses did not appreciate the significance of nursing theory, or could not relate to it, and therefore, did not re-

TABLE 38–5. QUESTIONNAIRE COMMENTS

Area	Question	Comment
Rehab	1—What is nursing?	Caring!
Management	1—What is nursing?	Compassion, understanding, and empathy
	1—What is nursing?	Should include preventative measures
Medical-Surgical	2—Nursing Actions	Response "a"—in some cases patients cannot set goals or communicate
	3—What is a person?	Response "g"—makes a person sound like a microbe!
	3—What is a person?	Response "g"—may define patient but not person
	4—What is health?	Response "b"—some people are poor physically but have healthy attitudes; thus they are healthier than those with physical problems
Operating Room	Other	Being created by God with spiritual needs as well as physical, psycho-social, and economic needs

spond. Further research into this possible relationship and a follow-up as to the reasons for the low percent response might be interesting.

In summary, when viewed by categories, systems theories had the highest response, with 49 percent. The interactional theories were second with 40 percent. Developmental theories were last with 11 percent. However, there was not the same balance of choices for the developmental theories as there were for the other two categories. This is a criticism of the study. In future studies it would be advisable to equalize the number of choices for each of the three categories, or in the analysis of the data to weigh the top three priority responses. This was not done in this part of the study but was done in the next, as will now be described.

PROBLEM-SOLVING STYLE AND NURSING THEORY

In the same hospital setting another relationship was tested. The management group of the nursing department was given a questionnaire based on Jung's theory of problem-solving. This theory focuses on how individuals gather information and how they evaluate information from the world around them (Hellriegel, Slocum, & Woodman, 1983). Individuals perceive the world either by sensation or by intuition, and they respond to their perceptions, or reach decisions, by thinking or feeling. Individuals are a combination of these types. Everyone has each type to some degree; however, a dominent characteristic usually exists for perceiving the environment—that is, sensation or intuition—and a dominent characteristic for responding to those perceptions—thinking or feeling.

Those who perceive their environment by sensation gather information through their senses. The information that they collect is very concrete; that is, it is information that can be processed through the senses. Sensation-type personalities are pragmatic people. Their time focus is in the present, and they work better with what they can actually see.

The intuitive type, which is the other approach to perception, is characterized by the use of imagination. This personality type perceives the world around them in terms of possibilities. They are the dreamers, the idealists, the entrepreneurs. These people are future-oriented. They see the world in terms of ideas, concepts, and long-range plans.

Feeling-type people approach decision making with human interaction as an emphasis. Feelings and emotions have a high priority. They are empathetic, probing people who are very good at drawing out the feelings of others. Thinking types, on the other hand, respond to their environment through logic, organization, analysis, and systematic inquiry. They are effective communicators who weigh alternatives and who are objective, rational, and analytical.

There is a lot of information in the literature on Jung's theory of problem-solving. The information discussed above is by no means comprehensive. It is included only to provide a brief definition of the terms. The purpose of this study was to investigate whether problem-solving styles had any relationship to the choice of a nursing theory. In this study the same results of the questionnaire on nursing theory were used.

Method and Treatment of Data

The management group of the nursing department was given a modified version of the Myers-Briggs type indicator, which is a test that identifies personality types according to Jung's theory (Briggs & Myers, 1962). The results were tallied and each person was identified as either sensation (S) or intuition (N), and, as thinking (T) or feeling (F). Four groups then existed: sensation-feeling (SF), sensation-thinking (ST), intuition-feeling (NF), and intuition-thinking (NT). The groups were then classified according to their choice of specific nurse theorists, and according to their choice of broad nursing theory categories of developmental, interactional and systems theory. Table 38–6 shows the relationship of problem-solving style to the choice of specific nurse theorists, and Table 38–7 shows the relationship of problem-solving style to the broad nursing theory categories. The numerical values from the nursing theory questionnaire were tallied for each person in each personality type (SF, ST, NF, and NT). These values were tallied for both the choice of a specific nurse theorist and for the broad nursing theory categories and a mean score was obtained.

TABLE 38-6. SPECIFIC NURSE THEORISTS CHOICES FROM THE QUESTIONNAIRE: RELATIONSHIP OF PROBLEM-SOLVING STYLE TO NURSING THEORY

Name	Nightingale	Orlando	Levine	Orem	Roy	Neuman	King
			Sensation-Feeling				
Rita	6	17	11	9	25	23	21
Kathy	10	15	18	10	22	23	14
Debbie	17	15	15	14	14	20	17
Karen	2	0	12	14	21	18	13
Barb	10	19	18	11	19	23	12
Roberta	14	26	14	14	16	17	11
Kim	13	14	18	14	18	21	14
Tammy	10	20	18	12	17	23	12
Josie	11	18	16	11	19	24	13
Judy	16	18	12	14	19	20	13
Mean	**11**	**16**	**15**	**12**	**19**	**21**	**14**
			Sensation-Thinking				
Terry	11	18	13	15	17	22	16
Anne	7	11	20	12	24	18	20
Mary	6	13	14	12	19	26	22
Susan	15	15	17	12	22	18	13
Betty	10	11	18	18	19	20	16
Fran	12	10	16	14	23	16	21
Jane	12	16	16	11	19	21	17
Mean	**10**	**13**	**16**	**13**	**20**	**20**	**18**
			Intuition-Feeling				
Sara	7	12	14	19	26	20	14
Nancy	21	10	21	14	12	23	11
Elizabeth	9	13	21	13	20	20	16
Janet	9	13	22	10	16	19	20
Heather	7	11	18	13	22	22	19
Mean	**11**	**12**	**19**	**14**	**19**	**21**	**16**
			Intuition-Thinking				
Pat	7	16	18	13	24	22	12
Audrey	12	20	17	12	16	20	15
Mean	**10**	**18**	**18**	**13**	**20**	**21**	**14**

TABLE 38–7. BROAD NURSING THEORY CHOICES FROM THE QUESTIONNAIRE: RELATIONSHIP OF PROBLEM-SOLVING STYLE TO NURSING THEORY

Name	Sensation-Feeling		
	Developmental	*Interaction*	*Systems*
Kathy	19	75	102
Rita	9	25	50
Debbie	6	8	14
Judy	2	13	13
Roberta	8	30	38
Tammy	24	87	109
Barb	7	23	46
Josie	12	59	69
Karen	14	48	78
Kim	8	33	40
Mean	**11**	**40**	**56**

Name	Sensation-Thinking		
	Developmental	*Interaction*	*Systems*
Terry	24	79	93
Anne	13	22	21
Mary	14	54	44
Susan	9	55	48
Betty	7	45	60
Fran	0	7	13
Jane	12	43	57
Mean	**11**	**44**	**48**

Name	Intuition-Feeling		
	Developmental	*Interaction*	*Systems*
Heather	2	12	14
Elizabeth	8	31	42
Nancy	26	65	77
Kathy	7	33	44
Janet	8	23	25
Mean	**10**	**33**	**40**

Name	Intuition-Thinking		
	Developmental	*Interaction*	*Systems*
Pat	7	47	58
Audrey	12	49	51
Mean	**10**	**48**	**55**

The mean scores of the data did not seem to show any significant patterns or relationships. Therefore a further step was added. The three highest choices for each participant were chosen. Each choice was given a numerical value. The first choice was given 30 points, the second 20 points, and the third 10 points. An example can be seen in Table 38–8, case one. In some cases the numerical values of the three highest choices were the same. In Table 38–8, case two, King and Nightingale had the same numerical values from the nursing theory questionnaire results. They were both considered the second choice and each was given 10 points. Another example is case three. In this instance, Orlando, Orem, and King were chosen for the third choice. The total points that were to be alloted were 10 and each received 3.3 points. After all the points were distributed and tallied, a mean score was then obtained for each nurse theorist in each of the personality types, as seen in Table 38–9 and for each of the broad nursing theory categories, as seen in Table 38–10.

Data Analysis

As seen in the first part of the study, systems theory had the highest response. Interactional theories had the next highest response, and developmental the

TABLE 38–8. POINT VALUE FOR PRIORITY CHOICES OF NURSE THEORISTS

Case #1

Priority	Nurse Theorist	Points Given
1st	Orlando	30
2nd	Neuman	20
3rd	Roy	10

Case #2

Priority	Nurse Theorist	Points Given
1st	Neuman	30
2nd	King	10
2nd	Nightingale	10
3rd	Orlando	5
3rd	Levine	5

Case #3

Priority	Nurse Theorist	Points Given
1st	Neuman	30
2nd	Roy	10
2nd	Levine	10
3rd	Orland	3.3
3rd	Orem	3.3
3rd	King	3.3

TABLE 38-9. PRIORITY CHOICES FOR SPECIFIC NURSE THEORISTS: RELATIONSHIP OF PROBLEM-SOLVING STYLE TO NURSING THEORY

Sensation-Feeling

Name	Nightingale	Orlando	Levine	Orem	Roy	Neuman	King
Rita					30	20	10
Kathy			10		20	30	
Debbie	10	5	5			30	10
Karen					30	20	10
Barb		10	10		10	30	
Roberta		30			10	20	
Kim		3.3	10	3.3	10	30	3.3
Tammy		20	10			30	
Josie		10			20	30	
Judy		10			20	30	
Mean	**1**	**8.83**	**4.5**	**0.33**	**15**	**27**	**3.33**

Sensation-Thinking

Name	Nightingale	Orlando	Levine	Orem	Roy	Neuman	King
Terry		20			10	30	
Anne		10	10		30		10
Mary					10	30	20
Susan			10		30	20	
Betty			5	5	20	30	
Fran			5		30	5	20
Jane					20	30	10
Mean	**0**	**4.2857**	**4.286**	**0.71**	**21**	**20.71**	**8.57**

Intuition-Feeling

Name	Nightingale	Orlando	Levine	Orem	Roy	Neuman	King
Sara				10	30	20	
Nancy	20		10			30	
Elizabeth			30		10	10	10
Janet			30			10	20
Heather			10		15	15	20
Mean	**4**	**0**	**16**	**2**	**11**	**17**	**10**

Intuition-Thinking

Name	Nightingale	Orlando	Levine	Orem	Roy	Neuman	King
Pat			10		30	20	
Audrey		15	20		10	15	
Mean	**0**	**8**	**15**	**0**	**20**	**18**	**0**

TABLE 38–10. PRIORITY CHOICES FOR BROAD NURSING THEORY CATEGORIES: RELATIONSHIP OF PROBLEM-SOLVING STYLE TO NURSING THEORY

Sensation-Feeling

Name	Developmental		Interaction		Systems	
Rita	0		0		60	
Kathy	0		10		50	
Debbie	10		10		40	
Karen	0		0		60	
Barb	0		20		40	
Roberta	0		30		30	
Kim	0		16.6		43.3	
Tammy	0		30		30	
Josie	0		10		50	
Judy	0		10		50	
Mean	**1.00**	**2%**	**13.66**	**23%**	**45.33**	**76%**

Sensation-Thinking

Name	Developmental		Interaction		Systems	
Terry	0		20		40	
Anne	0		20		40	
Mary	0		0		60	
Susan	0		10		50	
Betty	0		10		50	
Fran	0		5		55	
Jane	0		0		60	
Mean	**0.00**	**0%**	**9.29**	**15%**	**50.71**	**85%**

Intuition-Feeling

Name	Developmental		Interaction		Systems	
Sara	0		10		50	
Nancy	20		10		30	
Elizabeth	0		30		30	
Janet	0		30		30	
Heather	0		10		50	
Mean	**4**	**7%**	**18**	**30%**	**38**	**63%**

Intuition-Thinking

Name	Developmental		Interaction		Systems	
Pat	0		10		50	
Audrey	0		35		25	
Mean	**0**	**0%**	**22.5**	**38%**	**37.5**	**63%**

lowest; but developmental was only represented by one nurse theorist, and, as was stated previously, that was a limitation of the study.

When a mean score was obtained using all the points given to the seven theorists as seen in Table 38–6, no significant pattern evolved, nor did one evolve in Table 38–7 when the broad categories were used. However, when the priority method was used, relationships did exist between the data on the broad categories.

The sensation-feeling (SF) and sensation-thinking (ST) groups showed a strong preference for systems theory. The mean score for the SF group for systems theory was 45.3 (76 percent) of the participants' first three choices. For the ST group, the mean score for systems theory was 50.71 (85 percent). Together, the SF/ST problem-solving approach represented an 80 percent preference for systems theory. In the SF group, 13.66 (23 percent) used an interaction approach whereas 9.29 (15 percent) of the interactionalists were in the ST group. Together, this represented 19 percent of the problem solvers who utilized the interactional method in their approach to patient care. In the combined SF/ST group, only 1 percent favored developmental nursing theory in this study.

On the other hand, even though intuition-feeling (NF) and the intuition-thinking (NT) groups chose systems theory first, they did not show the same strong preference for systems theory as did the SF/ST group. Together and separately, the mean score for the NF/NT system group was 63 percent. For the NF/NT interaction group, the mean score was 34 percent, with 30 percent and 38 percent given respectively. Finally, there was a mean of 4 (7 percent) in the NF developmental group, and none in the NT developmental group.

Conclusion

The data pointed to the fact that systems theory was chosen more often by the nurses in this hospital setting. Personality types, however, seem to make a difference in the weight of the emphasis in systems theory. It seems from the results that the sensation type and the thinking type would strongly choose a systems approach because they both are practical, analytical, and rational. Because of these characteristics it is not surprising that they might choose a theory that has categories, compartments, and boundaries to it. On the other hand, the feeling type would probably move toward a theoretical approach that was more people- and relationship-oriented. They may have an appreciation for a developmental approach or an interactional approach. The intuitive type also may prefer developmental or interaction approaches because they see the world around them broadly and in terms or concepts, ideas, and long-range plans. They may not choose to fit into the structure of a systems approach.

Again, in this study, systems was the most frequent choice from the nurses in a hospital setting. This may be related to the fact that nursing in a hospital is structured, by necessity. It would be interesting in the future to explore other components of nursing to see if the same results surface. Also, age, experience, and education are factors that may influence the problem-solving styles and the choice of nursing theory, and these areas should be researched as well.

REFERENCES

Briggs, K., & Myers, I. (1962). *The Myers-Briggs type indicator.* Princeton: Educational Testing Service.

Campbell, C. (1984, October). Orem's story. *Nursing Mirror, 159*(13), 28–30.

Capers, C., O'Brian, C., Quinn, R., et al. (1985, May). The Neuman System Model in practice: Planning phase. *Journal of Nursing Administration, 15*(5), pp. 29–38.

Fitzpatrick, J., & Whall, A. L. (1983). *Conceptual models of nursing: Analysis and application.* Bowie, MD: Brady.

Hellriegel, D., Slocum, J., & Woodman, R. (1983). *Organizational behavior* (3rd ed.). New York: West Publishing.

Mastal, M., Hammond, H., & Roberts, M. (1982, June). Theory in hospital practice: A pilot implementation. *Journal of Nursing Administration, 12*, 9–15.

Riehl, J., & Roy, C. (1980). *Conceptual models for nursing practice* (2nd ed.). East Norwalk, CT: Appleton-Century-Crofts.

Riehl-Sisca, J. (1985). *The science and art of self-care.* East Norwalk, CT: Appleton-Century-Crofts.

Schmieding, N. (1984, June). Putting Orlando's theory into practice. *American Journal of Nursing, 6*, 759–761.

Stevens, B. (1980). *The nurse as executive.* Rockville, MD: Aspen.

Appendix 38-A _____

Nursing Theory Questionnaire

The following is a questionnaire on nursing theory. The purpose of the questionnaire is to identify if there are any threads of a nursing theory or theories presently operating in the nursing department of your hospital. All registered nurses are asked to participate.

In the questionnaire you will find four questions: What is your definition of nursing? What situations or events determine your nursing interventions? What is your view or definition of "person"? What does health mean to you? Each of the questions has seven responses. These are responses of seven actual theorists as stated in the book *Conceptual Models of Nursing: Analysis and Application* by Joyce Fitzpatrick and Ann Whall (1983). Please read the choices and rate them according to how you personally would respond to the questions. More specific directions will appear below. In answering the questionnaire there are no "right" or "wrong" answers.

The seven theorist's responses were arbitrarily chosen. There are, however, more than seven nurse theorists. If you would respond differently than any of the stated choices, your response may reflect another theorist, so please state your ideas in the designated areas for comments.

It would be appreciated if you would identify yourself by name and by your nursing area so that commonalities can be identified.

Results of the study will be given to the nursing department when the study is completed.

Thank you for participating.

Doris J. Wiegand, RN, MS. C.

DIRECTIONS: The following questions have choices from A to G. Please rate your responses to the choices with numbers from 1 to 7, with 1 being the most favored response and 7 the least favored. If you do not choose any of the responses mark "other" with an *X*. If you choose "other" please explain. Feel free to comment if there are other responses to the statements that you would like to make.

1. WHAT IS YOUR DEFINITION OF NURSING?

_____ A. Nursing is a unique profession concerned with the total person, that is, all the variables affecting an individual's response to stressors.

_____ B. Human interaction; incorporates scientific principles in the use of the nursing process.

_____ C. A profession for women, the goal of which is to discover and use nature's laws governing health in the service of humanity.

_____ D. A process of analyses and action related to the care of the ill or potentially ill person.

_____ E. Interaction with a patient who has a need, involving patient validation with both the need and the help provided, in order to improve the patient's health.

_____ F. The process of human interaction between nurse and client.

_____ G. A human service designed to overcome human limitations in self-care action for health related reasons.

_____ OTHER

COMMENTS:

2. WHAT SITUATIONS OR EVENTS DETERMINE YOUR NURSING INTERVENTIONS?

_____ A. Nurse and client perceive each other and the situation, communicate information, mutually set goals, and take action to attain goals.

_____ B. Holostic care individualized to each person's needs; nurse supports the person's adaptation.

_____ C. To put the person in the best condition for nature to restore or preserve health, and to prevent or cure disease and injury.

_____ D. The formal object of nursing practice rests with the inabilities of individuals to engage in self-care because of health or health-related reasons.

_____ E. Patient needs determine nursing actions.

_____ F. Nursing activity derives from the model which prescribes a process of assessment and intervention. Nursing intervention is carried out within the context of the nursing process and involves manipulation of stimuli.

_____ G. The nurse is seen as the "actor" or intervener who attempts to reduce an individual's encounter with certain stressors or attempts to minimize the effect of certain stressors.

_____ OTHER

COMMENTS:

3. WHAT IS YOUR VIEW OR DEFINITION OF "PERSON"?

_____ A. Complex individual in interaction with internal and external environment.

_____ B. A bio-psycho-social being in constant interaction with a changing environment. The person is an open, adaptive system.

_____ C. Man is a integrated whole, functioning biologically, symbolically, and socially.

_____ D. A person is a physiological, psychological, sociocultural, and developmental being. The person must be viewed as a whole; the wholeness concept is related to the dynamic interrelationship of variables.

_____ E. Comprised of physical, intellectual, and metaphysical attributes and potentialities.

_____ F. A open system exhibiting permeable boundaries permitting an exchange of matter, energy, and information with the environment.

_____ G. Behaving human organism: (patients) are persons under medical supervision or treatment.

_____ OTHER

COMMENTS:

4. WHAT DOES "HEALTH" MEAN TO YOU?

_____ A. A person's health is a state of wellness or illness which is determined by the four variables: physiological, psychological, sociocultural, and developmental. Health is relative and in a dynamic state of flux.

_____ B. Free of disease and to be able to use one's own power to the fullest.

_____ C. A state of wholeness or integrity of the individual.

_____ D. The health-illness continuum is a continuous line representing states of degrees of health or illness that a person might experience at a given time. Health-illness is an inevitable dimension of the person's life (example of continuum: "illness _____ wellness").

_____ E. Man seeking a balance between disease and health in order to be a "whole" person.

_____ F. Mental and physical comfort, sense of adequacy and well-being.

_____ G. Dynamic adjustment to stressors in the internal and external environment through optimum uses of resources to achieve maximum potential for daily living.

_____ OTHER

COMMENTS:

NAME _____   NURSING AREA _____

Self-Concept of the Child with Diabetes:

Its Relationship to Control of Blood Glucose

Linda R. Stumpf

Middle childhood spans the years 6 through 12 and has been described as a period of latency and sexual tranquility, a contrast to the early years of rapid growth and development and also to prepubescence and adolescence. According to Whaley and Wong (1979) it has now been found that the middle childhood period contributes greatly to one's sociocultural achievements and self-concept development—that is, one's personality.

Self-concept is formed as a result of environmental feedback to the child about bodily appearance and behavior. The child appraises the information and reacts to self and others, and through these actions the personality of the individual can be assessed.

A healthy child can have a difficult time during this period of life, but a child with a defect must contend with an additional burden, especially in the development of the self-concept.

The child with diabetes mellitus does not have an obvious handicap but the condition is life threatening if not treated with dietary adherence and daily injections of insulin.

Most children that are diagnosed as having diabetes mellitus are 12 years of age or younger and in the middle childhood period, a critical time in the formation of self-concept.

The child with diabetes mellitus between the ages of 6 and 12 years has a twofold task to accomplish. Normal maturation—a growth process for that age range—and diabetes management must be achieved. The latter task ranks equally important with the first in that the quality of a diabetic's life greatly depends on the degree of control exercised over the diabetic condition. The person with diabetes strives to avoid long-term complications that may surface in later years and greatly reduce the life span of the individual.

Literature Review

Diabetes mellitus occurs when the endocrine portion of the pancreas, called the Islets of Langerhans, no longer produces insulin. Glucose molecules remain in the blood instead of entering the cells of the body, thus causing the blood glucose measurement to rise. The nondiabetic blood glucose level is between 80 and 120 mg/dl whereas the accepted blood glucose range for the diabetic person is 80 to 180 mg/dl. Children with diabetes can monitor their daily blood glucose levels using a home monitoring device or by having a glycosylated hemoglobin test drawn every 3 months. The latter test is also known as the hemoglobin A_{1c} ($HgbA_{1c}$). The fraction of the hemoglobin called $HgbA_{1c}$ is hemoglobin that has combined with glucose on the A_{1c} fraction of the red blood cell. The $HgbA_{1c}$ level changes slowly over a period of several weeks rather than fluctuating like the daily blood sugar level. Because a red blood cell's life span is approximately 120 days, the $HgbA_{1c}$ reading will reflect a 3-month history of blood glucose control. This measurement cannot be altered by fasting before the blood test is drawn.

Diabetes mellitus is treated by balancing diet, exercise, and insulin injections with blood glucose levels. Each person's treatment regimen must be tailored to the individual's needs so that blood glucose control is achieved. The diets used for diabetes are basically all low in carbohydrate content. This means that the intake of sugars and starches is drastically reduced, and therefore so are desserts, snacks, and many other sugar-sweetened food products. It is also important that the diet is appropriately balanced between fats, proteins, and carbohydrates. Foods can then be most advantageously metabolized without an unusual rise in the blood glucose.

The treatment for diabetes—insulin, diet, and exercise—can be life threatening if not used correctly. Control of diabetes and its therapeutic modalities are complex tasks to master, especially for a child.

There is a paucity of literature about the child with diabetes in the middle childhood stage. The school age child with "the ugly duckling" appearance develops ideas about his or her body image from environmental feedback of parents and friends. Van der Velde (1985) states that body images serve as mental outlines for social behavior, thus forming the foundation for self-concept. He further contends that the personality develops during the first 12 years of life and influences individual behaviors and personality traits displayed in adulthood.

Johnson and Rosenbloom (1982) discovered that in some children during childhood and adolescence the feelings of being "different" resulted in lowered self-esteem. Research by Sullivan (1979) and Bennett (1978) suggests that diabetes and its management affect the childrens' self-esteem, their relationship with family and friends, and their performance in school.

When a child is diagnosed with diabetes mellitus there is an impact on each family member. Johnson and Rosenbloom (1982) found a relationship between behavior and diabetes control in a group of childhood and adolescent diabetic children. Better control occurred in children with stable families, low-stress environments, low anxiety levels in parent, and little interpersonal conflict between parents and child. Minuchin et. al. (1975, 1978) demonstrated a positive correlation in a functional family pattern, low stress, and diabetes control.

Swift, Seidman, and Stein (1966) compared 50 juvenile diabetics with 50 matched controls and found that an adequate self-concept was related to good control. The poorer the self-concept, the worse the diabetes control.

The literature supports the view that the formation of a child's self-concept develops from experiences and interactions with others that are internalized and integrated as part of the concept. The resulting behavior of a child with diabetes in terms of successful management indicates that a desirable self-concept has been formed.

The Riehl Interaction Model, an evolving nursing theory, provided the framework for this study (Riehl, 1980). The foundation for Riehl's model is symbolic interactionism, a psycho-social approach to self-concept theory (Wells & Marwell, 1976). A basic premise is that self-concept is the key element between behavior and the social organization to which the individual belongs. In this study the behavior was the child's management of the diabetes and the social organization was the family.

Implicit in Riehl's model are the concepts of role, communication, locus of control, and change. The role of the patient and family, the nurse, and the sub-concepts of role relationship and role-taking are identified at every level of Riehl's model. Role-taking is used by the nurse and encouraged to be used by the patient and family members so that each may understand the position of the other.

Learning takes place through communication. Words, symbols, and bodily gestures are all means of communication through which people learn many meanings and values that guide their behavior. Communication skills are necessary to teach clients in all levels of Riehl's model as change is achieved.

The movement from an external locus of control to one of internal control is the major change identified in the model. As the process of change is evolving, roles are changing and role relationships are altered. Ultimately, the locus of control resides in the patient or family and the nurse's role is one of a support person.

The child and family have a problem when confronted with the diagnosis of diabetes mellitus, and are dependent on the health care provider, in this case the nurse. The nurse, first as health care provider and then as educator, is the primary source of the external locus of control. Moreover, the nurse provides care for the child, problem solving for the family, and assistance with the development of appropriate adjustment and coping mechanisms.

The patient and family continue to learn about the management of the diabetes, which includes the medical aspect and the daily activities of regular exercise and diet control. As they become knowledgeable and more comfortable with the condition the blood glucose can usually be regulated within an acceptable range of control. The nurse then moves to a consulting role, facilitating the shift of the locus of control from an external source to the internal source, where control resides within the patient and family. In the process, the patient and family begin to perceive their ability to control the diabetes and direct their lives. Ultimately, the patient and family will be able to set and achieve their own short- and long-range goals, which include daily and life-long diabetes management with the support of the nurse. At this point the nurse remains a friend and advocate to clients who have reached an optimal level of function.

Internal locus of control occurs with the formation of an adequate self-concept. It is at this stage that control of the blood glucose is usually achieved. The literature supports this observation with studies of adolescents that correlate self-concept and diabetes control. It has been revealed that an adequate self-concept is usually found in adolescents with acceptable blood glucose results, but there is a scarcity of information about the middle childhood stage. This study addresses this age group and the issue of whether there is a relationship between self-concept and blood glucose control.

Study Purpose

The purpose of this study was to investigate the self-concept of children with diabetes in the age range of 8 to 12 years to determine if an adequate self-concept has been formed, and if the condition has been accepted by the child as demonstrated by acceptable blood glucose control. A hypothesis was developed, which stated that there would be a positive correlation between an adequate self-concept and acceptance of the diabetic condition, as evidenced by acceptable blood glucose control in children with diabetes.

Definition of Terms

CHILD WITH DIABETES: A child, regardless of sex, between the ages of 8 and 12 years, with diabetes mellitus for at least 6 months.

SELF-CONCEPT: The view one holds of self as a result of real-life experiences with others.

ADEQUATE SELF-CONCEPT: A child with diabetes obtaining a raw score between 45 and 55 on the Piers-Harris children's self-concept scale.

ACCEPTANCE OF THE DIABETIC CONDITION: A child with diabetes having a hemoglobin $_{A1c}$ within the range of 8 to 12 in the 6 months prior to the self-concept testing.

POSITIVE CORRELATION: A relationship between the self-concept and blood glucose control such that as one increases so does the other.

ACCEPTABLE BLOOD GLUCOSE CONTROL: The amount of glucose contained in the blood of a child with diabetes as measured by the $HgbA_{1c}$ test. The accepted range of control measurement for the $HgbA_{1c}$:

- < 7.0 Nondiabetic range.
- 8–10.9 Excellent glucose control.
- 11–12.9 Fair glucose control.
- > 13.0 Poor glucose control.

Research Design

The research design of this investigation was a type of interrelational study called a correlational study. According to LoBiondo-Wood and Haber (1986) the correlational design is employed when trying to determine if a change in one variable results in a related change in the other variable. The principal interest in this design was quantifying the strength of the relationship between the variables.

In this study the independent variable (X) was the self-concept scores and the dependent variable (Y) was the blood glucose results. The intent of this investigation was to test the hypothesis, which states that there is a positive correlation between an adequate self-concept and acceptance of the diabetic condition as evidenced by acceptable blood sugar control in diabetic children.

Study Sample

A convenience sample was used in this study. The sample of volunteers consited of a group of diabetic children, male and female, between the ages of 8 and 12 years who had been diagnosed with diabetes for a period of longer than 6 months. This criteria was chosen to eliminate the newly diagnosed child who may not be insulin regulated and could still be undergoing daily or weekly dosage adjustments. Also, a $HgbA_{1c}$ test during the first 6 months could reflect the high blood sugar from the months before the diagnosis of diabetes was made and the treatment initiated. The reading would not be representative of the child's control of his or her condition at the time of the study.

Any diabetic child meeting the specified criteria was encouraged to participate in order to secure a sample of at least 30 children. The sample under study was obtained using three approaches. First, the researcher made personal contact with families attending diabetic support group meetings. Second, referrals from nurses, families of children with diabetes, and physicians were obtained. Third, phone calls to families were made to solicit participation in the project.

Permission from parents or guardians was obtained on a prepared form before the child could participate. The most recent $HgbA_{1c}$ test result within the previous 6 months was recorded on the permission slip.

Setting

The setting for the study was rural and urban areas of southwestern Pennsylvania covering a 100-mile area in all. Diabetic self-help and support groups, clinics, physicians, and seminars held in this area were considered as sources of potential candidates. Private physician offices were avoided; however, on one occasion a child was administered the self-concept scale in a private office at the mother's request. Permission of the physician was obtained beforehand to administer the test. Individual homes were also the setting of several testings. Appointments for these sessions were scheduled in advance at a mutually agreeable time. Although contact was made with many people, only 24 of the children met criteria for the investigation.

On two occasions a group of children was given the self-concept scale, but the number of participants did not exceed 5. All other testing was conducted on an individual basis.

The Piers-Harris self-concept scale was administered to the participants by the researcher to avoid inconsistency in providing directions or other variables that might influence the testing situation. The same introductory paragraph was read to each child before the scale was administered. The children read the statements and responded to them, except on three occasions where the children could not read the sentences. The researcher read each statement to the three individuals in a calm, nonexpressive voice to avoid influencing any responses.

The data collection for this research began in March 1986 and continued into July of the same year. This span of time was necessary to network through people to obtain the necessary access to the study sample and administer and complete the testing of the sample.

Instrumentation

The Piers-Harris children's self-concept scale (Piers & Harris, 1969), entitled "The Way I Feel About Myself," is an 80-item, self-report scale designed to assess how children between the ages of 8 and 18 years perceive themselves. Self-concept, as assessed by this instrument, is defined as a relatively stable set of self-attitudes reflecting both a description and an evaluation of one's own behavior and attributes. Piers (1984) explains that the items on the scale are scored in either a positive or negative direction to reflect this self-evaluative dimension. A high score on the scale suggests a positive self-evaluation whereas a low score suggests a negative self-evaluation. This test focuses on children's conscious self-perceptions, rather than attempting to infer how they feel about themselves from their behaviors or the attribution of others.

The Piers-Harris scale appears to be a highly reliable instrument. A number of studies have investigated the test-retest stability of the Piers-Harris scale, according to Piers (1984), with demonstrated coefficients ranging from 0.42 to 0.96. Internal consistency, a measure of the average correlation among items within a test, revealed estimates for the total score ranging from 0.88 to 0.93. The reliability figures compare favorably with other measures used to assess personality traits in children. The Piers-Harris scale has adequate temporal stability and good internal consistency.

It has been questioned whether young children have a stable self-concept that can be measured in any consistent fashion. It is felt by Piers (1984) that this may be true for preschoolers, but the results of the internal consistency studies showed that self-attitudes are reasonably stable by age 7 or 8.

The Piers-Harris scale is not intended to be used as a diagnostic test but as a screening instrument. A limitation of the scale is that the child can be influenced by the reference gorup that was involved in his or her self-concept formation. Thus, children from a setting different from the Piers-Harris norm group may interpret the test items differently, and as a result the responses may not correspond to those on the answer key. The number of answers inconsistent with the key is subtracted from 80, the total number of responses on the scale. An overall assessment of self-concept is reflected in the total score. It is the single most reliable measure for the Piers-Harris scale. This measure has the best research support and is the indicator used in this study. A high total score is associated with a favorable self-concept and a lower score is associated with a lower self-concept. However, scores greater than 70 should be interpreted cautiously. Scores this high may accurately represent a child's positive self-evaluation or may reflect a need to appear supremely self-confident or a lack of critical self-evaluation. Piers ranks 45 to 60 as average.

Once the adequacy of the child's self-concept was determined to be normal, above normal, or below normal, this information was compared to the child's blood glucose results. These results were graphed to determine if the hypothesis was supported—that is, whether the self-concept positively correlated with blood glucose control.

FINDINGS

This study investigated the level of self-concept development in 24 children with diabetes and the degree of their blood glucose control to determine if a positive correlation existed.

The sample consisted of 24 children who made up a convenience or incidental sample. According to Knapp (1978) this sample is so named because children who happened to be in a particular place at a particular time were selected. It is also a nonprobability sample as described by Kerlinger (1973). He further comments that the weakness of this sampling can be somewhat mitigated by using knowledge, expertise, and care in selecting samples and by replicating studies with different samples. The 24 children who make up the sample consisted of 11 females and 13 males, aged 8 through 12 years, and diagnosed with diabetes for at least 6 months. The mean age was 10.0 years. The raw scores from the Piers-Harris self-concept scale were the independent variable (X), while the HgbA$_{1c}$ test results were the dependent variable (Y). This bivariate data was plotted on a scatter diagram to determine if a correlation existed—that is, to see if as (X) increased there would be a definite shift in the value of (Y).

The coefficient of linear correlation, r, or Pearson's product moment r, is the measure of strength of linear relationship between two variables. Coefficient r will have a value of zero when there is no linear correlation, whereas values close to -1 or $+1$ will be considered a high correlation. Somewhere between 0 and 1.0, and 0 and -1.0 there is a value where the conclusion changes. Johnson (1976) relates that these are decision points and are determined by the size of the sample, which in this investigation was n = 24 with a decision point of 0.404. Any value calculated at less than 0.404 would be considered no correlation. The value of the calculated linear correlation coefficient in this study was r = -0.06. This indicated that a linear correlation did not exist between (X) and (Y), the level of self-concept and blood glucose control in this study sample. The hypothesis stating that there would be a positive correlation between an adequate self-concept and acceptance of the diabetic condition as evidenced by blood glucose control in children with diabetes was not supported.

DISCUSSION

It is interesting to note that 17 of the 24 children, or 71 percent of the sample, had an adequate self-concept score and acceptable HgbA$_{1c}$ results. It seems that the adequate self-concept and acceptable blood glucose control are related but do not demonstrate linear correlation (*see* Table 39–1).

An analysis of the study reveals that the small size of the sample may have been a factor. The area on the scatter diagram covered by the ordered pairs is very diverse.

From the children's record of the grade into which they had passed it was noted that five of the children were just moving from the first grade into the second. The comprehension level must be considered as a possible problem with the use of this scale. The researcher read three of the self-concept scales for the participants who could not read well enough to respond to the statements; therefore a question arises concerning comprehension skills. As noted earlier the scale was designed for children aged 8 through 18 years and in grades 4 through 12, which this researcher questions as to the congruency of age 8 years and grade 4.

The testing environment should be consistent for each child and established parameters explained to all participants. The presence of a person other than the test monitor should not be allowed, so that the child will be encouraged to be truthful in responding to the statements. The test monitor can better determine if the child can adequately read the statements and understand the meaning if a predetermined reading and grade level were established.

The original norms of the Piers-Harris test are based on data from one

TABLE 39-1. DEMOGRAPHIC DATA AND SELF-CONCEPT AND BLOOD SUGAR RESULTS

Client Number	Sex	Age	Grade	Self-Concept Score	HgbA$_{1c}$
1	M	10	4	46	14.6
2	F	10	4	72	6.7
3	F	10	4	80	10.7
4	F	11	5	60	9.0
5	F	10.5	5	74	11.1
6	M	10	3	71	11.8
7	F	11	5	56	13.2
8	M	12	6	68	8.3
9	M	8	2	67	8.1
10	M	11	5	56	10.7
11	F	11	4	56	11.9
12	M	10	5	77	11.0
13	F	12	6	43	9.8
14	F	8	2	73	11.4
15	F	8.5	2	53	13.5
16	M	12	7	70	10.6
17	M	8	2	45	10.5
18	M	8	2	50	9.2
19	F	10.5	5	53	7.5
20	M	12	5	69	13.3
21	M	10	4	73	9.0
22	M	10.5	6	41	11.0
23	M	10	5	32	8.8
24	F	9.5	4	56	9.8

F = 11.
M = 13.

Pennsylvania school district. Although subsequent studies suggest that these results generalize to more diverse school populations in the United States, comparability of the normative or other psychometric data for other populations should not be assumed. This is particularly true for younger children or those whose background differs significantly from the standardization sample. This study sample consisted exclusively of children with diabetes. The statements on the self-concept test could have a different meaning to them than to a non-diabetic child; therefore the answers could have a different interpretation. Statements such as "I cause trouble to my family" could be interpreted in terms of the extra activities, such as diet, planning, various restrictions, and continual monitoring of the diabetes by means of blood sugars. Several of the statements that are included on more than one cluster scale present similarly, such as:

- I like being the way I am.
- I feel left out of things.
- I wish I were different.
- I am unhappy.
- I am different from other people.

To reflect the self-concept, the right questions must be asked. The self-concept tool used for a normal sample may not be adequate for testing a study sample that is exclusively diabetic.

The Piers-Harris self-concept scale norms are based on a normal school population. The population composed entirely of children with diabetes is a different population. It is recommended that the Piers-Harris scale be administered in conjuction with another test, such as the Sullivan diabetic adjustment scale, which measures a child's adjustment to diabetes rather than self-concept. The scores from both tests could be compared for similarity and then correlated to the blood glucose readings.

The Piers-Harris mean raw score was 51.84. Six participants in this study group fell below this mean and 18 scored higher. The mean for this study sample was 60. The mean $HgbA_{1c}$ of the study group was 10.5, which is in the excellent control range for children with diabetes. Only four children had $HgbA_{1c}$ results in the poor glucose control range—that is, readings greater than 13.0.

These observations seem to warrant the conclusion that this study group was above average in both self-concept scores and blood glucose control although a linear correlation between the two did not exist.

An analysis of the children who were not within the acceptable ranges reveals that 7 children, or 29 percent of the sample, did not have a positive relationship between their self-concept scores and the $HgbA_{1c}$ results (see Table 39–2). As in the total sample, the sex distribution was almost equally divided, with males slightly outnumbering females. Of the seven children in Table 39-2, the female

TABLE 39–2. NONCORRELATING SELF-CONCEPT SCORES AND BLOOD GLUCOSE RESULTS

Client Number	Sex	Age	Grade	Self-Concept Scores	$HgbA_{1c}$
1	F	8.5	2	53	13.5*
2	F	11	5	56	13.2*
3	F	12	6	43*	9.8
4	M	10	4	46	14.6*
5	M	10	5	32*	8.8
6	M	10.5	6	41*	11.0
7	M	12	5	69	13.3*

M = male.
F = female.
* = out of range.

clients 1 and 2 have adequate self-concept scores but poor blood glucose control, whereas female client 3 had excellent blood glucose control and a self-concept score just below the defined adequate range. Male clients 4 and 7 had poor glucose control and adequate self-concept scores, whereas clients 5 and 6 fell below the defined adequate self-concept range yet maintained excellent and fair glucose control, respectively.

The literature review revealed that this age range, from 8 through 12 years, is one in which physical growth occurs rapidly at times. When children with diabetes experience a growth spurt, the body's demand for insulin increases, so that a child who normally does not run a high blood glucose level may experience difficulty achieving control.

During these periods, the child with diabetes may need support and guidance from the nurse. If the child has a low self-concept with an external locus of control, the nurse will need to function in the role of educator. A physical assessment of the child and the entire diabetes treatment regimen is necessary to work toward stablization of the blood glucose within an acceptable range. It is also important to examine the family and peer relationships to determine if these areas need improvement to enhance the child's self-esteem. The nurse encourages the use of role-taking by the client and family members so that each may understand the position of the other. Parental supervision may also need to be reviewed with the child and family members to determine both the individual and collective impact upon the family unit.

Communication, both verbal and nonverbal, with the child and family members must take place so that problem resolution can occur. The nurse must be able to understand the situation as it is perceived by the clients in order to facilitate learning and effect a change from an external to an internal locus of control. At this point the client and family will have become their own support system and the nurse will function as an advocate and friend. The primary goal throughout is an improved level of health or functioning at the optimal level for client and family.

A recommendation for further research is a longitudinal study of a group of children with diabetes using self-concept and diabetes adjustment scales. Variables to be considered might be the following:

- The effects of family interactions on diabetes management.
- The sibling position of the child with diabetes in the family.
- The length of time the child has been diagnosed with the condition.

A final recommendation would be the replication of this study to refute or validate the findings. There is little in the literature to directly compare the results. Obtaining a larger study population may yield a better correlation when used in conjuction with the previous recommendations to correct the problems encountered in this study. In this age group, with sporadic physical growth periods and emotional maturation, blood glucose stabilization is difficult to achieve even under stable conditions. The analysis seems to indicate that a correlation to one factor, such as self-concept, may not be possible.

REFERENCES

Bennett, D. L. (1978). The adolescent with diabetes mellitus. *Pediatric Annual, 7,* 626–632.

Johnson, R. (1976). *Elementary statistics* (2nd ed.). North Scituate, MA: Duxbury.

Johnson, S. B, & Rosenbloom, A. L. (1982). Behavioral aspects of diabetes mellitus in childhood and adolescence. *Psychiatric Clinics of North America, 5,* 357–369.

Kerlinger, F. N. (1973). *Foundations of behavioral research* (2nd ed.). New York: Holt, Rinehart & Winston.

Knapp, R. G. (1978). *Basic statistics for nurses.* New York: Wiley.

LoBiondo-Wood, G., & Haber, J. (1986). *Nursing research: Critical appraisal and utilization.* St. Louis: Mosby.

Minuchin, S., Baker, L., Rosman, B., et al. (1975). *Archives of General Psychiatry, 32,* 1031–1038.

Minuchin, S., Rosman, B., & Baker, L. (1978). *Psychosomatic families.* Cambridge, MA: Harvard University Press.

Piers, E. V. (1984). *Revised manual for Piers-Harris children's self-concept scale.* Los Angeles: Western Psychological Services.

Piers, E. V., & Harris, D. B. (1969). *Piers-Harris children's self-concept scale.* Los Angeles: Western Psychological Services.

Riehl, J. P. (1980). The Riehl Interaction Model. In J. P. Riehl & C. Roy (Eds.), *Conceptual models for nursing practice* (2nd ed.). New York: Appleton-Century-Crofts.

Sullivan, B. J. (1979). I. Adjustment in diabetic adolescent girls. II. Adjustment, self-esteem and depression in diabetic adolescent girls. *Psychosomatic Medicine, 42,* 127–138.

Swift, C. R., Siedman, F., & Stein, H. (1966). Adjustment problems in juvenile diabetes. *Psychosomatic Medicine, 29,* 555–571.

Van der Velde, C. D. (1985). Body images of one's self and others: Developmental and clinical significance. *American Journal of Psychiatry, 142,* 527–537.

Wells, L. E., & Marwell, G. (1976). *Self-esteem: its conceptualization and measurement.* Beverly Hills: Sage.

Whaley, L. F., & Wong, D. L. (1979). *Nursing care of infants and children.* St. Louis: Mosby.

The Nursing Role, Symbolic Interactionism, and the Patient's Personal Space

Rose Marie Foster

THE PROBLEM

Years of observing patients who repositioned the chair that they occupy at the side of the desk in examination rooms led to an interest in, and pursuit of knowledge about, spatial behavior. This behavior was so pervasive that it simply demanded attention.

Professional nurses would be wise to consider the implications of this concept for their interpersonal relationships with both patients and families. If patients are made actuely uncomfortable by the presence of the nurse within their personal space, this discomfort will interfere with the nursing process. Conversely, if nurses are granted spatial privilege because of the nursing role, then they must be cognizant of this privilege and not abuse it.

Although patients are necessary to the survival of the health care delivery system, they are often only passively involved in it. They frequently remain on the periphery and are subjected to intervention by a vast array of health care personnel. It is the nurse, as patient advocate, who fills this gap between the patient and the system. The role of the nurse comprises that cluster of norms and values that direct nursing behavior within the health care delivery system. It forms a reciprocal and complementary role with that of the patient.

Riehl (1980) defined role taking as a psycho-social concept that is "a mental or cognitive activity (not overt behavior) (p. 352)." In this context action is initiated only after trying, through insight, to understand another's behavior.

It is precisely through this role-taking process that the nurse is able to assess culturally based beliefs of the patient that might impede response to treatment. This assessment, along with identification of other social, cultural, and psychological variables pertinent to patient response, forms the foundation of the

475

nursing role of advocacy. Through the mental or cognitive activity of role taking, the nurse fulfills the prescribed imperative of the American Nurses' Association Social Policy Statement (1980). This statement directs nurses to "diagnose and treat human responses to actual or potential health problems (p. 9)."

The policy statement further declares that "nursing care is provided in an interpersonal relationship process of nurse-with-a-patient, nurse-with-a-family, nurse-with-a-group (p. 18.)." The meaning of the concept of nursing arises in the process of interaction with others. This meaning is a social product. If it were more clearly defined, the context of this interpersonal process would further expand knowledge of the meaning and effect of the nursing role on the status of the patient.

Symbolic interactionism is a theory that has been proposed, alon with psychoanalytic theory, to supplement those of the behaviorist and the Gestaltist. It addresses those aspects of humans that makes them inherently different from other vertebrates.

Rose (1980) defined a symbol as "a stimulus that has a learned meaning and value for people (p. 39)." He also stated that a person responds to a symbol "in terms of its meaning and value rather than in terms of its physical stimulation of his sense organs (p. 39)." Rose described the meaning and value of a chair as the support it provides to one who sits on it rather than as its ability to stimulate the sense organs.

Symbols can be transmitted through gestures, motions, and objects, but people usually express them verbally. Symbols exist in human repertoire primarily because of our ability to store meanings and values in a complex nervous system but also because they can communicate using a unique vocal apparatus. These abilities allow human beings to live in a symbolic as well as a physical environment. The meaning and value of symbols is culturally determined.

Riehl (1980, p. 351) listed five analytic assumptions that underlie the Riehl model:

1. Humans live in a symbolic as well as in a physical environment and can be stimulated to act by symbols as well as by physical stimuli.
2. Through symbols, people have the capacity to stimulate others in ways other than those in which they are stimulated themselves.
3. Through communication of symbols, humans can learn large numbers of meanings and values—and hence ways of acting—from other people.
4. The symbols—and the meanings and values to which they refer—do not occur in isolated bits, but in large and complex clusters.
5. Thinking is the process by which possible symbolic solutions and other future courses of action are examined, assessed for their relative advantages in terms of the values of the individal, and chosen for action or rejected.

These assumptions enumerate the steps of the mental or cognitive process which is central to symbolic interactionism. They are pertinent to nursing interaction with patients. The first two assumptions will be emphasized because of their centrality to the use of symbolic interactionism and the nonverbal communication of the meaning and use of space.

Hall (1969) coined the term *proxemics* and defined it as "the interrelated observations and theories of man's use of space as a specialized elaboration of culture (p. 1)." He described humans "as surrounded by a series of expanding and contracting fields which provide information of many kinds (p. 115)." This information includes subtle changes in observable behavior of the other person as he or she responds to what is said or done. The cultural influence on the observational power of the individual is such that people of different cultures could conceivably inhabit different perceptual worlds. The physical space over which patients have jurisdiction becomes an extension of themselves and is organized so as to facilitate their functioning. It is proposed that information provided by these fields represents symbols that impact on interaction of the nursing role with that of the patient. The meaning and significance of the nurse's use of space will be explored in the context of its effect on the patient.

Purpose

The purpose of the study was to determine whether the nurse, from the perspective of symbolic interactionism, can intrude into the intimate space of patients without causing stress. Stress in the context of patient care has a negative impact on the interaction between the nurse and the patient.

Research Questions

1. Will intrusion by the nurse into the patient's intimate space increase the subject's anxiety score?
2. Will intrusion by the nurse into the patient's intimate space increase the subject's heart rate?
3. Will intrusion by the nurse into the patient's intimate space correlate with withdrawal behavior?

Hypothesis

From the symbolic interactionism perspective, the nurse in the professional role cannot intrude into the patient's intimate space without producing stress.

Definition of Terms

From the perspective of symbolic interactionism, the nurse was not presumed to have spatial privilege because of her professional role. Inherent in this nursing approach is the act of taking on the role of the patient and noting, interpreting, and analyzing the situation as he or she believes the patient sees it. Taking the role of the patient then guides the nurses's actions in the patient-care setting and includes behaviors that are supportive and nurturing. If intrusion into the intimate space of the patient produces no significant stress, increased heart rate, or withdrawal behavior on the part of the patient, it will be presumed that the nursing role assumes primacy over the need of patients to protect themselves from the intrusion.

Anxiety was defined as consisting of two types. The first is trait anxiety, or a relatively stable level of anxiety that is an integral part of the personality. The second type is state anxiety, which occurs in response to a specific stimulus. Most of the current instruments for measuring anxiety include a measure for both types. Trait anxiety was used as a baseline, and state anxiety was presumed to have been caused by the specific intrusion.

Stress was measured by three parameters: (1) the psychological, or the difference between trait and state anxiety scores; (2) the physiological measurement of changes in the heart rate during the intrusion; and (3) the sociological, or observation for withdrawal behavior during the intrusion. These three dependent variables—anxiety scores, heart rate and withdrawal behavior—comprise the three measures of stress. The effect of the independent variable, intrusion into the intimate space of the patient by the nurse, was measured in these three areas.

Intimate space was defined according to Hall (1969) to be within 18 inches of the patient's body. Intrusion was for the nurse to place his or her head between the patient's upper arm and face while attaching the blood pressure cuff. The blood pressure reading was of no interest other than to provide the opportunity to intrude into the intimate space of the patient.

Research Design

This was a quasi-experimental design using a convenience sample of patients in a hospital-sponsored ambulatory service. Subjects were assigned on an alternating basis to either the study or comparison group. After obtaining consent and collecting demographic data, each subject was asked to complete a trait anxiety scale. Three heart rate readings were recorded at one-minute intervals. These were averaged to obtain the baseline reading. The intrusion as described above was implemented with the study group, whereas the blood pressure was taken from the normal distance, without intruding into the intimate space of patients in the comparison group. While appearing to read the blood pressure, the biofeedback digital reader was observed for the maximum reading during the intrusion. If subjects asked what the blood pressure reading was, they were told that the investigator forgot one of the numbers and it was taken again and results given as requested. All subjects then completed the state anxiety questionnaire. While they did this, three heart rate readings were again recorded. These readings were averaged to obtain the post heart rate. All of the encounters were videotaped for later scoring of withdrawal behavior. A cohort turned the recorder on when the blood pressure cuff was removed from its holder and recorded until the investigator replaced it in the holder.

REVIEW OF THE LITERATURE ON SYMBOLIC INTERACTIONISM

Nursing is concerned with the quality of life as it relates to the attainment or maintenance of health. Nursing is practiced within the context of interpersonal relationships and is presently attempting to define its concepts by moving away from behavioristic and medical models. They are being replaced with holistic, humanistic models. One of these is symbolic interactionism, an approach introduced in the work of Mead, Rose, Blumer, and others. Blumer (1969) proposed five philosophical premises that are considered to have significance for nursing. Riehl based her model on the key factors of this theory—the basic assumptions, definitions and concepts of symbolic interactionism (Riehl, 1980). She felt that the analytic assumptions (cited earlier in this chapter) include all ages of humans except socialization of the child, which was subsumed under Blumer's (1969) genetic assumptions. Riehl also said that these assumptions complement other theories and she used Erickson's eight ages of man as an example.

The first of Riehl's philosophical premises is that human conduct is based on the meaning of the situation for the person. This means that the nurse, through role taking, must understand meaning within the client's frame of reference in order to arrive at the common ground of authentic communication. The second premise is that meanings are social products derived through interpersonal processes. It is through the use of self in interpersonal interaction that the nurse can help the client to define his or her experience in more satisfying ways. The third premise is that people interpret and modify meanings in terms of what they consider important about a situation. They use these interpretations and meanings to direct their actions in specific situations. Nurses must look to these premises as a basis for interaction rather than defining behavior as a medical problem or a symptom.

Blumer (1969) proposed that "symbolic interactionism is that which occurs between human beings who interpret or define each other's actions instead of just reacting to them. Their responses are based on the meanings they attach to each action. Social action is lodged in the acting individuals (pp. 2–3)."

Spatial Behavior

Communication is an integral part of interpersonal relationships. Communication as a process involves three levels of interaction—verbal, kinesic, and proxemic. Therapeutic communication involves understanding both the process of communication and the influence of culture on that process.

Verbal communication is spoken language, the words we use and how we use them. Nonverbal communication includes kinesics or the way we use body parts, and proxemics, which is the way we use the space around our bodies. Proxemics involves two concepts of space. The first is territoriality, or a state that is characterized by possessiveness, control, and authority over an area of physical space (Hayter, 1981). Territoriality was studied in animals between the early 1900s and the 1960s. It was during the 1960s that Hall did his work on proxemics (Scheflen & Ashcraft, 1976). The second concept of space subsumed under proxemics is personal space. Hall (1969) visualized people as surrounded by expanding and contracting perceptual fields that at all times provide them with information. He stated that people interact in four spatial zones: intimate, personal, social, and public.

The intimate zone is the zone of physical contact. It is the area within 18 inches of the body. It is the zone of love-making and comforting. Sight is blurred or distorted at this distance. The perception of odors, heat, and breath from another's body is heightened. The voice is kept to a whisper if used at all. Americans feel uncomfortable if forced into the intimate zone of a stranger. They respond by becoming immobile, holding their arms at their sides, staring into space, and tensing their bodies.

The personal zone comprises the area from 18 inches to 4 feet from the body. This area is sometimes visualized as a bubble that a person keeps between himself and others. The bubble expands and contracts according to circumstances. At a small personal distance one can hold and touch another. At a greater personal distance one is just within reach when both parties extend their arms. One can see the texture of hair, the pores of the skin, and the three-dimensional qualities of objects. One cannot feel the breath or body heat of the other and the voice level is moderate. This is the space where most nurse-client interaction takes place, probably at the inner limit.

Social distance is from 4 to 12 feet. At this distance people cannot touch. This is the distance appropriate for business and student-teacher interactions.

Hall (1969) stated that as one moves from personal and social areas to public distance, important sensory shifts occur. Public distance has two phases, close at 12 to 25 feet and far at 25 feet or more. This is a formal distance wherein all forms of expression change in charater. The alert subject can also flee danger successfully at this distance.

Anxiety

There seems to be no precise definition for anxiety, although many writers have attempted to operationalize the term. Many studies claim to arouse anxiety for the purpose of studying it. Except in textbooks on psychiatric nursing there is little available that focuses on everyday behaviors that evoke an anxiety response in patients. Wilson and Kneisl (1979) claimed that anxiety is subjective and caused by personal fear rather than by actual danger. They defined it as a form of energy or tension often described as unexplained discomfort, a subjectively painful warning of impending danger that motivates the individual to stop the pain (p. 187).

Zuckerman and Lubin's (1985) multiple affect adjective checklist-revised (MAACL-R), both the general (trait) and the today (state) forms was used in this study to measure anxiety. Data on the revised MAACL indicate its use with a variety of normal and patient samples. In a comparison of the MAACL-R scores for anxiety and depression with clinical ratings of anxiety, the MAACL-R scores were significantly related. Correlations of the anxiety scale with self-ratings were 0.43, $p < .001$ for 10 state hospital patients; 0.51 and 0.52, $p < 0.001$, for community clinics 1 and 2, $n = 62$ and 118. College students' correlations with self-ratings were 0.52, $p < .001$, $n = 104$. As would be expected with the trait-state model, state scales have low retest reliabilities in contrast to trait scales. Validity studies are reported for populations including normal adolescents and adults, counseling clients, and patients in clinics and state hospitals. When comparing peer ratings with MAACL-R scores, convergent validities of 0.55 for trait and 0.13 for state anxiety are found. This compares favorably with the internal consistency of 0.85.

Heart Rate

According to Holden and Barlow (1986), skin resistance seems to be subject to very rapid habituation, thus reducing its power as a discriminator. They also stated that skin resistance frequently seems to be confounded by levels of activity. Holden and Barlow affirmed that there is considerable evidence favoring heart rate as the preferred measure when multiple responses cannot be recorded. Heart rate therefore was used in this study as physiological evidence of stress.

Research

The concept of personal space has been tested in many settings and with different age groups. Kinzel (1970) studied prisoners. He concluded that the need for a large personal zone in a violent prisoner may reflect a pathological body image. He also concluded that body buffer zone measurement could be used in the detection, treatment, and prognosis of individuals predisposed to violent behavior. Hildreth, Derogatis, and McCusker (1971) also studied inmates in a prison. They found that sensitivity to physical closeness correlates with aggressive behavior. They added that both aggressive and nonaggressive inmates were more sensitive to approach from the rear than from the front.

Allekian (1973) studied hospitalized patients. She concluded that patients apparently anticipate physical contact on admission to a hospital and are psychologically prepared for these intrusions. Actions of caregivers that were shown to evoke anxiety including treatment to personal areas of the body, rearranging personal articles in the bedside stand without permission, and regulating air and light (opening or closing windows and raising or lowering shades) without first assessing the needs and desires of the patient. Allekian suggested that territorial intrusion may be seen as reducing the patient's personal control, individuality, and identity. Stillman (1978) affirmed the need for nurses to assess and communicate the patient's preference regarding the use of space to other health team members.

A new aspect of territoriality was introduced by Hayter (1981). She described a territory of expertise or role (p. 84) and enumerated implications of illness as they embody threats to roles or areas of expertise of the patient. Hayter suggested that to reinforce all aspects of the patient's role or expertise is therapeutic, because this strengthens the patient's territorial image.

Louis (1981), stating a need for studies of older adults and their use of space, found a three-way interaction effect with the independent variables of sex, type, and angle of approach. She suggested that in future research, the reaction time of elderly participants should be included, because she felt that this might have been a confounding variable in her study.

In an article on the boundaries of personal space, Meisenhelder (1982) suggested that personal space may be the only remaining evidence of identity and integrity for the hospitalized individual. She felt that nurses' knowledge about the patient's reaction to intrusions into his or her space would reduce anxiety, facilitate healing, and increase the individual's trust in caretakers.

Personal space preferences of hospitalized adults were also studied by Geden and Begeman (1981). Silhouettes representing self, doctor, nurse, family member, and stranger were placed by patients where they would prefer them in proximity to themselves. Support was found for smaller space preferences in the hospital than in the home. The authors also discovered that patients referred to doctors as specific persons but to nurses as a class. They summarized that the identification of nurses may be dependent on the method of assignment—for example, team nursing—in which case the patient cannot claim to have "a nurse."

Ricci (1981) studied white males between the ages of 17 and 72 in an ambulatory setting. She defined personal space as that contiguous to the subject and extending to a distance of 18 inches. She placed a chair according to tape on the floor at 18 inches. In the invasion condition she sat with her chair on this line and her feet inside the space. In the second, noninvasion condition, the interviewer sat with her toes on the tape, thus extending the distance to 24 to 28 inches. Ricci used Spielberger's A-trait and A-state scales to measure anxiety. The third measure was a recording of electrodermal skin responses per unit of time. Ricci reported finding no support for either hypothesis, one dealing with increased emotional response and the other with anxiety scores. The patients in this study were referred to a cardiologist because they were thought to have developed cardiac disease. Ricci questioned whether their denial behaviors, the youth of some of the subjects, or her definition of personal space were confounding variables.

Summary

This investigation differed from Ricci's in several respects. In order to eliminate the confounding effects of youth and old age, the current subjects were limited to those between 25 and 65 years of age. Because attending to markers on the floor and the placement of chairs could prove distracting, intrusion was confined to intimate space, or to within 18 inches of the body as defined by Hall. One person completed the intervention without leaving the room. These procedures were implemented to reduce distraction that could have caused stress.

There seems to be ample evidence to support the need to study the nursing role as it relates to the personal space needs of the patient in a clinical setting. Symbolic interactionism, which clearly describes the nursing imperative for understanding interpersonal processes and establishing authentic communication between self and patient, is a valid theory for use with the concept of personal space. Because personal space is symbolic in meaning, nurses need to become familiar with its significance. If, as several investigators have proposed, intrusion into the patient's personal space causes stress, the interaction of the nurse and patient could have an adverse effect on healing and the individual's trust in caretakers, as well as on patient education, which is becoming increasingly important. Considering patients from a holistic point of view, and treating them in a humanistic manner—in all of their dimensions—is the goal toward which this work aspires.

METHODOLOGY

Setting

The setting for the study was a hospital-sponsored ambulatory care facility located within a community hospital.

Study Sample

Because it is generally recommended that 20 to 30 subjects be selected for each cell of an experimental design, 20 subjects were included in both the study and comparison groups. Because the sample was chosen from scheduled appointments at the researcher's place of work, it must be considered a convenience sample. The type of sample must be kept in mind because it will affect the generalizability of the results. Because all patients have the opportunity to schedule in any given appointment slot, there was an element of randomness for this particular group. Because the use of space is believed to be influenced by age, subjects were limited to those between 25 and 65 years of age.

Subjects' participation was solicited when they arrived for their scheduled appointments and were determined to be in the proper age group. As the encounter began, subjects were alternately assigned to either the study or the comparison group. Intervention proceeded according to which group they were assigned.

The community in which the study was conducted has a highly ethnic population primarily from central and eastern Europe. Because spatial behavior is culturally determined, only native-born Americans were included. Blacks have been reported to use space differently and so were eliminated from this study. Many patients in this setting come from a facility for the mentally retarded. These clients were eliminated for obvious reasons.

Instrumentation

Three measures of stress were obtained from all subjects: (1) anxiety scores (trait and state); (2) heart rate; and (3) scores from withdrawal behavior.

Anxiety scores were obtained by using the MAACL-R. Whether one measures trait or state anxiety is determined by instructions given to subjects before they complete the checklists. They were told to check items as rapidly as possible and to list words describing either how they generally feel (trait) or how they felt while the blood pressure was being taken (state).

The heart rate was measured using a heart rate monitor with digital readout manufactured by Thought Technology, Ltd. of Montreal. According to their catalog description, it can detect changes as small as ½ beat per minute. The average of three readings was computed both before and after the intrusion. These and the maximum rate during the intrusion were manually recorded. Statistically, this was treated as a repeated measures design.

The intrusions were videotaped. The reason for taping the intrusions was so that they could later be scored for withdrawal behavior. This score was the third measure of stress, the sociological act of withdrawing because of discomfort when the intimate space was intruded upon. The tapes were scored by three raters to control for interrater reliability. In cases where the raters did not agree, the tapes were reviewed repeatedly until a consensus was reached.

Procedure

After selection and assignment to groups as described above, the participants were escorted to an examination room where their medical appointment was completed. They had previously been asked to remain after the doctor finished in order to participate in the study. The investigator met them in the examination room and proceeded with the study as described above. Patients in this facility have already signed consent for videotaping.

To avoid having the nurse intrude prematurely into the subjects' intimate space, they were asked to attach the biofeedback electrode to the middle finger of the nondominant hand so that heart rate could be recorded. The electrode is entirely covered and is attached by using a velcro fastener. The baseline heart rate was manually recorded at one-minute intervals while subjects completed the trait anxiety check list.

The intrusion consisted of taking the blood pressure from the normal distance in the comparison group. The blood pressure is normally taken with the nurse seated at the desk and the patient in a chair beside the desk. In the study group, the intrusion consisted of having the nurse stand and place her head between the patient's upper arm and face while attaching the blood pressure cuff. Again, it should be noted that there was no interest in the blood pressure except to provide the opportunity to intrude. During this time the heart rate monitor was observed and the maximum rate was recorded as the intrusion heart rate.

The blood pressure cuff was removed and subjects were asked to complete the state anxiety checklist. During this time, the three post heart rate readings were recorded. The purpose of these readings was to observe for the return of the heart rate to baseline values. Although the end value might not have returned to baseline, a trend was presumed to be evident at this point that would at least distinguish it from the intrusion heart rate. The biofeedback electrode was removed. The investigator thanked the subjects for participating and left the room.

Data Collection

The data were collected over a 2-month period during the winter. The length of time was influenced by scheduling and the ability to find a sufficient number of willing subjects.

DATA AND ANALYSIS

The purpose of this study was to determine whether the nurse, from the symbolic interactionism perspective, would increase patients' stress by intruding into their intimate space. There were three study questions:

1. Will intrusion by the nurse into the patient's intimate space increase the subject's anxiety scores?
2. Will intrusion by the nurse into the patient's intimate space increase the subject's heart rate?
3. Will intrusion by the nurse into the patient's intimate space correlate with withdrawal behavior?

Anxiety

Pearson correlation coefficients (SPSS-X), including all variables, found no correlation higher than 0.473. Testing standard T scores for anxiety produced the results given in Table 40-1.

TABLE 40–1. GROUP MEANS AND STANDARD DEVIATIONS FOR ANXIETY SCORES

	Mean	Std. Dev.	Minimum	Maximum	No.
Study group					
Trait	56.789	19.153	42	113	19
State	49.789	13.024	37	92	19
Comparison group					
Trait	57.316	14.918	42	95	19
State	56.368	14.408	45	92	19

Heart Rate

Heart rate measures were tested using Student-Newman-Keuls (SNK) procedure (Dowdy & Wearden, 1983). This test uses different range values for different size subunits. In tests involving the same number of means it holds the experiment-wise error rate to alpha for each step of the testing procedure. See Table 40–2 for these results.

Withdrawal Behavior

Withdrawal behavior scores were tested using the Fisher exact test. The results are presented in Table 40–3.

SUMMARY AND RECOMMENDATIONS

Factors found in this study to be directly related to intrusion into the patient's intimate space were an increase in heart rate and in withdrawal behavior. Changes in anxiety scores were not statistically significant. Lack of significant change in anxiety scores can probably be attributed to several factors. The first is that paper-and-pencil tests and self-report measures of psychological states are not sensitive enough to exhibit small changes. The small group size also influenced these scores. Secondly, almost all subjects reacted emotionally when asked to complete the state anxiety check list. They said things such as: "Again!", "The whole thing?", and "Do I have to?" It goes without saying that no one was coerced, but they all agreed to complete it. However, most of the anxiety scores decreased. This is reflected in the mean scores of 56.789 and 49.789 for trait and state anxiety, respectively, in the study group, and mean scores of 57.316 and 56.368 for trait and state anxiety, respectively, in the comparison group. Zuckerman and Lubin (1980) suggested that a decrease in response set can in itself be an indicator of anxiety. Ricci (1981) noted this response but suggested that, although not statistically significant, this trend may have indicated that the invasion condition had a "calming rather than an arousing effect (p. 215)." Mean scores in this study decreased by 7 points in the study group and

TABLE 40–2. STUDENT-NEWMAN-KEUL'S TABLE OF DIFFERENCES BETWEEN GROUPS' MEAN SCORES FOR HEART RATE

		PO 2	P 1	PO 1	I 2	I 1
		74.84	75.37	77.37	78.42	90.89
P 2	72.63	2.21	2.74	4.74	5.79*	18.26†
PO 2	74.84		0.5	2.53	3.58	16.05†
P 1	75.37			2.07	3.05	15.52†
PO 1	77.37				1.05	13.52†
I 2	78.42					12.47†

*$p < .05$.
†$p < .01$.
Note: P1 is baseline heart rate, study group.
    I 1 is intrustion heart rate, study group.
    PO 1 is post heart rate, study group.
    P 2 is baseline heart rate, comparison group.
    I 2 is intervention pulse rate, comparison group.
    PO 2 is post heart rate, comparison group.

only by 0.948 in the comparison group. This would seem to indicate that, although not statistically significant, scores reflect a greater change in response set in the study group and therefore reflect more stress in this group.

No other study cited measured heart rate as an indicator of stress during intrusion into intimate space. The statistical significance of this change seems to confirm Holden and Barlow's (1986) findings regarding the strength of heart rate as a single physiological measure.

Both study and comparison groups exhibited a considerable amount of withdrawal behavior. This would appear to indicate that almost all patients were uncomfortable when the nurse moved closer to attach the blood pressure cuff. Taking the blood pressure could itself have some unknown significance for patients. Although no record was kept of the exact number, many patients asked what the reading was. Coupling this response with the popularity of blood pressure screening programs and the number of patients who present at this facility to have the nurse take the pressure in the absence of any history of hypertension raises some interesting questions. This could be the subject of a future study.

TABLE 40–3. FISHER EXACT TEST SCORES FOR WITHDRAWAL BEHAVIOR

Study group	.:18, 1
Comparison group	.:12, 7

The probability of 18 or more successes in 19 attempts given a total of 30 successes in 38 attempts is .0211223.*

*$p < .05$.

The groups in this study were small. They started with 20 subjects in each. Zuckerman and Lubin instruct that forms with more than 92 items checked on the trait form and more than 93 on the state form should be considered invalid. One subject in each group was eliminated for these reasons. Because of the small size of the groups and the lack of randomization, it would be interesting to see the results of a study without these limiting factors.

Overall, this study seems to provide support, within its limitations, for the hypothesis that from the perspective of symbolic interactionism, a nurse cannot intrude into the patient's intimate space without causing stress. When the patient experiences stress, he or she is motivated to stop the discomfort caused by stress. Surely this impacts negatively on the patient's ability to learn. This is another area that warrants further study. The discomfort probably also could impact negatively on the patient's impression of health care providers. Psychological stress certainly is not an emotional state conducive to healing. Nursing interventions that are planned with these facts in mind will most likely be more effective in meeting the patient's goal of improving his or her state of health or level of functioning.

REFERENCES

Allekian, C. I. (1973). Intrusions of territory and personal space: An anxiety-inducing factor for hospitalized persons—An exploratory study. *Nursing Research, 22*(3), 236–241.

American Nurses' Association. (1980). *Nursing: A social policy statement.* Kansas City, MO: AUTHOR.

Blumer, H. (1969). *Symbolic interactionism: Perspective and method.* Englewood Cliffs, NJ: Prentice-Hall.

Dowdy, S., & Wearden, S. (1983). *Statistics for research.* New York: Wiley.

Geden, E. A., & Begeman, A. V. (1981). Personal space preferences of hospitalized adults. *Research in Nursing and Health, 4,* 237–241.

Hall, E. T. (1969). *The Hidden Dimension.* Garden City, NY: Doubleday.

Hayter, K. (1981). Territoriality as a universal need. *Journal of Advanced Nursing, 6,* 79–85.

Hildreth, A. M., Durogatis, L. R., & McCusker, K. (1971). Body buffer zone and violence: A reassessment and confirmation. *American Journal of Psychiatry, 127*(12), 1641–1645.

Holden, A., Jr., & Barlow, D. H. (1986). Heart rate and heart rate variability recorded in vivo in agoraphobics and nonphobics. *Behavior Therapy, 17,* 26–42.

Kinzel, A. F. (1970). Body buffer zone in violent prisoners. *American Journal of Psychiatry, 127*(1), 59–64.

Louis, M. (1981). Personal space boundary needs of elderly persons: An empirical study. *Journal of Gerontological Nursing, 7*(7), 395–400.

Meisenhelder, J. B. (1982). Boundaries of personal space. *Image, 14*(1), 16–19.

Ricci, M. S. (1981). An experiment with personal-space invasion in the nurse-patient relationship and its effect on anxiety. *Images in Mental Health Nursing, 3,* 203–218.

Riehl, J. P. (1980). The Riehl Interaction Model. In J. P. Riehl, & C. Roy (Eds.), *Conceptual models for nursing practice* (2nd ed.). East Norwalk, CT: Appleton-Century-Crofts.

Rose, A. M. (1980). A systematic summary of symbolic interaction theory. In J. P. Riehl, & C. Roy (Eds.), *Conceptual models for nursing practice* (2nd ed.). East Norwalk, CT: Appleton-Century-Crofts.

Scheflen, A. E., & Ashcraft, N. (1976). *Human territories: How we behave in space-time.* Englewood Cliffs, NJ: Prentice-Hall.

Stillman, M. J. (1978). Territoriality and personal space. *American Journal of Nursing, 10,* 1670–1672.

Wilson, H. S., & Kneisl, C. R. (1979). *Psychiatric Nursing.* Menlo Park, CA: Addison-Wesley.

Zuckerman, M., & Lubin, B. (1980). *Manual for the multiple affect adjective checklist.* San Diego: Educational & Industrial Testing Service.

Future Implications for Developing Nursing Theory

Joan Riehl-Sisca

In gathering data for a book of this nature, it was important to present different views of nurse theorists and the thoughts expressed in their models. Some are more controversial than others, but different perspectives are healthy. They should provide challenge and thoughtful consideration before being summarily discarded. Those that do not withstand the test of time will be set aside.

Undoubtedly there is more than one school of thought in all professional fields and philosophical positions. And so it is in nursing. In contemplating this seriously and becoming more cognizant of the varied and legitimate perspectives, the position of suggesting a unified model for nursing has been tabled at this time as premature. This proposal appeared in the first two editions of this text. However, with the rapid knowledge explosion evident today, it tends to limit the extensive breadth needed for nursing to remain extant and grow.

Briefly reviewing the development of nursing model history, it seems evident that some first steps were away from and others closely related to the field of medicine. This vacillating process seems to be determined by the philosophy and the choice of mentors of each nurse theorist. Models classified as logistic are often related to a systems methodology with the medical model strongly evident. This is true of some early models as we know them today—those developed late in the 1960s and early 1970s. Their popularity may well be based on their medical model inclusion because this model is so familiar to nurses.

Other frameworks have not been strongly influenced by the medical model but have been independently developed based on the unmet needs of clients or patients and families. Nightingale was the first nurse theorist in this group. After her contribution, there was a void in progress until recently. Another distinguishing characteristic of the models in this group is that their frameworks have generally been influenced by a broader perspective, with several mentors contributing to the theorist's thinking. Reading diversity, philosophy, experience, and creative imagination are the ingredients that complete the shaping of these theorists' perspectives. The theorists fitting these categories represent nursing's true pioneers, whereas those who have key components that are obviously from the medical model formulate a bridge between medicine and nursing.

Because nursing is a young science, it is far too early to reach a point of closure by accepting one model to the exclusion of others. It is advisable for beginning nursing students to study one model to learn patient care from a nursing perspective, but they need to be aware that several frameworks exist and others are being developed. In fact, they may contribute to this process and should be encouraged to do so. In the basic and social sciences, several sub-specialty fields exist. This paradigm has withstood the test of time and naturally applies to nursing. Although there are basic ethical, legal, and political dimensions to consider, with latitude sanctioned the science of nursing will more rapidly become a reality.

Research is necessarily an integral part of this endeavor. Interest and accomplishment in nursing research is evidenced by the newly established National Center for Nursing Research in Washington, D.C.; by full days of scientific sessions at national nursing conferences; and by the increasing number of nurses receiving their doctorates. However, this is just the beginning. Research articles were sought on the models presented in this text, but few had been written so they were hard to find. This is undoubtedly true in all areas of nursing. Greater progress will be made in nursing theory when all nurse educators require a conceptual framework in all research done by their students. This probably will occur when all nurse educators are themselves knowledgeable in this area.

Continued development, knowledge, and sharing of conceptual maps with national input and central monitoring will help unify research efforts in nursing. The maps should be broad in scope and yet sufficiently definitive to capture the essence of our science. Input should be derived from the nursing practice, administration, and education fields. The program activities identified by the National Center for Nursing Research have a semblance of three broad conceptual map categories: (1) health promotion and disease prevention; (2) acute and chronic illness; and (3) nursing systems and special programs. The latter includes nursing care delivery, models, and research emanating from these perspectives. Channeling our research efforts has begun. Continual networking will assure success in establishing our science of nursing.

Index